The Mathematics of Computerized Tomography

The Mathematics of Computerized Tomography

F. Natterer
University of Münster
Federal Republic of Germany

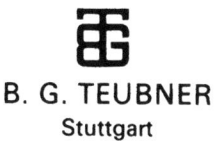

B. G. TEUBNER
Stuttgart

JOHN WILEY & SONS
Chichester · New York · Brisbane · Toronto · Singapore

ISBN 978-3-519-02103-2   ISBN 978-3-663-01409-6 (eBook)
DOI 10.1007/978-3-663-01409-6
Softcover reprint of the hardcover 1st edition 1986

Copyright © 1986 by John Wiley & Sons Ltd and
B G Teubner, Stuttgart

All rights reserved

No part of this book may be reproduced by any means, or transmitted, or translated into a machine language without the written permission of the publisher.

Library of Congress Cataloging-in-Publication Data:

Natterer, F. (Frank), 1941–
 The mathematics of computerized tomography.

  Bibliography:
  Includes index.
  1. Tomography—Mathematics.   I. Title.
RC78.7.T6N37   1986   616.07'572   85–29591

British Library Cataloguing in Publication Data:

Natterer, F.
 The mathematics of computerized tomography.
 1. Tomography—Data processing   2. Electronic data processing—Mathematics
 621.36' 73   RC78.7.T6

CIP-Kurztitelaufnahme der Deutschen Bibliothek

Natterer, Frank:
The mathematics of computerized tomography
/ F. Natterer.—Stuttgart: Teubner;
Chichester; New York; Brisbane; Toronto;
Singapore: Wiley, 1986.

Typeset by Macmillan India Ltd, Bangalore 25.

Contents

Preface   vii
Glossary of Symbols   ix

I. Computerized Tomography   **1**
I.1   The basic example: transmission computerized tomography   1
I.2   Other applications   3
I.3   Bibliographical notes   8

II. The Radon Transform and Related Transforms   **9**
II.1   Definition and elementary properties of some integral operators   9
II.2   Inversion formulas   18
II.3   Uniqueness   30
II.4   The ranges   36
II.5   Sobolev space estimates   42
II.6   The attenuated Radon transform   46
II.7   Bibliographical notes   52

III. Sampling and Resolution   **54**
III.1   The sampling theorem   54
III.2   Resolution   64
III.3   Some two-dimensional sampling schemes   71
III.4   Bibliographical notes   84

IV. Ill-posedness and Accuracy   **85**
IV.1   Ill-posed problems   85
IV.2   Error estimates   92
IV.3   The singular value decomposition of the Radon transform   95
IV.4   Bibliographical notes   101

V. Reconstruction Algorithms   **102**
V.1   Filtered backprojection   102
V.2   Fourier reconstruction   119
V.3   Kaczmarz's method   128

V.4	Algebraic reconstruction technique (ART)	137
V.5	Direct algebraic methods	146
V.6	Other reconstruction methods	150
V.7	Bibliographical notes	155

VI. Incomplete Data — **158**
VI.1	General remarks	158
VI.2	The limited angle problem	160
VI.3	The exterior problem	166
VI.4	The interior problem	169
VI.5	The restricted source problem	174
VI.6	Reconstruction of homogeneous objects	176
VI.7	Bibliographical notes	178

VII. Mathematical Tools — **180**
VII.1	Fourier analysis	180
VII.2	Integration over spheres	186
VII.3	Special functions	193
VII.4	Sobolev spaces	200
VII.5	The discrete Fourier transform	206

References — **213**

Index — 221

Preface

By computerized tomography (CT) we mean the reconstruction of a function from its line or plane integrals, irrespective of the field where this technique is applied. In the early 1970s CT was introduced in diagnostic radiology and since then, many other applications of CT have become known, some of them preceding the application in radiology by many years.

In this book I have made an attempt to collect some mathematics which is of possible interest both to the research mathematician who wants to understand the theory and algorithms of CT and to the practitioner who wants to apply CT in his special field of interest. I also want to present the state of the art of the mathematical theory of CT as it has developed from 1970 on. It seems that essential parts of the theory are now well understood.

In the selection of the material I restricted myself—with very few exceptions—to the original problem of CT, even though extensions to other problems of integral geometry, such as reconstruction from integrals over arbitrary manifolds are possible in some cases. This is because the field is presently developing rapidly and its final shape is not yet visible. Another glaring omission is the statistical side of CT which is very important in practice and which we touch on only occasionally.

The book is intended to be self-contained and the necessary mathematical background is briefly reviewed in an appendix (Chapter VII). A familiarity with the material of that chapter is required throughout the book. In the main text I have tried to be mathematically rigorous in the statement and proof of the theorems, but I do not hesitate in giving a loose interpretation of mathematical facts when this helps to understand its practical relevance.

The book arose from courses on the mathematics of CT I taught at the Universities of Saarbrücken and Münster. I owe much to the enthusiasm and diligence of my students, many of whom did their diploma thesis with me. Thanks are due to D. C. Solmon and E. T. Quinto, who, during their stay in Münster which has been made possible by the Humboldt-Stiftung, not only read critically parts of the manuscript and suggested major improvements but also gave their advice in the preparation of the book. I gratefully acknowledge the help of A. Faridani, U. Heike and H. Kruse without whose support the book would never have been finished. Last but not least I want to thank Mrs I. Berg for her excellent typing.

Münster, July 1985   Frank Natterer

Glossary of Symbols

Symbol	Explanation	References
$\mathbb{R}^n$	n-dimensional euclidean space	
Ω^n	unit ball of $\mathbb{R}^n$	
S^{n-1}	unit sphere in $\mathbb{R}^n$	
Z	unit cylinder in $\mathbb{R}^{n+1}$	II.1
T	tangent bundle to S^{n-1}	II.1
$\theta^\perp$	subspace or unit vector perpendicular to θ	
D^l	derivative of order $l = (l_1, \ldots, l_n)$	
$x \cdot \theta$	inner product	
$|x|$	euclidean norm	
$\mathbb{C}^n$	complex n-dimensional space	
$\hat{f}, \check{f}$	Fourier transform and its inverse	VII.1
C_l^λ	Gegenbauer polynomials, normed by $C_l^\lambda(1) = 1$	VII.3
Y_l	spherical harmonics of degree l	VII.3
$N(n, l)$	number of linearly independent spherical harmonics of degree l	VII.3
J_k	Bessel function of the first kind	VII.3
U_k, T_k	Chebyshev polynomials	VII.3
δ, δ_x	Dirac's δ-function	VII.1
sinc_b	sinc function	III.1
$\eta(\vartheta, b)$	exponentially decaying function	III.2
Γ	Gamma function	
$0(M)$	Quantity of order M	
$\mathscr{S}$	Schwartz space on $\mathbb{R}^n$	VII.1
	Schwartz space on Z, T	II.1
$\mathscr{S}'$	tempered distributions	VII.1
C^m	m times continuously differentiable functions	
C^∞	infinitely differentiable functions	
C_0^∞	functions in C^∞ with compact support	
H^α, H_0^α	Sobolev spaces of order α on $\Omega \subseteq \mathbb{R}^n$	VII.4
	Sobolev spaces of order α on Z, T	II.5

$L_p(\Omega)$	space with norm $\left(\int_\Omega |f|^p \, dx\right)^{1/2}$	
$L_p(\Omega, w)$	same as $L_p(\Omega)$ but with weight w	
$\langle u_1, \ldots, u_m \rangle$	span of $u_1, \ldots, u_m$	
R, **R**$_\theta$	Radon transform	II.1
P, **P**$_\theta$	X-ray transform	II.1
D$_a$	divergent beam transform	II.1
R$^\#$ etc.	dual of **R**, etc.	II.1
I^α	Riesz potential	II.2
R$_\mu$	attenuated Radon transform	II.6
T$_\mu$	exponential Radon transform	II.6
A^*	adjoint of operator A	
A^T	transpose of matrix A	
$\mathbb{Z}^n$	n-tupels of integers	
$\mathbb{Z}^n_+$	n-tupels of non-negative integers	
$f \perp g$	f perpendicular to g	
H	Hilbert transform	VII.1
M	Mellin transform	VII.3
$\square$	end of proof	

I
Computerized Tomography

In this chapter we describe a few typical applications of CT. The purpose is to give an idea of the scope and limitations of CT and to motivate the mathematical apparatus we are going to develop in the following chapters.

In Section I.1 we give a short description of CT in diagnostic radiology. This will serve as a standard example throughout the book. In Section I.2 we consider more examples and discuss very briefly some physical principles which lead to CT.

I.1 The Basic Example: Transmission Computerized Tomography

The most prominent example of CT is still transmission CT in diagnostic radiology. Here, a cross-section of the human body is scanned by a thin X-ray beam whose intensity loss is recorded by a detector and processed by a computer to produce a two-dimensional image which in turn is displayed on a screen. We recommend Herman (1979, 1980), Brooks and Di Chiro (1976), Scudder (1978), Shepp and Kruskal (1978), Deans (1983) as introductory reading and Gambarelli et al., (1977), Koritké and Sick (1982) for the medical background.

A simple physical model is as follows. Let $f(x)$ be the X-ray attenuation coefficient of the tissue at the point x, i.e. X-rays traversing a small distance Δx at x suffer the relative intensity loss

$$\Delta I / I = f(x) \Delta x. \tag{1.1}$$

Let I_0 be the initial intensity of the beam L which we think of as a straight line, and let I_1 be its intensity after having passed the body. It follows from (1.1) that

$$I_1/I_0 = \exp\left\{-\int_L f(x)\,dx\right\}, \tag{1.2}$$

i.e. the scanning process provides us with the line integral of the function f along each of the lines L. From all these integrals we have to reconstruct f.

The transform which maps a function on $\mathbb{R}^2$ into the set of its line integrals is called the (two-dimensional) Radon transform. Thus the reconstruction problem of CT simply calls for the inversion of the Radon transform in $\mathbb{R}^2$. In principle, this has been done as early as 1917 by Radon who gave an explicit inversion formula, cf. II, Section 2. However, we shall see that Radon's formula is of limited value for practical calculations and solves only part of the problem.

In practice the integrals can be measured only for a finite number of lines L. Their arrangement, which we refer to as scanning geometry, is determined by the design of the scanner. There are basically two scanning geometries in use (Fig. I.1). In the parallel scanning geometry a set of equally spaced parallel lines are taken for a number of equally distributed directions. It requires a single source and a single detector which move in parallel and rotate during the scanning process. In the fan-beam scanning geometry the source runs on a circle around the body, firing a whole fan of X-rays which are recorded by a linear detector array simultaneously for each source position. Parallel scanning has been used in A. Cormack's 1963 scanner and in the first commercial scanner developed by G. Hounsfield from EMI. It has been given up in favour of fan-beam scanning to speed up the scanning process.

Mathematics of Computerized Tomography

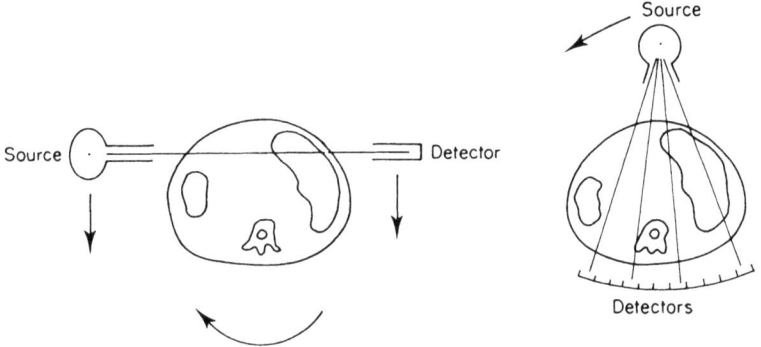

FIG. I.1 Principle of transmission CT. Cross-section of the abdomen shows spine, liver and spleen. Left: parallel scanning. Right: fan-beam scanning.

So the real problem in CT is to reconstruct f from a finite number of its line integrals, and the reconstruction procedure has to be adapted to the scanning geometry. The impact of finite sampling and scanning geometry on resolution and accuracy is one of the major themes in CT.

Sometimes it is not possible or not desirable to scan the whole cross-section. If one is interested only in a small part (the region of interest) of the body it seems reasonable not to expose the rest of the body to radiation. This means that only lines which hit the region of interest or which pass close by are measured. The opposite case occurs if an opaque implant is present. We then have to reconstruct f outside the implant with the line integrals through the implant missing. Finally it may happen that only directions in an angular range less than 180° are available. In all these cases we speak of incomplete data problems. A close investigation of uniqueness and stability and the development of reconstruction methods for incomplete data problems is indispensable for a serious study of CT.

So far we have considered only the two-dimensional problem. In order to obtain a three-dimensional image one scans the body layer by layer. If this is too time consuming (e.g. in an examination of the beating heart) this reduction to a series of two-dimensional problems is no longer possible. One then has to deal with the fully three-dimensional problem in which line integrals through all parts of the body have to be processed simultaneously. Since it is virtually impossible to scan a patient from head to toe, incomplete data problems are the rule rather than the exception in three-dimensional CT. As an example we mention only the cone beam scanning geometry, which is the three-dimensional analog of fan-beam scanning. In cone beam scanning, the source spins around the object on a circle, sending out a cone of X-rays which are recorded by a two-dimensional detector array. Even in the hypothetical case of an infinite number of source positions, only those lines which meet the source curve are measured in this way. Since these lines form only a small fraction of the set of all lines meeting the object the data set is extremely incomplete.

The problems we have mentioned so far are clearly mathematical in nature, and they can be solved or clarified by mathematical tools. This is what this book is trying to do. It will be concerned with questions such as uniqueness, stability, accuracy, resolution, and, of course, with reconstruction algorithms.

There is a bulk of other problems resulting from insufficient modelling which we shall not deal with. We mention only beam hardening: in reality, the function f does not only depend on x but also on the energy E of the X-rays. Assuming $T(E)$ to be the energy spectrum of the X-ray source, (1.2) has to be replaced by

$$I_1/I_0 = \int T(E) \exp\left\{-\int_L f(x, E)\,dx\right\} dE. \qquad (1.3)$$

Using (1.2) instead of (1.3) causes artefacts in the reconstructed image. More specifically we have approximately (see Stonestrom *et al.*, 1981)

$$f(x, E) = E^{-3} f_1(x) + C(E) f_2(x) \qquad (1.4)$$

with C the Klein–Nishina function which varies only little in the relevant energy range. Therefore the beam hardening effect is more pronounced at low energies.

I.2 Other Applications

From the foregoing it should be clear that CT occurs whenever the internal structure of an object is examined by exposing it to some kind of radiation which propagates along straight lines, the intensity loss being determined by (1.1). There are many applications of this type. We mention only electron microscopy since it is a typical example for incomplete data of the limited angle type. In transmission electron microscopy (Hoppe and Hegerl, 1980) an electron beam passes through a planar specimen under several incidence angles. Since the beam has to traverse the specimen more or less transversally, the incidence angle is restricted to an interval less than 180°, typically 120°.

In other applications the radiating sources are inside the object and it is the distribution of sources which is sought for. An example is emission CT in nuclear medicine (Budinger *et al.*, 1979). Here one wants to find the distribution f of a radiopharmaceutical in a cross-section of the body from measuring the radiation outside the body. If μ is the attenuation of the body (μ now plays the role of f in Section I.1) and assuming the same law as in (1.1) to be valid, the intensity I outside the body measured by a detector which is collimated so as to pick up only radiation along the straight line L (single particle emission computerized tomography: SPECT) is given by

$$I = \int_L f(x)\exp\left\{-\int_{L(x)} \mu(y)\,dy\right\}dx \qquad (2.1)$$

where $L(x)$ is the section of L between x and the detector.

If μ is negligible, then I is essentially the line integral of f and we end up with standard CT. However, in practice μ is not small. That means that we have to reconstruct f from weighted line integrals, the weight function being determined by the attenuation μ. The relevant integral transform is now a generalization of the Radon transform which we call attenuated Radon transform.

An important special case arises if the sources eject the particles pairwise in opposite directions and if the radiation in opposite directions is measured in coincidence, i.e. only events with two particles arriving at opposite detectors at the same time are counted (positron emission tomography: PET). Then, (2.1) has to be replaced by

$$I = \int_L f(x)\exp\left\{-\int_{L_+(x)} \mu(y)\,dy - \int_{L_-(x)} \mu(y)\,dy\right\}dx$$

where $L_+(x)$, $L_-(x)$ are the two half-lines of L with endpoint x. Since the exponent adds up to the integral over L we obtain

$$I = \exp\left\{-\int_L \mu(y)\,dy\right\}\int_L f(x)\,dx \qquad (2.2)$$

which does not lead to a new transform.

In SPECT as well as in PET we are interested in f, not in μ. Nevertheless, since μ enters the integral equation for f we have to determine it anyway, be it by additional measurements (e.g. a transmission scan) or by mathematical tools.

Another source of CT-type problems is ultrasound tomography in the geometrical acoustics approximation. Here the relevant quantity is the refractive index n of the object under examination. In the simplest case the travel time $T(x, y)$ of a sound signal travelling between two points x and y lying on the surface of the object is measured. The path of the signal is the geodesic $\Gamma_n(x, y)$ with respect to the metric $ds = n\sqrt{(dx_1^2 + dx_2^2 + dx_3^2)}$ joining x and y. We have

$$T(x, y) = \int_{\Gamma_n(x,y)} n \, ds. \qquad (2.3)$$

Knowing $T(x, y)$ for many emitter–receiver pairs x, y we want to compute n. Equation (2.3) is a nonlinear integral equation for n. Schomberg(1978) developed an algorithm for the nonlinear problem. Linearizing by assuming $n = n_0 + f$ with n_0 known and f small we obtain approximately

$$T(x, y) - \int_{\Gamma_{n_0}(x,y)} n_0 \, ds = \int_{\Gamma_{n_0}(x,y)} f \, ds \qquad (2.4)$$

and we have to reconstruct f from its integrals over the curves $\Gamma_{n_0}(x, y)$. This is the problem of integral geometry in the sense of Gelfand et al. (1965). Inversion formulas for special families of curves have been derived by Cormack (1981), Cormack and Quinto (1980) and Helgason (1980). In seismology the curves are circles, see Anderson (1984). If n_0 is constant, the geodesics are straight lines and we end up with the problem of CT.

It is well known that inverse problems for hyperbolic differential equations sometimes can be reduced to a problem in integral geometry, see Romanov (1974). As an example we derive the basic equation of diffraction tomography and show that CT is a limiting case of diffraction tomography.

Consider a scattering object in $\mathbb{R}^2$ which we describe by its refractive index $n(x) = (1 + f(x))^{1/2}$ where f vanishes outside the unit ball of $\mathbb{R}^2$, i.e. the object is contained in the unit circle. This object is exposed to a time harmonic 'incoming wave'

$$e^{-ikt} u_I(x)$$

with frequency k. We consider only plane waves, i.e.

$$u_I(x) = e^{ik\theta \cdot x}, \qquad (2.4)$$

the unit vector $\theta \in S^1$ being the direction of propagation.

In (direct) scattering (Courant and Hilbert (1962), ch. IV, Section 5) one finds for f given, a scattered wave

$$e^{-ikt} u_S(x)$$

such that $u = u_I + u_S$ satisfies the reduced wave equation

$$\Delta u + k^2 (1 + f) u = 0, \qquad (2.5)$$

Δ the Laplacian, and a boundary condition at infinity. In order to solve (2.5) within the Rytov approximation (Tatarski, 1961, ch. 7.2) we put in (2.5)

$$u = u_I e^{kw}$$

where the factor k has been introduced for convenience. We obtain

$$k\Delta w + 2ik^2\theta\cdot\nabla w + k^2|\nabla w|^2 = -k^2 f$$

with ∇ the gradient. The Rytov approximation u_R to u is obtained by neglecting $|\nabla w|^2$, i.e.

$$u_R = u_I e^{kw_R}$$

where w_R satisfies

$$\nabla w_R + 2ik\theta\cdot\nabla w_R = -kf \tag{2.6}$$

or

$$\Delta(u_I w_R) + k^2(u_I w_R) = -kfu_I. \tag{2.7}$$

This differential equation can be solved using an appropriate Green's function which in our case happens to be $H_0(k|x|)$ with $4iH_0$ the zero order Hankel function of the first kind. All we need to know about H_0 is the integral representation

$$H_0(k|x|) = \frac{-i}{4\pi}\int_{R^1} e^{i(|x_1|a(\sigma) + x_2\sigma)}\frac{d\sigma}{a(\sigma)} \tag{2.8}$$

where $a(\sigma) = \sqrt{(k^2 - \sigma^2)}$ (Morse and Feshbach, 1953, p. 823). The solution of (2.7) can now be written as

$$u_I w_R(x) = -k\int_{R^2} H_0(k|x - y|)f(y)u_I(y)dy. \tag{2.9}$$

This solves—within the Rytov approximation—the direct scattering problem.

In inverse scattering (see e.g. Sleeman (1982) for a survey) we have to compute f from a knowledge of u_S outside the scattering object. If the Rytov approximation is used, the inverse scattering problem can be solved simply by solving (2.9) for f, using as data

$$g(\theta, s) = w_R(r\theta + s\theta^\perp)$$

where r is a fixed number > 1, i.e. w_R is measured outside a circle of radius r. Inserting u_I from (2.4) and H_0 from (2.8) into (2.9) yields

$$g(\theta, s) = -ke^{-ikr}\int_{R^1}\int_{R^1} H_0(k((r-r')^2 + (s-s')^2)^{1/2})f(r'\theta + s'\theta^\perp)e^{ikr'}dr'ds'$$

$$= \frac{ik}{4\pi}e^{-ikr}\int_{R^1}\int_{R^1}\int_{R^1} e^{i(|r-r'|a(\sigma) + (s-s')\sigma)}\frac{d\sigma}{a(\sigma)}f(r'\theta + s'\theta^\perp)e^{ikr'}dr'ds'.$$

Since $r > 1$ and $f(r'\theta + s'\theta^\perp) = 0$ for $|r'| > 1$ we can drop the absolute value in $|r - r'|$. Interchanging the order of integration we get

$$g(\theta, s) = \frac{ik}{4\pi}e^{-ikr}\int_{R^1} e^{is\sigma}\frac{e^{ira(\sigma)}}{a(\sigma)}\int_{R^1}\int_{R^1} e^{-i(r'(a(\sigma) - k) + s'\sigma)}f(r'\theta + s'\theta^\perp)dr'ds'd\sigma.$$

The integration with respect to $y = r'\theta + s'\theta^\perp$ is a Fourier transform in $\mathbb{R}^2$, hence

$$g(\theta, s) = \frac{ik}{2} e^{-ikr} \int_{\mathbb{R}^1} e^{is\sigma} \frac{e^{ira(\sigma)}}{a(\sigma)} \hat{f}((a(\sigma) - k)\theta + \sigma\theta^\perp) d\sigma.$$

The integration with respect to σ is an inverse Fourier transform in $\mathbb{R}^1$. From the Fourier inversion theorem we obtain

$$\hat{f}((a(\sigma) - k)\theta + \sigma\theta^\perp) = -\left(\frac{2}{\pi}\right)^{1/2} i \frac{a(\sigma)}{k} e^{ir(k - a(\sigma))} \hat{g}(\theta, \sigma) \qquad (2.10)$$

where $\hat{g}$ is the one-dimensional Fourier transform with respect to the second argument. If σ runs over the interval $[-k, k]$, then

$$(a(\sigma) - k)\theta + \sigma\theta^\perp = \sqrt{(k^2 - \sigma^2)}\theta + \sigma\theta^\perp - k\theta$$

runs over the half-circle around $-k\theta$ with top at the origin, see Fig. I.2. Hence, if θ varies over S^1, f is given by (2.10) in a circle of radius at least k. Assuming that we are not interested in frequencies beyond k (i.e. that we are satisfied with a finite resolution in the sense of the sampling theorem, cf. Chapter III.1) and that the Rytov approximation is valid, (2.10) solves in principle the inverse scattering problem. In fact (2.10) is the starting point of diffraction tomography as suggested by Mueller *et al.* (1979), see also Devaney (1982), Ball *et al.* (1980).

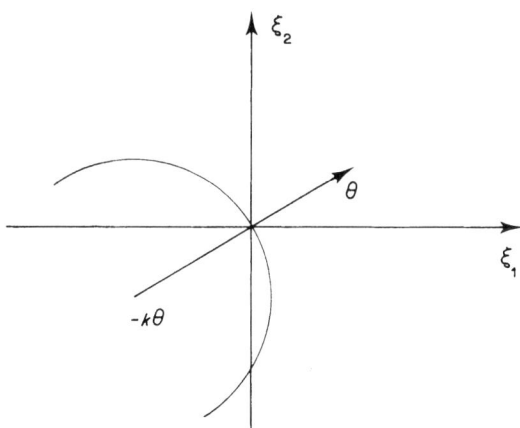

FIG. I.2. Half-circle on which $\hat{f}$ is given by (2.10).

If we let $k \to \infty$ then $a(\sigma)/k \to 1$, $a(\sigma) - k \to 0$, hence (2.10) becomes

$$\hat{f}(\sigma\theta^\perp) = -\left(\frac{2}{\pi}\right)^{1/2} i\hat{g}(\theta, \sigma), \qquad (2.11)$$

i.e. the circles on which f is given turn into lines. Later we shall see (cf. Theorem II.1.1) that

$$\hat{f}(\sigma\theta) = (2\pi)^{-1/2} (\mathbf{R}f)\hat{\,}(\theta, \sigma)$$

where

$$\mathbf{R}f(\theta, s) = \int_{\theta \cdot x = s} f(x)\,dx$$

is the Radon transform. Comparing this with (2.11) we find that

$$\mathbf{R}f(\theta^\perp, s) = -2i\,g(\theta, s)$$

or

$$\int_{\theta \cdot x = s} f(x)\,dx = -2i w_R (r\theta + s\theta^\perp) \qquad (2.12)$$

for $r > 1$. Thus, for large frequencies and within the Rytov approximation, the line integrals of f are given by the scattered field outside the scattering object, i.e. CT is a limiting case of the inverse scattering problem of the wave equation. Of course (2.12) follows also directly from (2.6) by letting $k \to \infty$.

A similar treatment of the inverse problem in electromagnetic scattering shows that the target ramp response in radar theory provides the radar silhouette area of the target along the radar line of incidence, see Das and Boerner (1978). This means that identifying the shape of the target is equivalent to reconstructing the characteristic function of the target from its integrals along planes in $\mathbb{R}^3$. This is an instance of CT in $\mathbb{R}^3$ involving the three-dimensional Radon transform, though with very incomplete data. Complete sampling of the three-dimensional Radon transform occurs in NMR imaging (Hinshaw and Lent, 1983). Even though the formulation in terms of the Radon transform is possible and has been used in practice, (Marr et al., 1981), the present trend is to deal with the NMR problem entirely in terms of Fourier transforms.

I.3 Bibliographical Notes

'Tomography' is derived from the greek word $\tau o\mu o\sigma$ = slice. It stands for several different techniques in diagnostic radiology permitting the imaging of cross-sections of the human body. Simple focusing techniques for singling out a specific layer have been used before the advent of CT, which sometimes has been called reconstructive tomography to distinguish it from other kinds of tomography. See Littleton (1976) for the early history of tomography and Klotz et al. (1974) for refined versions employing coded apertures.

The literature on CT has grown tremendously in the last few years, and we do not try to give an exhaustive list of references. We rather refer to the reasonably complete bibliography in Deans (1983); this book also gives an excellent survey on the applications of CT. A state-of-the-art review is contained in the March 1983 issue of the *Proceedings of the IEEE* which is devoted to CT. The conference proceedings Marr (1974a), Gordon (1975), Herman and Natterer (1981) give an impression of the exciting period of CT in the 1970s.

II
The Radon Transform and Related Transforms

In this chapter we introduce and study various integral transforms from a theoretical point of view. As general reference we recommend Helgason (1980). The material of this chapter serves as the theoretical basis for the rest of the book. It contains complete proofs, referring only to Chapter VII.

II.1 Definition and Elementary Properties of some Integral Operators

The (n-dimensional) Radon transform **R** maps a function on $\mathbb{R}^n$ into the set of its integrals over the hyperplanes of $\mathbb{R}^n$. More specifically, if $\theta \in S^{n-1}$ and $s \in \mathbb{R}^1$, then

$$\mathbf{R}f(\theta, s) = \int_{x \cdot \theta = s} f(x)\, dx = \int_{\theta^\perp} f(s\theta + y)\, dy$$

is the integral of $f \in \mathscr{S}(\mathbb{R}^n)$, the Schwartz space, over the hyperplane perpendicular to θ with (signed) distance s from the origin. For the Schwartz space and other notions not explained here see Chapter VII. Obviously, $\mathbf{R}f$ is an even function on the unit cylinder $Z = S^{n-1} \times \mathbb{R}^1$ of $\mathbb{R}^{n+1}$, i.e. $\mathbf{R}f(-\theta, -s) = \mathbf{R}f(\theta, s)$. We also write

$$\mathbf{R}_\theta f(s) = \mathbf{R}f(\theta, s).$$

The (n-dimensional) X-ray transform **P** maps a function on $\mathbb{R}^n$ into the set of its line integrals. More specifically, if $\theta \in S^{n-1}$ and $x \in \mathbb{R}^n$, then

$$\mathbf{P}f(\theta, x) = \int_{-\infty}^{+\infty} f(x + t\theta)\, dt$$

is the integral of $f \in \mathscr{S}(\mathbb{R}^n)$ over the straight line through x with direction θ. Obviously, $\mathbf{P}f(\theta, x)$ does not change if x is moved in the direction θ. We therefore normally restrict x to $\theta^\perp$ which makes $\mathbf{P}f$ a function on the tangent bundle

$$T = \{(\theta, x) : \theta \in S^{n-1}, x \in \theta^\perp\}$$

to S^{n-1}. We also write
$$\mathbf{P}_\theta f(x) = \mathbf{P} f(\theta, x).$$

$\mathbf{P}_\theta f$ is sometimes called the projection of f on to $\theta^\perp$. For $n = 2$, $\mathbf{P}$ and $\mathbf{R}$ coincide except for the notation of the arguments. Of course it is possible to express $\mathbf{R} f(\omega, s)$ as an integral over $\mathbf{P} f$: for any $\theta \in S^{n-1}$ with $\theta \perp \omega$ we have

$$\mathbf{R} f(\omega, s) = \int_{x \in \theta^\perp, \, x \cdot \omega = s} \mathbf{P} f(\theta, x) \, dx. \tag{1.1}$$

The divergent beam (in two dimensions also fan-beam) transform is defined by

$$\mathbf{D} f(a, \theta) = \int_0^\infty f(a + t\theta) \, dt.$$

This is the integral of f along the half-line with endpoint $a \in \mathbb{R}^n$ and direction $\theta \in S^{n-1}$. We also write
$$\mathbf{D}_a f(\theta) = \mathbf{D} f(a, \theta).$$

If $f \in \mathscr{S}(\mathbb{R}^n)$, then $\mathbf{R}_\theta f$, $\mathbf{P}_\theta f$, $\mathbf{R} f$, $\mathbf{P} f$ are in the Schwartz spaces on $\mathbb{R}^1$, $\theta^\perp$, Z, T respectively, the latter ones being defined either by local coordinates or simply by restricting the functions in $\mathscr{S}(\mathbb{R}^{n+1})$ to Z, those in $\mathscr{S}(\mathbb{R}^{2n})$ to T.

Many important properties of the integral transforms introduced above follow from formulas involving convolutions and Fourier transforms. Whenever convolutions or Fourier transforms of functions on Z or T are used they are to be taken with respect to the second variable, i.e.

$$h * g(\theta, s) = \int_{\mathbb{R}^1} h(\theta, s - t) g(\theta, t) \, dt,$$

$$\hat{h}(\theta, \sigma) = (2\pi)^{-1/2} \int_{\mathbb{R}^1} e^{-is\sigma} h(\theta, s) \, ds$$

for $h, g \in \mathscr{S}(Z)$ and

$$h * g(\theta, x) = \int_{\theta^\perp} h(\theta, x - y) g(\theta, y) \, dy, \qquad x \in \theta^\perp,$$

$$\hat{h}(\theta, \xi) = (2\pi)^{(1-n)/2} \int_{\theta^\perp} e^{-ix \cdot \xi} h(\theta, x) \, dx, \qquad \xi \in \theta^\perp$$

for $h, g \in \mathscr{S}(T)$.

We begin with the so-called 'projection theorem' or 'Fourier slice theorem'

THEOREM 1.1 For $f \in \mathscr{S}(\mathbb{R}^n)$ we have
$$(\mathbf{R}_\theta f)\,\hat{}\,(\sigma) = (2\pi)^{(n-1)/2}\,\hat{f}(\sigma\theta), \qquad \sigma \in \mathbb{R}^1,$$
$$(\mathbf{P}_\theta f)\,\hat{}\,(\eta) = (2\pi)^{1/2}\,\hat{f}(\eta), \qquad \eta \in \theta^\perp.$$

Proof We have
$$(\mathbf{R}_\theta f)\,\hat{}\,(\sigma) = (2\pi)^{-1/2} \int_{\mathbb{R}^1} e^{-i\sigma s}\, \mathbf{R}_\theta f(s)\, ds$$
$$= (2\pi)^{-1/2} \int_{\mathbb{R}^1} e^{-i\sigma s} \int_{\theta^\perp} f(s\theta + y)\, dy\, ds.$$

With $x = s\theta + y$ the new variable of integration we have $s = \theta \cdot x$, $dx = dy\, ds$, hence
$$(\mathbf{R}_\theta f)\,\hat{}\,(\sigma) = (2\pi)^{-1/2} \int_{\mathbb{R}^n} e^{-i\sigma\theta \cdot x} f(x)\, dx$$
$$= (2\pi)^{(n-1)/2}\,\hat{f}(\sigma\theta).$$

Similarly,
$$(\mathbf{P}_\theta f)\,\hat{}\,(\eta) = (2\pi)^{-(n-1)/2} \int_{\theta^\perp} e^{-i\eta \cdot y}\, \mathbf{P}_\theta f(y)\, dy$$
$$= (2\pi)^{-(n-1)/2} \int_{\theta^\perp} e^{-i\eta \cdot y} \int_{\mathbb{R}^1} f(y + t\theta)\, dt\, dy$$
$$= (2\pi)^{-(n-1)/2} \int_{\mathbb{R}^n} e^{-i\eta \cdot x} f(x)\, dx$$
$$= (2\pi)^{1/2}\,\hat{f}(\eta). \qquad \square$$

As a simple application we derive the formula
$$\mathbf{R}_\theta D^\alpha f = \theta^\alpha\, D^{|\alpha|}\, \mathbf{R}_\theta f \tag{1.2}$$
where $D^{|\alpha|}$ acts on the second variable of $\mathbf{R}f$. For the proof we use Theorem 1.1, R3 in VII.1 and the fact that the Fourier transform is invertible on $\mathscr{S}(\mathbb{R}^1)$, obtaining
$$(\mathbf{R}_\theta D^\alpha f)\,\hat{}\,(\sigma) = (2\pi)^{(n-1)/2}\, (D^\alpha f)\,\hat{}\,(\sigma\theta)$$
$$= (2\pi)^{(n-1)/2}\, i^{|\alpha|} \sigma^{|\alpha|} \theta^\alpha\, \hat{f}(\sigma\theta)$$
$$= i^{|\alpha|} \sigma^{|\alpha|} \theta^\alpha (\mathbf{R}_\theta f)\,\hat{}\,(\sigma)$$
$$= \theta^\alpha (D^{|\alpha|} \mathbf{R}_\theta f)\,\hat{}\,(\sigma).$$

In order to derive a formula for the derivatives of $\mathbf{R}f$ with respect to θ we give a second equivalent definition of the Radon transform in terms of the one-dimensional δ-function. Putting

$$\delta^b(t) = \frac{1}{2\pi} \int_{-b}^{b} e^{i(t-s)}\, ds$$

we know from VII.1 that $\delta^b \to \delta$ pointwise in $\mathscr{S}'$. Hence, for $f \in \mathscr{S}$,

$$\lim_{b \to \infty} \int_{\mathbb{R}^n} f(x)\delta^b(s - x\cdot\theta)\, dx = \lim_{b \to \infty} \int_{\mathbb{R}^1}\int_{\theta^\perp} f(t\theta + y)\, dy\, \delta^b(s - t)\, dt$$

$$= \int_{\theta^\perp} f(s\theta + y)\, dy.$$

In this sense we write

$$\mathbf{R}f(\theta, s) = \int_{\mathbb{R}^n} f(x)\delta(s - x\cdot\theta)\, dx. \tag{1.3}$$

(1.3) provides a natural extension of $\mathbf{R}f$ to $(\mathbb{R}^n - \{0\}) \times \mathbb{R}^1$ since, for $r > 0$,

$$\mathbf{R}f(r\theta, rs) = \int_{\mathbb{R}^n} f(x)\delta(rs - rx\cdot\theta)\, dx$$

$$= r^{-1}\int_{\mathbb{R}^n} f(x)\delta(s - x\cdot\theta)\, dx$$

$$= r^{-1}\mathbf{R}f(\theta, s). \tag{1.4}$$

i.e. $\mathbf{R}f$ is extended as a function homogeneous of degree -1. This function can be differentiated with respect to its first variable and we obtain

$$\frac{\partial}{\partial \theta_k}\mathbf{R}f(\theta, s) = \int_{\mathbb{R}^n} f(x)\frac{\partial}{\partial \theta_k}\delta(s - x\cdot\theta)\, dx$$

$$= -\int_{\mathbb{R}^n} f(x)x_k\delta'(s - x\cdot\theta)\, dx$$

$$= -\frac{\partial}{\partial s}\int_{\mathbb{R}^n} f(x)x_k\delta(s - x\cdot\theta)\, dx$$

$$= -\frac{\partial}{\partial s}(\mathbf{R}(x_k f))(\theta, s)$$

This formal procedure as well as the derivation of (1.4) can be justified by using the approximate δ-function δ^b. For k a multi-index we get

$$D_\theta^k \mathbf{R} f = (-1)^{|k|} \frac{\partial^{|k|}}{\partial s^{|k|}} \mathbf{R}(x^k f) \tag{1.5}$$

where D_θ denotes the derivative with respect to θ.

As an immediate consequence from R4 of VII.1 and Theorem 1.1, or by direct calculation as in the preceding proof, we obtain

THEOREM 1.2 For $f, g \in \mathscr{S}(\mathbb{R}^n)$ we have

$$\mathbf{R}_\theta(f * g) = \mathbf{R}_\theta f * \mathbf{R}_\theta g,$$
$$\mathbf{P}_\theta(f * g) = \mathbf{P}_\theta f * \mathbf{P}_\theta g.$$

In the following we want to define dual operators $\mathbf{R}_\theta^\#$, $\mathbf{R}^\#$, $\mathbf{P}_\theta^\#$, $\mathbf{P}^\#$. We start out from

$$\int_{\mathbb{R}^1} \mathbf{R}_\theta f(s) g(s) \, ds = \int_{\mathbb{R}^1} \int_{\theta^\perp} f(s\theta + y) g(s) \, dy \, ds$$

$$= \int_{\mathbb{R}^n} f(x) g(x \cdot \theta) \, dx.$$

Defining

$$\mathbf{R}_\theta^\# g(x) = g(x \cdot \theta)$$

we thus have

$$\int_{\mathbb{R}^1} \mathbf{R}_\theta f(s) g(s) \, ds = \int_{\mathbb{R}^n} f(x) \mathbf{R}_\theta^\# g(x) \, dx. \tag{1.6}$$

Integrating over S^{n-1} we obtain

$$\int_{S^{n-1}} \int_{\mathbb{R}^1} \mathbf{R} f(\theta, s) g(\theta, s) \, ds \, d\theta = \int_{\mathbb{R}^n} f(x) \mathbf{R}^\# g(x) \, dx, \tag{1.7}$$

$$\mathbf{R}^\# g(x) = \int_{S^{n-1}} g(\theta, x \cdot \theta) \, dx.$$

Similarly,

$$\int_{\theta^\perp} \mathbf{P}_\theta f(x) g(x) \, dx = \int_{\mathbb{R}^n} f(x) \mathbf{P}_\theta^\# g(x) \, dx, \tag{1.8}$$

$$\int_{S^{n-1}} \int_{\theta^\perp} \mathbf{P} f(x) g(x) \, dx \, d\theta = \int_{\mathbb{R}^n} f(x) \mathbf{P}^\# g(x) \, dx \tag{1.9}$$

where

$$\mathbf{P}_\theta^\# g(x) = g(\theta, E_\theta x)$$

$$\mathbf{P}^\# g(x) = \int_{S^{n-1}} g(\theta, E_\theta x)\, d\theta$$

with E_θ the orthogonal projection on $\theta^\perp$.

Note that $\mathbf{R}, \mathbf{R}^\#$ form a dual pair in the sense of integral geometry: while $\mathbf{R}$ integrates over all points in a plane, $\mathbf{R}^\#$ integrates over all planes through a point. This is the starting point of a far-reaching generalization of the Radon transform, see Helgason (1980). The same applies to $\mathbf{P}, \mathbf{P}^\#$.

THEOREM 1.3 For $f \in \mathscr{S}(\mathbb{R}^n)$ and $g \in \mathscr{S}(Z), \mathscr{S}(T)$ respectively we have

$$(\mathbf{R}^\# g) * f = \mathbf{R}^\# (g * \mathbf{R}f),$$
$$(\mathbf{P}^\# g) * f = \mathbf{P}^\# (g * \mathbf{P}f).$$

Proof We have

$$\mathbf{R}^\# g * f(x) = \int_{\mathbb{R}^n} \mathbf{R}^\# g(x - y) f(y)\, dy$$

$$= \int_{\mathbb{R}^n} \int_{S^{n-1}} g(\theta, (x - y) \cdot \theta)\, d\theta\, f(y)\, dy$$

$$= \int_{S^{n-1}} \int_{\mathbb{R}^n} g(\theta, (x - y) \cdot \theta) f(y)\, dy\, d\theta.$$

Making the substitution $y = s\theta + z$, $z \in \theta^\perp$ in the inner integral we obtain

$$\mathbf{R}^\# g * f(x) = \int_{S^{n-1}} \int_{\mathbb{R}^1} \int_{\theta^\perp} g(\theta, x \cdot \theta - s) f(s\theta + z)\, dz\, ds\, d\theta$$

$$= \int_{S^{n-1}} \int_{\mathbb{R}^1} g(\theta, x \cdot \theta - s) \mathbf{R}f(\theta, s)\, ds\, d\theta$$

$$= \int_{S^{n-1}} (g * \mathbf{R}f)(\theta, x \cdot \theta)\, d\theta$$

$$= \mathbf{R}^\# (g * \mathbf{R}f)(x).$$

$\mathbf{P}$ is dealt with in the same way. □

THEOREM 1.4 For $g \in \mathscr{S}(Z)$ we have

$$(\mathbf{R}^* g)\hat{}(\xi) = (2\pi)^{(n-1)/2}|\xi|^{1-n}\left(\hat{g}\left(\frac{\xi}{|\xi|}, |\xi|\right) + \hat{g}\left(-\frac{\xi}{|\xi|}, -|\xi|\right)\right).$$

Proof For $w \in \mathscr{S}(\mathbb{R}^n)$ we obtain from the definition of $\mathbf{R}^*$ as dual of $\mathbf{R}$

$$\int_{\mathbb{R}^n} \mathbf{R}^* g \hat{w} \, dx = \int_{S^{n-1}} \int_{\mathbb{R}^1} g(\theta, s) \mathbf{R}\hat{w}(\theta, s) \, ds \, d\theta$$

$$= \int_{S^{n-1}} \int_{\mathbb{R}^1} \hat{g}(\theta, \sigma)(\mathbf{R}\hat{w})\check{}(\theta, \sigma) \, d\sigma \, d\theta$$

where we have made use of Rule 5 of VII.1 in the inner integral. By Theorem 1.1,

hence $\qquad (\mathbf{R}\hat{w})\check{}(\theta, \sigma) = (2\pi)^{(n-1)/2} w(\sigma\theta),$

$$\int_{\mathbb{R}^n} \mathbf{R}^* g \hat{w} \, dx = (2\pi)^{(n-1)/2} \int_{S^{n-1}} \int_{\mathbb{R}^1} \hat{g}(\theta, \sigma) w(\sigma\theta) \, d\sigma \, d\theta$$

$$= (2\pi)^{(n-1)/2} \int_{\mathbb{R}^n} \left(\hat{g}\left(\frac{\xi}{|\xi|}, |\xi|\right) + \hat{g}\left(-\frac{\xi}{|\xi|}, -|\xi|\right)\right)|\xi|^{1-n} w(\xi) \, d\xi$$

where we have put $\xi = \sigma\theta$ separately for $\sigma > 0$ and $\sigma < 0$. This shows that the distribution $(\mathbf{R}^* g)\hat{}$ is in fact represented by the function

$$(2\pi)^{(n-1)/2}\left(\hat{g}\left(\frac{\xi}{|\xi|}, |\xi|\right) + \hat{g}\left(-\frac{\xi}{|\xi|}, -|\xi|\right)\right)|\xi|^{1-n}. \qquad \square$$

THEOREM 1.5 For $f \in \mathscr{S}(\mathbb{R}^n)$ we have

$$\mathbf{R}^* \mathbf{R} f = |S^{n-2}||x|^{-1} * f,$$
$$\mathbf{P}^* \mathbf{P} f = 2|x|^{1-n} * f,$$

$|S^{m-1}|$ is the surface of the unit sphere S^{m-1} in $\mathbb{R}^m$, see VII.2.

Proof We have

$$\mathbf{R}^* \mathbf{R} f(x) = \int_{S^{n-1}} (\mathbf{R}f)(\theta, x \cdot \theta) \, d\theta$$

$$= \int_{S^{n-1}} \int_{\theta^\perp} f((x \cdot \theta)\theta + y) \, dy \, d\theta$$

$$= \int_{S^{n-1}} \int_{\theta^\perp} f(x + y) \, dy \, d\theta$$

since $x - (x \cdot \theta)\theta \in \theta^\perp$. Using (VII.2.8) with $f(x)$ replaced by $f(x+y)$ we obtain

$$\int_{S^{n-1}} \int_{\theta^\perp} f(x+y) \, dy \, d\theta = |S^{n-2}| \int_{\mathbf{R}^n} |y|^{-1} f(x+y) \, dy$$

hence

$$\mathbf{R}^* \mathbf{R} f(x) = |S^{n-2}| \int_{\mathbf{R}^n} |x-y|^{-1} f(y) \, dy.$$

Similarly,

$$\mathbf{P}^* \mathbf{P} f(x) = \int_{S^{n-1}} \mathbf{P} f(\theta, E_\theta x) \, d\theta$$

$$= \int_{S^{n-1}} \int_{\mathbf{R}^1} f(E_\theta x + t\theta) \, dt \, d\theta$$

$$= \int_{S^{n-1}} \int_{\mathbf{R}^1} f(x + t\theta) \, dt \, d\theta$$

since $x - E_\theta x = (x \cdot \theta)\theta$ is a multiple of θ. Breaking the inner integral into positive and negative part we obtain

$$\mathbf{P}^* \mathbf{P} f(x) = 2 \int_{S^{n-1}} \int_0^\infty f(x + t\theta) \, dt \, d\theta$$

$$= 2 \int_{\mathbf{R}^n} f(x+y) |y|^{1-n} \, dy$$

upon setting $y = t\theta$. This proves the second formula. $\square$

So far we have considered the integral transforms only on $\mathscr{S}(\mathbf{R}^n)$. Since

$$\int_{\mathbf{R}^1} |\mathbf{R}_\theta f(s)| \, ds \le \int_{\mathbf{R}^n} |f(x)| \, dx,$$

$$\int_{\theta^\perp} |\mathbf{P}_\theta f(x)| \, dx \le \int_{\mathbf{R}^n} |f(x)| \, dx,$$

$$\int_{S^{n-1}} |\mathbf{D}_a f(\theta)| \, d\theta \le \int_{\mathbf{R}^n} |f(x)| \, |x-a|^{1-n} \, dx,$$

the operators $\mathbf{R}_\theta$, $\mathbf{P}_\theta$ are easily extended to $L_1(\mathbb{R}^n)$, $\mathbf{D}_a$ to $L_1(\mathbb{R}^n, |x-a|^{1-n})$. Whenever we apply this operators to functions other than $\mathscr{S}$ we tacitly assume that the extended operators are meant. The duality relations (1.6), (1.7) hold whenever either of the functions $(\mathbf{R}|f|)g$, $f(\mathbf{R}^*|g|)$ is integrable, and correspondingly for (1.8), (1.9).

The Hilbert spaces $L_2(Z)$, $L_2(T)$ are defined quite naturally by the inner products

$$(g, h)_{L_2(Z)} = \int_{S^{n-1}} \int_{\mathbb{R}^1} g(\theta, s)\overline{h}(\theta, s)\,ds\,d\theta,$$

$$(g, h)_{L_2(T)} = \int_{S^{n-1}} \int_{\theta^\perp} g(\theta, x)\overline{h}(\theta, x)\,dx\,d\theta.$$

We have the following continuity result.

THEOREM 1.6 Let Ω^n be the unit ball in $\mathbb{R}^n$. Then, the operators

$$\mathbf{R}_\theta: L_2(\Omega^n) \to L_2([-1, +1], (1-s^2)^{(1-n)/2}),$$

$$\mathbf{P}_\theta: L_2(\Omega^n) \to L_2(\theta^\perp, (1-|x|^2)^{-1/2}),$$

$$\mathbf{R}: L_2(\Omega^n) \to L_2(Z, (1-s^2)^{(1-n)/2}),$$

$$\mathbf{P}: L_2(\Omega^n) \to L_2(T, (1-|x|^2)^{-1/2}),$$

$$\mathbf{D}_a: L_2(\Omega^n) \to L_2(S^{n-1}), \qquad (|a| > 1)$$

are continuous.

Proof For $f \in \mathscr{S}$ with support in Ω^n we have from the Cauchy–Schwarz inequality

$$|\mathbf{R}_\theta f(s)|^2 = \left| \int_{y \in \theta^\perp, |y| \leq (1-s^2)^{1/2}} f(s\theta + y)\,dy \right|^2$$

$$\leq (1-s^2)^{(n-1)/2} |\Omega^{n-1}| \int_{\theta^\perp} |f(s\theta + y)|^2\,dy$$

with $|\Omega^n|$ the volume of the unit ball Ω^n of $\mathbb{R}^n$, hence

$$\int_{\mathbb{R}^1} (1-s^2)^{(1-n)/2} |\mathbf{R}_\theta f(s)|^2\,ds \leq |\Omega^{n-1}| \int_{\mathbb{R}^1} \int_{\theta^\perp} |f(s\theta + y)|^2\,dy\,ds$$

$$= |\Omega^{n-1}| \int_{\mathbb{R}^n} |f(x)|^2\,dx.$$

This settles the case of $\mathbf{R}_\theta$. Integrating over S^{n-1} gives the continuity of $\mathbf{R}$. $\mathbf{P}_\theta$, $\mathbf{P}$ are dealt with in the same way. For $\mathbf{D}_a$ we have

$$|\mathbf{D}_a f(\theta)|^2 = \left|\int_0^\infty f(a+t\theta)\,dt\right|^2$$

$$\leq 2\int_0^\infty |f(a+t\theta)|^2\,dt$$

hence

$$\int_{S^{n-1}} |\mathbf{D}_a f(\theta)|^2\,d\theta \leq 2\int_{S^{n-1}}\int_0^\infty |f(a+t\theta)|^2\,dt\,d\theta$$

$$= 2\int_{\mathbb{R}^n} |f(a+y)|^2\,|y|^{1-n}\,dy$$

$$\leq 2(|a|-1)^{1-n}\int_\Omega |f(x)|^2\,dx. \quad \square$$

From Theorem 1.6 it follows that the operators $\mathbf{R}_\theta$, $\mathbf{P}_\theta$, $\mathbf{R}$, $\mathbf{P}$, $\mathbf{D}_a$ have continuous adjoints. For instance

$$\mathbf{R}_\theta^* : L_2([-1,+1],(1-s^2)^{(1-n)/2}) \to L_2(\Omega^n)$$

is given by

$$\mathbf{R}_\theta^* g(x) = \mathbf{R}_\theta^\# ((1-s^2)^{(1-n)/2} g).$$

II.2 Inversion Formulas

Explicit inversion formulas for the integral transforms are not only of obvious significance for the development of inversion algorithms, but play also an important role in the study of the local dependence of the solution on the data. In the following we derive inversion formulas for $\mathbf{R}$ and $\mathbf{P}$.

For $\alpha < n$ we define the linear operator $\mathbf{I}^\alpha$ by

$$(\mathbf{I}^\alpha f)\hat{\,}(\xi) = |\xi|^{-\alpha} \hat{f}(\xi).$$

$\mathbf{I}^\alpha$ is called the Riesz potential. If $\mathbf{I}^\alpha$ is applied to functions on Z or T it acts on the second variable. For $f \in \mathcal{S}$, $(\mathbf{I}^\alpha f)\hat{\,} \in L_1(\mathbb{R}^n)$, hence $\mathbf{I}^\alpha f$ makes sense and $\mathbf{I}^{-\alpha}\mathbf{I}^\alpha f = f$.

THEOREM 2.1   Let $f \in \mathcal{S}(\mathbb{R}^n)$. Then, for any $\alpha < n$, we have

$$f = \tfrac{1}{2}(2\pi)^{1-n}\mathbf{I}^{-\alpha}\mathbf{R}^* \mathbf{I}^{\alpha-n+1} g, \qquad g = \mathbf{R}f, \tag{2.1}$$

$$f = \frac{1}{|S^{n-2}|}(2\pi)^{-1}\mathbf{I}^{-\alpha}\mathbf{P}^{\#}\,\mathbf{I}^{\alpha-1}g, \qquad g = \mathbf{P}f. \tag{2.2}$$

Proof We start out from the Fourier inversion formula

$$\mathbf{I}^{\alpha}f(x) = (2\pi)^{-n/2}\int_{\mathbf{R}^n} e^{ix\cdot\xi}|\xi|^{-\alpha}\hat{f}(\xi)\,d\xi. \tag{2.3}$$

Introducing polar coordinates $\xi = \sigma\theta$ yields

$$\mathbf{I}^{\alpha}f(x) = (2\pi)^{-n/2}\int_{S^{n-1}}\int_0^{\infty} e^{i\sigma x\cdot\theta}\sigma^{n-1-\alpha}\hat{f}(\sigma\theta)\,d\sigma\,d\theta.$$

Here we express $\hat{f}$ by $(\mathbf{R}f)\hat{\ }$ using Theorem 1.1. We obtain

$$(\mathbf{I}^{\alpha}f)(x) = (2\pi)^{-n+1/2}\int_{S^{n-1}}\int_0^{\infty} e^{i\sigma x\cdot\theta}|\sigma|^{n-1-\alpha}(\mathbf{R}f)\hat{\ }(\theta,\sigma)\,d\sigma\,d\theta.$$

Replacing θ by $-\theta$ and σ by $-\sigma$ and using that $(\mathbf{R}f)\hat{\ }$ is even yields the same formula with the integral over $(0,\infty)$ replaced by the integral over $(-\infty,0)$. Adding both formulas leads to

$$\mathbf{I}^{\alpha}f(x) = \tfrac{1}{2}(2\pi)^{-n+1/2}\int_{S^{n-1}}\int_{-\infty}^{+\infty} e^{i\sigma x\cdot\theta}|\sigma|^{n-1-\alpha}(\mathbf{R}f)\hat{\ }(\theta,\sigma)\,d\sigma\,d\theta.$$

The inner integral can be expressed by the Riesz potential, hence

$$\mathbf{I}^{\alpha}f(x) = \tfrac{1}{2}(2\pi)^{-n+1}\int_{S^{n-1}}\mathbf{I}^{\alpha+1-n}\mathbf{R}f(\theta, x\cdot\theta)\,d\theta$$

$$= \tfrac{1}{2}(2\pi)^{-n+1}\mathbf{R}^{\#}\mathbf{I}^{\alpha+1-n}\mathbf{R}f(x)$$

and the inversion formula for $\mathbf{R}$ follows by applying $\mathbf{I}^{-\alpha}$.

For the second inversion formula we also start out from (2.3). Using the integral formula (VII.2.8).

$$\int_{\mathbf{R}^n} h(\xi)\,d\xi = \frac{1}{|S^{n-2}|}\int_{S^{n-1}}\int_{\theta^{\perp}}|\eta|h(\eta)\,d\eta\,d\theta$$

for the integral in (2.3) we obtain

$$\mathbf{I}^{\alpha}f(x) = (2\pi)^{-n/2}\frac{1}{|S^{n-2}|}\int_{S^{n-1}}\int_{\theta^{\perp}} e^{ix\cdot\eta}|\eta|^{1-\alpha}\hat{f}(\eta)\,d\eta\,d\theta.$$

Here we express $\hat{f}$ by $(Pf)^{\wedge}$ using Theorem 1.1. We obtain

$$I^{\alpha} f(x) = (2\pi)^{-(n+1)/2} \frac{1}{|S^{n-2}|} \int_{S^{n-1}} \int_{\theta^{\perp}} e^{ix\cdot\eta} |\eta|^{1-\alpha} (Pf)^{\wedge}(\eta) \, d\eta \, d\theta.$$

The inner integral can be expressed by the Riesz potential, hence

$$I^{\alpha} f(x) = (2\pi)^{-1} \frac{1}{|S^{n-2}|} \int_{S^{n-1}} I^{\alpha-1} Pf(\theta, E_{\theta} x) \, d\theta$$

$$= (2\pi)^{-1} \frac{1}{|S^{n-2}|} P^{*} I^{\alpha-1} Pf(x)$$

and the inversion formula for **P** follows. □

We want to make a few remarks.

(1) Putting $\alpha = 0$ in (2.1) yields

$$f = \tfrac{1}{2}(2\pi)^{1-n} \mathbf{R}^{*} \mathbf{I}^{1-n} g$$

where $\mathbf{I}^{1-n}$ acts on a function in $\mathbb{R}^1$. Since for $h \in \mathscr{S}(\mathbb{R}^1)$

$$(\mathbf{I}^{1-n} h)^{\wedge}(\sigma) = |\sigma|^{n-1} \hat{h}(\sigma)$$

$$= (\operatorname{sgn}(\sigma))^{n-1} \sigma^{n-1} \hat{h}(\sigma)$$

and since the Hilbert transform **H** can be defined by

$$(\mathbf{H} h)^{\wedge}(\sigma) = -i \operatorname{sgn}(\sigma) \hat{h}(\sigma),$$

see (VII.1.11), we can write

$$\mathbf{I}^{1-n} h = \mathbf{H}^{n-1} h^{(n-1)},$$

hence

$$f = \tfrac{1}{2}(2\pi)^{1-n} \mathbf{R}^{*} \mathbf{H}^{n-1} g^{(n-1)} \tag{2.4}$$

where the $(n-1)$st derivative is taken with respect to the second argument. Using

$$\mathbf{H}^{n-1} = \begin{cases} (-1)^{(n-2)/2} \mathbf{H}, & n \text{ even}, \\ (-1)^{(n-1)/2}, & n \text{ odd} \end{cases}$$

and the explicit form of $\mathbf{R}^{*}$ from Section II.1, (2.4) can be written as

$$f(x) = \tfrac{1}{2}(2\pi)^{1-n} \begin{cases} (-1)^{(n-2)/2} \int_{S^{n-1}} \mathbf{H} g^{(n-1)}(\theta, x\cdot\theta) \, d\theta, & n \text{ even}, \\ (-1)^{(n-1)/2} \int_{S^{n-1}} g^{(n-1)}(\theta, x\cdot\theta) \, d\theta, & n \text{ odd}. \end{cases} \tag{2.5}$$

(2) The fact that **H** shows up in (2.5) only for n even has an important practical consequence. Remember that $g(\theta, x\cdot\theta)$ is the integral of f over the hyperplane perpendicular to θ containing x. For n odd, (2.5) can be evaluated if $g(\theta, y\cdot\theta)$ is known for $\theta \in S^{n-1}$ and y in a neighbourhood of x, i.e. if the integrals of f along all

hyperplanes meeting a neighbourhood of x are known. Thus we see that the problem of reconstructing a function from its integrals over hyperplanes is, for odd dimension, local in the following sense: the function is determined at some point by the integrals along the hyperplanes through a neighbourhood of that point. This is not true for even dimension, since the Hilbert transform

$$\mathbf{H}h(s) = \frac{1}{\pi} \int_{\mathbf{R}^1} \frac{h(t)}{s-t} dt \qquad (2.6)$$

(see VII.1.10) is not local. Thus the problem of reconstructing a function from its integrals over hyperplanes is, in even dimension, not local in the sense that computing the function at some point requires the integrals along all hyperplanes meeting the support of the function. Anticipating later discussions (see VI.4) we mention that locality can be restored only to a very limited extent.

(3) For n even we want to give an alternative form of (2.5). Expressing $\mathbf{H}$ in (2.5) by (2.6) we obtain

$$f(x) = (-1)^{n/2+1} (2\pi)^{-n} \int_{S^{n-1}} \int_{\mathbf{R}^1} \frac{g^{(n-1)}(\theta, t)}{x \cdot \theta - t} dt \, d\theta$$

$$= (-1)^{n/2} (2\pi)^{-n} \int_{S^{n-1}} \int_{\mathbf{R}^1} \frac{g^{(n-1)}(\theta, x \cdot \theta + q)}{q} dq \, d\theta \qquad (2.7)$$

where we have made the substitution $t = q + x \cdot \theta$. The inner integral, which is a Cauchy principal value integral, can be expressed as an ordinary integral as in (VII.1.9). We obtain

$$f(x) = (-1)^{n/2} (2\pi)^{-n} \frac{1}{2} \int_{S^{n-1}} \int_{\mathbf{R}^1} \frac{g^{(n-1)}(\theta, x \cdot \theta + q) - g^{(n-1)}(\theta, x \cdot \theta - q)}{q} dq \, d\theta.$$

Now interchanging the order of integration is permitted and yields

$$f(x) = (-1)^{n/2} (2\pi)^{-n} \frac{1}{2} \int_{\mathbf{R}^1} \frac{1}{q} \int_{S^{n-1}} (g^{(n-1)}(\theta, x \cdot \theta + q)$$

$$- g^{(n-1)}(\theta, x \cdot \theta - q)) \, d\theta \, dq. \qquad (2.8)$$

Since g is even and $n-1$ is odd, $g^{(n-1)}$ is odd. Making the substitution $\theta \to -\theta$ for the second term in the inner integral we see that the integrals are the same.
Thus (2.8) simplifies to

$$f(x) = c(n) \int_{-\infty}^{\infty} \frac{F_x^{(n-1)}(q)}{q} dq, \quad c(n) = (-1)^{n/2} (2\pi)^{-n} |S^{n-1}|,$$

$$F_x(q) = \frac{1}{|S^{n-1}|} \int_{S^{n-1}} g(\theta, x \cdot \theta + q) \, d\theta.$$

F_x is even because g is. Hence $F_x^{(n-1)}$ is odd and we obtain finally Radon's original inversion formula (Radon, 1917)

$$f(x) = 2c(n) \int_0^\infty \frac{1}{q} F_x^{(n-1)}(q) \, dq$$

which, for $n = 2$, he wrote as

$$f(x) = -\frac{1}{\pi} \int_0^\infty \frac{dF_x(q)}{q}. \tag{2.9}$$

This formula can be found on the cover of the *Journal for Computer Assisted Tomography*.

(4) Putting $\alpha = n - 1$ in (2.1) we obtain

$$f = \frac{1}{2}(2\pi)^{1-n} \mathbf{I}^{1-n} \mathbf{R}^\# g. \tag{2.10}$$

This is the basis for the ρ-filtered layergram algorithm, see V.6. For n odd, $\mathbf{I}^{1-n}$ is simply a differential operator

$$\mathbf{I}^{1-n} = (-\Delta)^{(n-1)/2}$$

with Δ the Laplacian. Specifically, for $n = 3$,

$$f(x) = -\frac{1}{8\pi^2} \Delta \int_{S^2} g(\theta, x \cdot \theta) \, d\theta$$

where Δ acts on the variable x. This has also been derived by Radon.

(5) If f is a radial function, i.e. $f(x) = f_0(|x|)$ with some function f_0 on $\mathbb{R}^1$, then $g(s) = Rf(\theta, s)$ is independent of θ and

$$\begin{aligned}
g(s) &= \int_{\mathbb{R}^{n-1}} f_0((s^2 + |y|^2)^{1/2}) \, dy \\
&= |S^{n-2}| \int_0^\infty r^{n-2} f_0((s^2 + r^2)^{1/2}) \, dr \tag{2.11} \\
&= |S^{n-2}| \int_s^\infty (t^2 - s^2)^{(n-3)/2} t f_0(t) \, dt.
\end{aligned}$$

Thus Radon's integral equation reduces for radial functions to an Abel type integral equation, which can be solved by the Mellin transform (what we will do in Theorem 2.3 below in a more general context) or by the following elementary procedure: integrating (2.11) against $s(s^2-r^2)^{(n-3)/2}$ from r to ∞ yields

$$\int_r^\infty s(s^2-r^2)^{(n-3)/2} g(s)\,ds = |S^{n-2}| \int_r^\infty \int_s^\infty s((s^2-r^2)(t^2-s^2))^{(n-3)/2} tf_0(t)\,dt\,ds$$

$$= |S^{n-2}| \int_r^\infty \int_r^t s((s^2-r^2)(t^2-s^2))^{(n-3)/2}\,ds\,tf_0(t)\,dt.$$

For the inner integral we obtain by the substitution

$$s' = \frac{r^2+t^2-2s^2}{r^2-t^2}$$

the value

$$c(n)(t^2-r^2)^{n-2}, \quad c(n) = 2^{1-n} \int_{-1}^{+1} (1-s'^2)^{(n-3)/2}\,ds',$$

hence

$$\int_r^\infty s(s^2-r^2)^{(n-3)/2} g(s)\,ds = |S^{n-2}|c(n) \int_r^\infty (t^2-r^2)^{n-2} tf_0(t)\,dt.$$

We have

$$\frac{1}{2r}\frac{d}{dr}\int_r^\infty (t^2-r^2)^{n-2} tf_0(t)\,dt = \begin{cases} -(n-2)\int_r^\infty (t^2-r^2)^{n-3} tf_0(t)\,dt, & n > 2, \\ -\tfrac{1}{2}f_0(r), & n = 2. \end{cases}$$

Applying the operator $(1/2r)(d/dr)$ $n-2$ more times yields

$$\left(\frac{1}{2r}\frac{d}{dr}\right)^{n-1} \int_r^\infty s(s^2-r^2)^{(n-3)/2} g(s)\,ds = |S^{n-2}|c(n)(-1)^{n-1}\frac{(n-2)!}{2}f_0(r)$$

and this is clearly an inversion formula for the Radon transform in the case of radial symmetry.

(6) We cannot resist sketching Radon's original direct and elegant proof of (2.9). It basically relies on two different evaluations of the integral

$$\int_{|x|>q} f(x)(|x|^2-q^2)^{-1/2}\,dx. \tag{2.12}$$

Substituting $x = q\theta + s\theta^\perp, \theta \in S^1, s > 0$ we have $(|x|^2 - q^2)^{-1/2} dx = ds\, d\theta$, hence (2.12) becomes

$$\int_{S^1}\int_0^\infty f(q\theta + s\theta^\perp)\,ds\,d\theta = \frac{1}{2}\int_{S^1}\int_{-\infty}^{+\infty} f(q\theta + s\theta^\perp)\,ds\,d\theta$$

$$= \frac{1}{2}\int_{S^1} g(\theta, q)\,d\theta$$

$$= \pi F_0(q)$$

with F_0 as in remark 3.

On the other hand, introducing $x = r\theta, \theta \in S^1$ in (2.12) yields

$$\int_q^\infty \int_{S^1} f(r\theta)(r^2 - q^2)^{-1/2} r\,d\theta\,dr = 2\pi \int_q^\infty \overline{f}(r)(1 - (q/r)^2)^{-1/2}\,dr$$

where

$$\overline{f}(r) = \frac{1}{2\pi}\int_{S^1} f(r\theta)\,d\theta.$$

Comparing the two expressions for (2.12) we obtain

$$\int_q^\infty \overline{f}(r)(1 - (q/r)^2)^{-1/2}\,dr = \frac{1}{2} F_0(q). \tag{2.13}$$

This is an Abel integral equation of type (2.11) for $n = 2$ which we have solved in the preceding remark by elementary means, but Radon decided to proceed more directly. Computing

$$-\frac{1}{\pi}\int_0^\infty \frac{dF_0(q)}{q} = -\frac{1}{\pi}\lim_{\varepsilon \to 0}\int_\varepsilon^\infty \frac{F_0'(q)}{q}\,dq = \frac{1}{\pi}\lim_{\varepsilon \to 0}\left\{\frac{F_0(\varepsilon)}{\varepsilon} - \int_\varepsilon^\infty \frac{F_0(q)}{q^2}\,dq\right\}$$

with F_0 from (2.13) gives

$$\frac{2}{\pi}\lim_{\varepsilon \to 0}\left\{\frac{1}{\varepsilon}\int_\varepsilon^\infty \overline{f}(r)(1 - (\varepsilon/r)^2)^{-1/2}\,dr - \int_\varepsilon^\infty\int_q^\infty \overline{f}(r)(1 - (q/r)^2)^{-1/2}\,dr\,\frac{dq}{q^2}\right\}$$

$$= \frac{2}{\pi}\lim_{\varepsilon \to 0}\left\{\frac{1}{\varepsilon}\int_\varepsilon^\infty \overline{f}(r)(1 - (\varepsilon/r)^2)^{-1/2}\,dr - \int_\varepsilon^\infty \overline{f}(r)\int_\varepsilon^r (1 - (q/r)^2)^{-1/2}\,\frac{dq}{q^2}\,dr\right\}$$

$$= \frac{2}{\pi} \lim_{\varepsilon \to 0} \left\{ \frac{1}{\varepsilon} \int_\varepsilon^\infty \overline{f}(r)(1-(\varepsilon/r)^2)^{-1/2}\, dr - \frac{1}{\varepsilon} \int_\varepsilon^\infty \overline{f}(r)(1-(\varepsilon/r)^2)^{1/2}\, dr \right\}$$

$$= \frac{2}{\pi} \lim_{\varepsilon \to 0} \varepsilon \int_\varepsilon^\infty \overline{f}(r)(1-(\varepsilon/r)^2)^{-1/2} \frac{dr}{r^2}$$

$$= \frac{2}{\pi} \lim_{\varepsilon \to 0} \left\{ \overline{f}(0) \varepsilon \int_\varepsilon^\infty (1-(\varepsilon/r)^2)^{-1/2} \frac{dr}{r^2} + \varepsilon \int_\varepsilon^\infty (\overline{f}(r) - \overline{f}(0))(1-(\varepsilon/r)^2)^{-1/2} \frac{dr}{r^2} \right\}$$

$$= \frac{2}{\pi} \lim_{\varepsilon \to 0} \left\{ \overline{f}(0) \int_0^1 (1-t^2)^{-1/2}\, dt + \varepsilon \int_\varepsilon^\infty (\overline{f}(r) - \overline{f}(0))(1-(\varepsilon/r)^2)^{-1/2} \frac{dr}{r^2} \right\}.$$

The first integral is $\pi/2$, and the second integral tends to zero as $\varepsilon \to 0$. Hence

$$-\frac{1}{\pi} \int_0^\infty \frac{dF_0(q)}{q} = \overline{f}(0) = f(0)$$

which is (2.9) for $x = 0$.

(7) The inversion formula for **P** coincides—up to notation—with the inversion formula for **R** if $n = 2$. For $n > 3$ it is virtually useless since it requires the knowledge of all line integrals while only a small fraction of the line integrals can be measured in practice. An inversion formula which meets the needs of practice much better will be derived in VI.5.

A completely different inversion formula for the Radon transform is derived by expanding f and $g = Rf$ in spherical harmonics, see VII.3, i.e.

$$f(x) = \sum_{l=0}^\infty \sum_{k=0}^{N(n,l)} f_{lk}(|x|) Y_{lk}(x/|x|),$$

$$g(\theta, s) = \sum_{l=0}^\infty \sum_{k=0}^{N(n,l)} g_{lk}(s) Y_{lk}(\theta).$$

The following theorem gives a relation between f_{lk} and g_{lk}.

THEOREM 2.2 Let $f \in \mathcal{S}(\mathbb{R}^n)$. Then we have for $s > 0$

$$g_{lk}(s) = |S^{n-2}| \int_s^\infty C_l^{(n-2)/2}\left(\frac{s}{r}\right) \left(1 - \frac{s^2}{r^2}\right)^{(n-3)/2} f_{lk}(r) r^{n-2}\, dr \qquad (2.14)$$

where $C_l^{(n-2)/2}$ is the (normalized) Gegenbauer polynomial of degree l, see VII.3.

Proof We can express integrals over $x \cdot \theta = s$ by integrals over the half-sphere

$\{\omega \in S^{n-1}: \omega \cdot \theta > 0\}$ by rotating the coordinate system in (VII.2.5). We obtain

$$\int_{x \cdot \theta = s} f(x)\,dx = \int_{\substack{S^{n-1} \\ \omega \cdot \theta > 0}} f\left(\frac{s}{\theta \cdot \omega}\omega\right) \frac{s^{n-1}}{(\theta \cdot \omega)^n}\,d\omega.$$

We apply this to the function $f(x) = f_{lk}(|x|) Y_{lk}(x/|x|)$, obtaining

$$\int_{x \cdot \theta = s} f_{lk}(|x|) Y_{lk}(x/|x|)\,dx = \int_{\substack{S^{n-1} \\ \theta \cdot \omega > 0}} f_{lk}\left(\frac{s}{\theta \cdot \omega}\right) Y_{lk}(\omega) \frac{s^{n-1}}{(\theta \cdot \omega)^n}\,d\omega.$$

Here we can apply the Funk–Hecke theorem (VII.3.12). Defining

$$h(t) = \begin{cases} f_{lk}\left(\dfrac{s}{t}\right) \dfrac{s^{n-1}}{t^n}, & t > 0 \\ 0 & \text{otherwise} \end{cases}$$

we get

$$\int_{x \cdot \theta = s} f_{lk}(|x|) Y_{lk}(x/|x|)\,dx = g_{lk}(s) Y_{lk}(\theta),$$

$$g_{lk}(s) = |S^{n-2}| \int_0^1 f_{lk}\left(\frac{s}{t}\right) \frac{s^{n-1}}{t^n} C_l^{(n-2)/2}(t)(1-t^2)^{(n-3)/2}\,dt.$$

We obtain (2.14) by putting $r = s/t$. □

The integral equation (2.14) is an Abel type integral equation; in fact it reduces to an Abel equation for $n = 2$ and $l = 0$. It can be solved by the Mellin transform. This leads to

THEOREM 2.3 Let $f \in \mathscr{S}(\mathbb{R}^n)$. Then we have for $r > 0$

$$f_{lk}(r) = c(n) r^{2-n} \int_r^\infty (s^2 - r^2)^{(n-3)/2} C_l^{(n-2)/2}\left(\frac{s}{r}\right) g_{lk}^{(n-1)}(s)\,ds,$$

$$c(n) = \frac{(-1)^{n-1}}{2\pi^{n/2}} \frac{\Gamma((n-2)/2)}{\Gamma(n-2)} \qquad (2.15)$$

(For $n = 2$ one has to take the limit $n \to 2$, i.e. $c(2) = -1/\pi$).

Proof Using the convolution as defined in VII.3. in connection with the Mellin transform we may write (2.14) in the form

$$g_{lk} = (r^{n-1} f_{lk}) * b,$$

$$b(x) = |S^{n-2}| \begin{cases} C_l^{(n-2)/2}(x)(1-x^2)^{(n-3)/2}, & 0 \leq x < 1, \\ 0 & \text{otherwise.} \end{cases} \qquad (2.16)$$

Taking the Mellin transform and making use of the rules (VII.3.8), (2.16) becomes

$$\mathbf{M}g_{lk} = \mathbf{M}(r^{n-1} f_{lk})\mathbf{M}b. \tag{2.17}$$

$\mathbf{M}b$ is obtained from (VII.3.9) with $\lambda = (n-2)/2$:

$$\mathbf{M}b(s) = c_1 \frac{\Gamma(s)2^{-s}}{\Gamma\left(\dfrac{l+s+n-1}{2}\right)\Gamma\left(\dfrac{s+1-l}{2}\right)}$$

$$c_1 = |S^{n-2}|\Gamma\left(\frac{1}{2}\right)\Gamma\left(\frac{n-1}{2}\right).$$

Writing

$$\frac{1}{\mathbf{M}b(s-1)} = \frac{1}{c_1} \frac{\Gamma\left(\dfrac{l+s+n-2}{2}\right)\Gamma\left(\dfrac{s-l}{2}\right)}{\Gamma(s-1)2^{-s+1}}$$

$$= \frac{1}{c_1} \frac{\Gamma(s+n-2)}{\Gamma(s-1)} \cdot \frac{2^{s-1}\Gamma\left(\dfrac{s+l}{2} + \dfrac{n-2}{2}\right)\Gamma\left(\dfrac{s-l}{2}\right)}{\Gamma(s+n-2)}$$

we see from (VII.3.10) with $\lambda = (n-2)/2$ that the last term is the Mellin transform of the function

$$a(x) = c_2 \begin{cases} (1-x^2)^{(n-3)/2} C_l^{(n-2)/2}\left(\dfrac{1}{x}\right), & 0 \leq x < 1 \\ 0 & \text{otherwise,} \end{cases}$$

$$c_2 = \frac{\Gamma((n-2)/2)}{\Gamma(n-2)}.$$

Here, we have to interpret c_2 as being 2 in the case $n = 2$, i.e. we have to take the limit $n \to 2$. Hence,

$$\frac{1}{\mathbf{M}b(s-1)} = \frac{1}{c_1} \frac{\Gamma(s+n-2)}{\Gamma(s-1)} \mathbf{M}a(s).$$

With the rules (VII.3.8) we obtain from (2.17) with s replaced by $s-1$

$$\mathbf{M}(r^{n-2} f_{lk})(s) = \mathbf{M}(r^{n-1} f_{lk})(s-1)$$

$$= \frac{\mathbf{M}g_{lk}(s-1)}{\mathbf{M}b(s-1)}$$

$$= \frac{1}{c_1} \mathbf{M}a(s) \frac{\Gamma(s+n-2)}{\Gamma(s-1)} \mathbf{M}g_{lk}(s-1)$$

$$= \frac{(-1)^{n-1}}{c_1} \mathbf{M}a(s)\mathbf{M}(t^{n-2} g_{lk}^{(n-1)})(s).$$

This is equivalent to

$$r^{n-2} f_{lk} = \frac{(-1)^{n-1}}{c_1} a * (t^{n-2} g_{lk}^{(n-1)})$$

where the convolution is to be understood in the sense of VII.3 again, i.e.

$$r^{n-2} f_{lk}(r) = \frac{(-1)^{n-1}}{c_1} \int_0^\infty a\left(\frac{r}{t}\right) t^{n-2} g^{(n-1)}(t) \frac{dt}{t}$$

$$= \frac{c_2(-1)^{n-1}}{c_1} \int_r^\infty \left(1 - \frac{r^2}{t^2}\right)^{(n-3)/2} C_l^{(n-2)/2}\left(\frac{t}{r}\right) t^{n-3} g^{(n-1)}(t) \, dt.$$

This is essentially (2.15). □

The relevance of (2.15) comes from the fact that it gives an explicit solution to the exterior problem, see VI.3. It is usually called Cormack's inversion formula since it has been derived for $n = 2$ in Cormack's (1963) pioneering paper. We remark that the assumption $f \in \mathscr{S}$ in Theorems 2.2 and 2.3 has been made to ensure that the integrals (2.14), (2.15) make sense. For functions which are not decaying fast enough at infinity the exterior problem is not uniquely solvable as is seen from the example following Theorem 3.1 below.

Let us have a closer look at the two-dimensional case. The expansions in spherical harmonics are simply Fourier series which, in a slightly different notation, read

$$f(r, \omega) = \sum_l f_l(r) e^{il\varphi},$$

$$\omega = \begin{pmatrix} \cos \varphi \\ \sin \varphi \end{pmatrix}.$$

$$g(\omega, s) = \sum_l g_l(s) e^{il\varphi},$$

Formulas (2.14), (2.15) can now be written as

$$g_l(s) = 2 \int_s^\infty T_{|l|}\left(\frac{s}{r}\right)\left(1 - \frac{s^2}{r^2}\right)^{-1/2} f_l(r) \, dr,$$

$$f_l(r) = -\frac{1}{\pi} \int_r^\infty (s^2 - r^2)^{-1/2} T_{|l|}\left(\frac{s}{r}\right) g_l'(s) \, ds \qquad (2.18)$$

with T_l the Chebyshev polynomials of the first kind, see VII.3. We will give an alternative form of (2.18). From Theorem 4.1 we know that

$$\int_{\mathbb{R}^1} s^m g'(\omega, s) \, ds = -m \int_{\mathbb{R}^1} s^{m-1} g(\omega, s) \, ds$$

is a polynomial of degree $m-1$ in ω, i.e.

$$\int_{\mathbb{R}^1} s^m g'(\omega, s) \, ds = \sum_{|k| < m} c_{mk} e^{ik\varphi}$$

with some constants c_{mk}. Then,

$$\int_{\mathbb{R}^1} s^m g'_l(s) \, ds = \frac{1}{2\pi} \int_{\mathbb{R}^1} s^m \int_0^{2\pi} e^{-il\varphi} g'(\omega, s) \, d\varphi \, ds$$

$$= \frac{1}{2\pi} \int_0^{2\pi} e^{-il\varphi} \int_{\mathbb{R}^1} s^m g'(\omega, s) \, ds \, d\varphi$$

$$= \frac{1}{2\pi} \int_0^{2\pi} e^{-il\varphi} \sum_{|k| < m} c_{mk} e^{ik\varphi} \, d\varphi$$

$$= 0$$

for $m \leq |l|$ because of the orthogonality properties of the exponential functions. Since g is even, $g'_l(-s) = (-1)^{l+1} g'_l(s)$. Thus, if $Q_{|l|}$ is a polynomial of degree $< |l|$ which is even for l odd and odd for l even, then

$$\int_0^\infty Q_{|l|}(s) g'_l(s) \, ds = 0.$$

Therefore we can rewrite (2.18) as

$$f_l(r) = -\frac{1}{\pi r} \Bigg\{ \int_r^\infty \left(\left(\frac{s^2}{r^2} - 1 \right)^{-1/2} T_{|l|}\left(\frac{s}{r}\right) - Q_{|l|}\left(\frac{s}{r}\right) \right)$$

$$\times g'_l(s) \, ds - \int_0^r Q_{|l|}\left(\frac{s}{r}\right) g'_l(s) \, ds \Bigg\}. \qquad (2.19)$$

Now we want to choose $Q_{|l|}$ so as to make the factor of g'_l in the first integral small, improving in this way the stability properties of the formula. From (VII.3.4) we know that for $x \geq 1$

$$(x^2 - 1)^{-1/2} T_{|l|}(x) = \frac{\cosh(|l| \operatorname{arc\,cosh} x)}{\sinh(\operatorname{arc\,cosh} x)}.$$

If we choose

$$Q_{|l|}(x) = \frac{\sinh(|l| \operatorname{arc\,cosh} x)}{\sinh(\operatorname{arc\,cosh} x)} = U_{|l|-1}(x)$$

with U_l the Chebyshev polynomials of the second kind, then

$$(x^2 - 1)^{-1/2} T_{|l|}(x) - Q_{|l|}(x) = \frac{e^{-|l|\operatorname{arc\,cosh} x}}{\sinh(\operatorname{arc\,cosh} x)}$$

$$= \frac{(x + \sqrt{(x^2 - 1)})^{-|l|}}{\sqrt{(x^2 - 1)}}.$$

If we use this in (2.19) with $x = s/r$ we obtain

$$f_l(r) = -\frac{1}{\pi r} \left\{ \int_r^\infty \left(\frac{s^2}{r^2} - 1\right)^{-1/2} \left[\frac{s}{r} + \sqrt{\left(\frac{s^2}{r^2} - 1\right)}\right]^{-|l|} \right.$$

$$\left. \times g_l'(s)\, ds - \int_0^r U_{|l|-1}\left(\frac{s}{r}\right) g_l'(s)\, ds \right\} \tag{2.20}$$

where we define $U_{-1} = 0$. The practical usefulness of formulas (2.18) and (2.20) will be discussed in VI.3 and V.6.

II.3 Uniqueness

From the inversion formulas in Section 2 we know that $f \in \mathscr{S}$ is uniquely determined by either of the functions Rf, Pf. In many practical situations we know these functions only on a subset of their domain. The question arises if this partial information still determines f uniquely.

The following 'hole theorem' follows immediately from Theorem 2.3.

THEOREM 3.1 Let $f \in \mathscr{S}$, and let K be a convex compact set ('the hole') in $\mathbb{R}^n$. If $Rf(\theta, s) = 0$ for every plane $x \cdot \theta = s$ not meeting K, then $f = 0$ outside K.

Proof For K a ball the theorem follows immediately from Theorem 2.3. In the general case we can find for each $x \notin K$ a ball containing K but not x. Applying the theorem to that ball we conclude that $f(x) = 0$, hence the theorem for K. □

Since the integrals over planes can be expressed in terms of integrals over lines we obtain immediately the corresponding theorem for P:

THEOREM 3.2 Let f, K be as in Theorem 3.1. If $Pf(\theta, x) = 0$ for each line $x + t\theta$ not meeting K, then $f = 0$ outside K.

We see that the problem of recovering a function in the exterior of some ball from integrals over planes or lines outside that ball (exterior problem, see VI.3) is uniquely solvable, provided the function is decaying fast enough at infinity. This assumption cannot be dropped, as is seen from the following example in $\mathbb{R}^2$. Let $z = x_1 + ix_2$ and

$$f(x) = z^{-p}$$

with $p \geq 2$ an integer. We show that $\mathbf{R}f(\theta, s) = 0$ for $\theta \in S^1$ and $s > 0$. We have

$$\mathbf{R}f(\theta, s) = \int_{\mathbf{R}^1} f(s\theta + t\theta^\perp)\,dt$$

$$= (-\theta_2 + i\theta_1)^{-1} \int_L z^{-p}\,dz, \qquad \theta = \begin{pmatrix} \theta_1 \\ \theta_2 \end{pmatrix},$$

where L is the straight line $x \cdot \theta = s$. Putting $w = 1/z$ we get

$$\int_L z^{-p}\,dz = -\int_C w^{p-2}\,dw$$

where the image C of L under $w = 1/z$ is a finite circle since L does not meet 0. By Cauchy's theorem, the integral over C vanishes for $p \geq 2$, hence $\mathbf{R}f(\theta, s) = 0$ for $s > 0$ and $p \geq 2$.

Much more can be said if f is known to have compact support. The following theorem is given in terms of the divergent beam transform $\mathbf{D}$.

THEOREM 3.3 Let S be an open set on S^{n-1}, and let A be a continuously differentiable curve. Let $\Omega \subseteq \mathbf{R}^n$ be bounded and open. Assume that for each $\theta \in S$ there is an $a \in A$ such that the half-line $a + t\theta$, $t \geq 0$ misses Ω. If $f \in C_0^\infty(\Omega)$ and $\mathbf{D}f(a, \theta) = 0$ for $a \in A$ and $\theta \in S$, then $f = 0$ in the 'measured region' $\{a + t\theta : a \in A, \theta \in S\}$.

Proof Define for each integer $k \geq 0$ and $a, x \in \mathbf{R}^n$

$$D_k f(a, x) = \int_0^\infty t^k f(a + tx)\,dt.$$

We shall prove that, under the hypothesis of the theorem,

$$D_k f(a, \theta) = 0, \qquad a \in A, \qquad \theta \in S \qquad (3.1)$$

for all $k \geq 0$. Since f has compact support, (3.1) clearly implies the theorem.

The proof of (3.1) is by induction. For $k = 0$, (3.1) follows from $\mathbf{D}f(a, \theta) = 0$, $a \in A$, $\theta \in S$. Let (3.1) be satisfied for some $k \geq 0$. Then,

$$D_k f(a, x) = 0, \qquad a \in A$$

for x in the open cone $C = \{x \neq 0 : x/|x| \in S\}$. Let $a = a(s)$ be a parametric representation of A. Then,

$$\frac{d}{ds} D_{k+1} f(a(s), x) = \frac{d}{ds} \int_0^\infty t^{k+1} f(a(s) + tx)\,dt$$

$$= \int_0^\infty t^{k+1} \sum_{i=1}^n a_i'(s) f_i(a(s) + tx)\,dt$$

with f_i the ith partial derivative of f,

$$= \int_0^\infty t^k \sum_{i=1}^n a_i'(s) \frac{\partial}{\partial x_i} f(a(s) + tx)\, dt$$

$$= \sum_{i=1}^n a_i'(s) \frac{\partial}{\partial x_i} D_k f(a(s), x)$$

$$= 0$$

for $x \in C$ since $D_k f(a(s), x)$ vanishes in the open set C. Thus, $D_{k+1} f(a, x)$ is constant along A for $x \in C$. Since, by the hypothesis of the theorem, $D_{k+1} f(a, x) = 0$ for at least one $a \in A$, $D_{k+1} f(a, x)$ must be zero on A for $x \in C$. This is (3.1) with k replaced by $k + 1$, hence the theorem. □

The assumption on the half-line missing Ω looks strange but cannot be dropped. This can be seen from the example in Fig. II.1, where Ω is the unit disk in $\mathbb{R}^2$ and f is a smoothed version of the function which is $+1$ in the upper strip and -1 in the lower strip and zero elsewhere. With A the arc ab and S given by the angle φ, the hypothesis of the theorem is not satisfied. In this case, f does not vanish in the measured region, even though $\mathbf{D}f$ is zero on $A \times S$. However, if A is chosen to be ac, then the hypothesis of the theorem is satisfied, but $\mathbf{D}f$ is no longer zero on $A \times S$.

A situation to which Theorem 3.3 applies occurs in three-dimensional tomography, see I.1. It tells us that, in principle, three-dimensional reconstruction of an object is possible if the X-ray sources run on a circle surrounding the object.

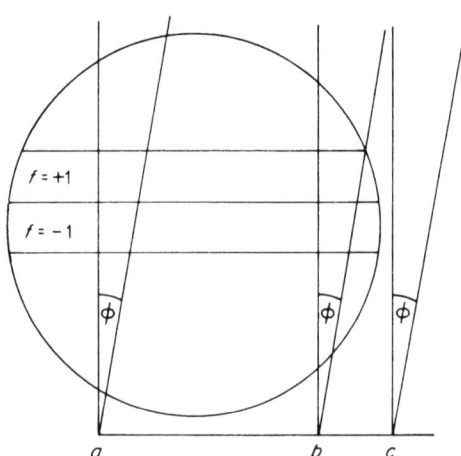

FIG. II.1 Example of non-uniqueness.

However, we shall see in VI.5 that the reconstruction problem is seriously ill-posed unless the curve satisfies a restrictive condition.

In the next two theorems we exploit the analyticity of the Fourier transform of functions with compact support.

THEOREM 3.4 Let A be a set of directions such that no non-trivial homogeneous polynomial vanishes on A. If $f \in C_0^\infty(\mathbb{R}^n)$ and $\mathbf{R}_\theta f = 0$ for $\theta \in A$, then $f = 0$.

Proof From Theorem 1.1 we have

$$\hat{f}(\sigma\theta) = (2\pi)^{(1-n)/2} (\mathbf{R}_\theta f)\hat{\ }(\sigma) = 0$$

for $\theta \in A$. Since f has compact support, $\hat{f}$ is an analytic function whose power series expansion can be written as

$$\hat{f}(\xi) = \sum_{k=0}^\infty a_k(\xi)$$

with homogeneous polynomials a_k of degree k. For $\xi = \sigma\theta$ we obtain

$$\hat{f}(\sigma\theta) = \sum_{k=0}^\infty \sigma^k a_k(\theta) = 0$$

for each σ and $\theta \in A$. It follows that $a_k(\theta)$ vanishes for $\theta \in A$, hence $a_k = 0$ and the theorem is proved. □

THEOREM 3.5 Let $f \in C_0^\infty(\mathbb{R}^n)$, and let $\mathbf{P}_\theta f = 0$ for an infinite number of directions. Then, $f = 0$.

Proof From Theorem 1.1 we have for infinitely many θ's

$$\hat{f}(\eta) = (2\pi)^{-1/2} (\mathbf{P}_\theta f)\hat{\ }(\eta) = 0$$

if $\eta \cdot \theta = 0$. Since $\hat{f}$ is an analytic function, $\hat{f}(\eta)$ must contain the factor $\eta \cdot \theta$ for each of the direction θ. Hence $\hat{f}$ has a zero of infinite order at 0 and hence vanishes identically.

For the divergent beam transform we have the following uniqueness theorem, which turns into Theorem 3.5 as the sources tend to infinity.

THEOREM 3.6 Let Ω^n be the unit ball in $\mathbb{R}^n$ and let A be an infinite set outside Ω^n. If $f \in C_0^\infty(\Omega^n)$ and $\mathbf{D}_a f = 0$ for $a \in A$ then $f = 0$.

Proof Let θ_0 be a limit point of $\{a/|a|: a \in A\}$. Choose $\varepsilon > 0$ such that $f(x) = 0$ for $|x| > 1 - 2\varepsilon$. After possibly removing some elements from A we may assume that, for a suitable neighbourhood $U(\theta_0)$ of θ_0 on S^{n-1},

$$a \cdot \theta > 1 - \varepsilon, \qquad a \in A, \, \theta \in U(\theta_0).$$

Now we compute

$$\int_{S^{n-1}} \mathbf{D}_a f(\omega)(\omega\cdot\theta)^{1-n}\,d\omega = \int_{S^{n-1}}\int_0^\infty f(a+t\omega)(\omega\cdot\theta)^{1-n}\,dt\,d\omega$$

$$= \int_{\mathbf{R}^n} f(a+y)(y\cdot\theta)^{1-n}\,dy$$

$$= \int_{|x|<1-2\varepsilon} f(x)(x\cdot\theta - a\cdot\theta)^{1-n}\,dx$$

where we have put $y = t\omega$ and $x = a+y$. Note that the last integral makes sense since for $f(x) \neq 0$

$$x\cdot\theta - a\cdot\theta < 1 - 2\varepsilon - (1-\varepsilon) = -\varepsilon.$$

Putting $x = s\theta + y$, $y \in \theta^\perp$ we obtain

$$\int_{S^{n-1}} \mathbf{D}_a f(\omega)(\omega\cdot\theta)^{1-n}\,d\omega = \int_{\mathbf{R}^1}\int_{\theta^\perp} f(s\theta+y)(s - a\cdot\theta)^{1-n}\,dy\,ds$$

$$= \int_{\mathbf{R}^1} \mathbf{R}f(\theta, s)(s - a\cdot\theta)^{1-n}\,ds.$$

Since $\mathbf{D}_a f = 0$ for $a \in A$ we have

$$\int_{|s|<1-2\varepsilon} \mathbf{R}f(\theta, s)(s - a\cdot\theta)^{1-n}\,ds = 0, \qquad a \in A,\ \theta \in U(\theta_0).$$

The power series

$$(s - a\cdot\theta)^{1-n} = \sum_{k=0}^\infty c_k(a\cdot\theta)^{1-n-k} s^k$$

converges uniformly in $|s| \le 1 - 2\varepsilon$ for each $a \in A$, $\theta \in U(\theta_0)$. All we need to know about the coefficients c_k is that they do not vanish. Hence

$$\sum_{k=0}^\infty c_k (a\cdot\theta)^{1-n-k} \int_{\mathbf{R}^1} \mathbf{R}f(\theta, s)s^k\,ds = 0$$

for $a \in A$, $\theta \in U(\theta_0)$. Anticipating Theorem 4.1 we have

$$\int_{\mathbf{R}^1} \mathbf{R}f(\theta, s) s^k\,ds = P_k(\theta)$$

where P_k is a homogeneous polynomial of degree k. It follows that

$$\sum_{k=0}^{\infty} c_k(a \cdot \theta)^{1-n-k} P_k(\theta) = 0$$

for $a \in A$ and $\theta \in U(\theta_0)$. Since the set of points $a \in A$ for which $a \cdot \theta$ assumes only finitely many values is contained in a $(n-1)$-dimensional set we can find an open subset $U' \subseteq U(\theta_0)$ such that $\{a \cdot \theta : a \in A\}$ is infinite for $\theta \in U'$. Then, varying a in A gives

$$P_k(\theta) = 0$$

for $\theta \in U'$ and each k, hence $P_k = 0$ for each k. Thus,

$$\int_{\mathbb{R}^1} \mathbf{R} f(\theta, s) s^k \, ds = 0$$

for each k. Since the monomials are dense in $L_2(-1, +1)$ we conclude $\mathbf{R}f = 0$, hence $f = 0$. □

It is not surprising that the last two theorems do not hold for finitely many directions or sources. However, the extent of non-uniqueness in the finite case is, in view of the applications, embarrassing. We consider only the case of finitely many directions in Theorem 3.4.

THEOREM 3.7 Let $\theta_1, \ldots, \theta_p \in S^{n-1}$, let $K \subseteq \mathbb{R}^n$ be compact, and let f be an arbitrary function in $C_0^{\infty}(K)$. Then, for each compact set K_0 which lies in the interior of K there is a function $f_0 \in C_0^{\infty}(K)$ which coincides with f on K_0 and for which $\mathbf{P}_{\theta_k} f_0 = 0$, $k = 1, \ldots, p$.

Proof Let

$$q(\xi) = \prod_{k=1}^{p} \theta_k \cdot \xi$$

and let Q be the differential operator obtained from $q(\xi)$ by replacing ξ_l by $-i \, \partial/\partial x_l$. We compute a solution h of $Qh = f$. For $p = 1$ this differential equation reads

$$-i\theta_1 \cdot \nabla h = f$$

with ∇ the gradient. Putting $x = s\theta_1 + y$, $y \in \theta_1^{\perp}$, a solution is

$$h(x) = i \int_0^s f(t\theta_1 + y) \, dt.$$

For $p > 1$ we repeat this construction. Now let $\Psi \in C_0^{\infty}(K)$ be 1 on K_0 and put $f_0 = Q\Psi h$. We have $f_0 \in C_0^{\infty}(K)$, and on K_0, $f_0 = Qh = f$. Also, by R3 from VII.1,

$$\hat{f}_0(\xi) = q(\xi)(\Psi h)\hat{}(\xi),$$

and, by Theorem 1.1,

$$(\mathbf{P}_\theta f_0)\hat{}(\eta) = (2\pi)^{1/2} \hat{f}_0(\eta) = (2\pi)^{1/2} q(\eta)(\Psi h)\hat{}(\eta)$$
$$= 0$$

for $\eta \in \theta_k^\perp$. It follows that $\mathbf{P}_{\theta_k} f_0 = 0$ and the theorem is proved. □

Loosely speaking Theorem 3.7 states that for each object there is another one differing from the first one only in an arbitrary small neighbourhood of its boundary and for which the projections in the directions $\theta_1, \ldots, \theta_p$ vanish. At a first glance this makes it appear impossible to recover a function from finitely many projections. A closer look at the proof of Theorem 3.7 reveals that f_0 is a highly oscillating function: Since q is a polynomial of degree p, $\hat{f}_0$ assumes large values for $|\xi| > 1$ fixed and p large. This means that for p large the second object behaves quite erratically in the thin boundary layer where it is different from the first one. In order to make up for this indeterminacy in the case of finitely many projections we have to put restrictions on the variation of the object. This is pursued further in Chapters III and IV.

II.4 The Ranges

In this section we shall see that the ranges of the operators introduced in Section II.1 are highly structured. This structure will find applications in the study of resolution, of algorithms and of problems in which the data are not fully specified.

THEOREM 4.1 Let $f \in \mathscr{S}$. Then, for $m = 0, 1, \ldots$

$$\int_{\mathbf{R}^1} s^m \mathbf{R}_\theta f(s) \, ds = p_m(\theta), \tag{4.1}$$

$$\int_{\theta^\perp} (x \cdot y)^m \mathbf{P}_\theta f(x) \, dx = q_m(y), \qquad y \perp \theta$$

with p_m, q_m homogeneous polynomials of degree m, q_m being independent of θ.

Proof We compute

$$\int_{\mathbf{R}^1} s^m \mathbf{R}_\theta f(s) \, ds = \int_{\mathbf{R}^1} s^m \int_{\theta^\perp} f(s\theta + y) \, dy \, ds$$

$$= \int_{\mathbf{R}^n} (x \cdot \theta)^m f(x) \, dx$$

where we have put $x = s\theta + y$. Obviously, this is a homogeneous polynomial of degree m in θ. Likewise,

$$\int_{\theta^\perp} (x \cdot y)^m \, \mathbf{P}_\theta f(x) \, dx = \int_{\theta^\perp} (x \cdot y)^m \int_{\mathbb{R}^1} f(x + t\theta) \, dt \, dx$$

$$= \int_{\mathbb{R}^n} (z \cdot y)^m f(z) \, dz$$

for $y \perp \theta$ where we have put $z = x + t\theta$. This is a homogeneous polynomial of degree m in y which is independent of θ. □

The condition (4.1) for the Radon transform has the following consequence which we shall use in later chapters. If $f \in C_0^\infty(\Omega^n)$ we can expand $\mathbf{R}f$ in terms of the products $C_l^\lambda Y_{kj}$, where C_l^λ are the Gegenbauer polynomials and Y_{kj} the spherical harmonics, see VII.3. These functions form a complete orthogonal system in $L_2(Z, (1-s^2)^{\lambda - 1/2})$. The expansions reads

$$\mathbf{R}f(\theta, s) = (1-s^2)^{\lambda - 1/2} \sum_{l=0}^{\infty} \sum_{k=0}^{\infty} \sum_{j} c_{lkj} C_l^\lambda(s) Y_{kj}(\theta)$$

where j runs over all $N(n, k)$ spherical harmonics of degree k. The C_l^λ are orthogonal in $[-1, +1]$ with respect to the weight function $(1-s^2)^{\lambda - 1/2}$, hence

$$\int_{-1}^{+1} C_l^\lambda(s) \mathbf{R}f(\theta, s) \, ds = \sum_{k=0}^{\infty} \sum_{j} c_{lkj} \int_{-1}^{+1} (1-s^2)^{\lambda - 1/2} (C_l^\lambda(s))^2 \, ds \, Y_{kj}(\theta).$$

According to (4.1), the left-hand side is a polynomial of degree l in θ which, due to the evenness of $\mathbf{R}f$, is even for l even and odd for l odd. Hence, $c_{lkj} \neq 0$ only for $k = l, l-2, \ldots$, and $\mathbf{R}f$ assumes the form

$$\mathbf{R}f(\theta, s) = (1-s^2)^{\lambda - 1/2} \sum_{l=0}^{\infty} C_l^\lambda(s) h_l(\theta) \tag{4.2}$$

where h_l is a linear combination of spherical harmonics of degree $l, l-2, \ldots$.

The conditions (4.1) are called the Helgason–Ludwig consistency conditions. They characterize the range of $\mathbf{R}, \mathbf{P}$ resp. in the following sense.

THEOREM 4.2 Let $g \in \mathscr{S}(Z)$ be even (i.e. $g(\theta, s) = g(-\theta, -s)$) and assume that for each $m = 0, 1, \ldots$

$$\int_{\mathbb{R}^1} s^m g(\theta, s) \, ds = p_m(\theta)$$

is a homogeneous polynomial of degree m in θ. Then, there is $f \in \mathscr{S}(\mathbb{R}^n)$ such that $g = \mathbf{R}f$. If, in addition, $g(\theta, s) = 0$ for $|s| \geq a$, then $f(x) = 0$ for $|x| \geq a$.

Proof In view of Theorem 1.1 it appears natural to define
$$\hat{f}(\sigma\theta) = (2\pi)^{(1-n)/2} \hat{g}(\theta, \sigma), \quad \sigma > 0.$$
$\hat{g}$ is even since g is, hence this is true for $\sigma < 0$, too. It suffices to show that $\hat{f} \in \mathscr{S}$. For in that case, $f \in \mathscr{S}$ and it follows from Theorem 1.1 that $g = \mathbf{R}f$.

The crucial point in the proof that $\hat{f} \in \mathscr{S}$ is smoothness at the origin. Here, the essential hypothesis of the theorem is needed. We start out from

$$e^{it} = \sum_{m=0}^{q-1} \frac{(it)^m}{m!} + e_q(t),$$

$$e_q(t) = \sum_{m=q}^{\infty} \frac{(it)^m}{m!}.$$

For f defined as above we obtain

$$\hat{f}(\sigma\theta) = (2\pi)^{-n/2} \int_{\mathbf{R}^1} e^{-is\sigma} g(\theta, s)\, ds$$

$$= (2\pi)^{-n/2} \left\{ \sum_{m=0}^{q-1} \frac{(-i\sigma)^m}{m!} \int_{\mathbf{R}^1} s^m g(\theta, s)\, ds + \int_{\mathbf{R}^1} e_q(-\sigma s) g(\theta, s)\, ds \right\}$$

$$= (2\pi)^{-n/2} \left\{ \sum_{m=0}^{q-1} \frac{(-i\sigma)^m}{m!} p_m(\theta) + \int_{\mathbf{R}^1} e_q(-\sigma s) g(\theta, s)\, ds \right\}$$

with p_m the polynomial of the theorem. Since p_m is homogeneous we have for $\xi = \sigma\theta$

$$\hat{f}(\xi) = (2\pi)^{-n/2} \left\{ \sum_{m=0}^{q-1} \frac{(-i)^m}{m!} p_m(\xi) + \int_{\mathbf{R}^1} e_q(-\sigma s) g(\theta, s)\, ds \right\}. \quad (4.3)$$

Let A_p be the class of expressions of the form

$$\sigma^p a(s\sigma) h(\theta, s)$$

where a and its derivatives are bounded C^∞-functions and $h \in \mathscr{S}(Z)$, or a finite linear combination thereof. We shall show that for derivatives D^α of order $|\alpha| \le q$ with respect to ξ, we have

$$D^\alpha e_q(\sigma s) g(\theta, s) \in A_{q-|\alpha|}. \quad (4.4)$$

For the proof we have to express $\partial/\partial \xi_j$ in terms of $\partial/\partial \sigma, \partial/\partial \theta_j$. We do the calculation in the spherical cap

$$\xi_i = \sigma \theta_i, \; i = 1, \ldots, n-1,$$
$$\xi_n = \sigma \sqrt{(1 - \theta_1^2 - \ldots - \theta_{n-1}^2)}, \; \theta_1^2 + \ldots + \theta_{n-1}^2 < 1, \sigma > 0.$$

From the chain rule we obtain

$$\frac{\partial}{\partial \xi_j} = \frac{\partial \sigma}{\partial \xi_j} \frac{\partial}{\partial \sigma} + \sum_{i=1}^{n-1} \frac{\partial \theta_i}{\partial \xi_j} \frac{\partial}{\partial \theta_i}.$$

Since

$$\sigma = (\xi_1^2 + \ldots + \xi_n^2)^{1/2}, \quad \theta_i = \frac{\xi_i}{\sigma}, \quad i = 1, \ldots, n-1$$

we obtain for $i = 1, \ldots, n-1$, $j = 1, \ldots, n$

$$\frac{\partial \sigma}{\partial \xi_j} = \theta_j, \quad \frac{\partial \theta_i}{\partial \xi_j} = \frac{1}{\sigma}(\delta_{ij} - \theta_i \cdot \theta_j)$$

with $\delta_{ij} = 1$ for $i = j$ and $\delta_{ij} = 0$ otherwise. Hence,

$$\frac{\partial}{\partial \xi_j} = \theta_j \frac{\partial}{\partial \sigma} + \frac{1}{\sigma} \sum_{i=1}^{n-1} (\delta_{ij} - \theta_i \cdot \theta_j) \frac{\partial}{\partial \theta_i}$$

$$= \theta_j \frac{\partial}{\partial \sigma} + \frac{1}{\sigma} D_\theta \tag{4.5}$$

where D_θ stands for a linear differential operator with respect to $\theta_1, \ldots, \theta_{n-1}$ which is of first order and which has C^∞-coefficients depending only on θ. Note that

$$\left(\theta_j \frac{\partial}{\partial \sigma} + \frac{1}{\sigma} D_\theta \right) A_p \subseteq A_{p-1}, \quad p = 1, 2, \ldots$$

as is easily seen from the definition of A_p. Doing this calculation in an arbitrary spherical cap we obtain globally

$$\frac{\partial}{\partial \xi_j} A_p \subseteq A_{p-1}, \quad p = 1, 2, \ldots \tag{4.6}$$

The proof of (4.4) is by induction. The case $|\alpha| = 0$ is obvious since $e_q(\sigma s) g(\theta, s) \in A_q$. Assume (4.4) to be correct for all derivatives up to some order $p < q$ and let $|\alpha| = p$. Then, from (4.5) and (4.6)

$$\frac{\partial}{\partial \xi_j} D^\alpha e_q(\sigma s) g(\theta, s) \in (\theta_j \frac{\partial}{\partial \sigma} + \frac{1}{\sigma} D_\theta) A_{q - |\alpha|}$$

$$\subseteq A_{q - |\alpha| - 1},$$

hence (4.4) holds also for derivatives of order $p + 1$. This proves (4.4).

Now let D^α be a derivative of order $|\alpha| = q$. From (4.3) we have for $|\xi| \neq 0$

$$D^\alpha \hat{f}(\xi) = (2\pi)^{-n/2} \int_{\mathbf{R}^1} D^\alpha e_q(-\sigma s) g(\theta, s) ds$$

and this is a continuous and bounded function of ξ in a punctured neighbourhood of 0 because of (4.4). Since q is arbitrary, $\hat{f} \in C^\infty$.

It remains to show that each derivative of $\hat{f}$ is decaying faster than any power of $|\xi|$ as $|\xi| \to \infty$. This follows immediately from repeated application of (4.5) to $\hat{g} \in \mathscr{S}(Z)$.

The remark on the supports of g and f follows immediately from Theorem 3.1. □

THEOREM 4.3 Let $g \in \mathscr{S}(T)$ and $g(\theta, x) = 0$ for $|x| \geq a$. Assume that for $m = 0, 1, \ldots$

$$\int_{\theta^\perp} (x \cdot y)^m g(\theta, x) \, dx = q_m(y), \qquad y \perp \theta$$

is a homogeneous polynomial of degree m in y which does not depend on θ. Then, there is $f \in \mathscr{S}(\mathbb{R}^n)$ with $f(x) = 0$ for $|x| \geq a$ and $g = \mathbf{P}f$.

Proof We want to reduce Theorem 4.3 to Theorem 4.2. If we already knew that $g = \mathbf{P}f$ we could express $\mathbf{R}f(\omega, s)$ in terms of $\mathbf{P}f$ by (1.1). Therefore we put for some $\theta \perp \omega$

$$h_\theta(\omega, s) = \int_{\substack{\theta^\perp \\ x \cdot \omega = s}} g(\theta, x) \, dx$$

and try to show that h_θ does not depend on the choice of θ and that $h_\theta = \mathbf{R}f$ for some $f \in \mathscr{S}(\mathbb{R}^n)$ with support in $|x| \leq a$.

To begin with, we compute

$$\int_{\mathbb{R}^1} s^m h_\theta(\omega, s) \, ds = \int_{\mathbb{R}^1} s^m \int_{\substack{\theta^\perp \\ x \cdot \omega = s}} g(\theta, x) \, dx \, ds$$

$$= \int_{\theta^\perp} (x \cdot \omega)^m g(\theta, x) \, dx \qquad (4.7)$$

$$= q_m(\omega)$$

where q_m is the polynomial of the theorem. Since q_m does not depend on θ, the integral on the left-hand side of (4.7) does not depend on θ either. $h_\theta(\omega, s)$ vanishes for $|s| \geq a$ because of $g(\theta, x) = 0$ for $|x| \geq a$. Since the polynomials are dense in $L_2(-a, a)$ it follows that h_θ does not depend on θ, and from (4.7) we see that $h = h_\theta$ satisfies the assumptions of Theorem 4.2. Hence $h = \mathbf{R}f$ for some $f \in \mathscr{S}(\mathbb{R}^n)$ with support in $|x| \leq a$.

For $n > 2$ we have to show that $g = \mathbf{P}f$. For θ fixed we shall show that the integrals of g and $\mathbf{P}f$ over arbitrary planes in $\theta^\perp$ coincide. If $\{x \in \theta^\perp : x \cdot \omega = s\}$ is such a plane where $\omega \in \theta^\perp$, the integral of g over this plane gives $h(\omega, s)$, and the integral of **P**f is

$$\int_{\substack{\theta^\perp \\ x\cdot\omega = s}} \mathbf{P}f(\theta, x)\,dx = \int_{\substack{\theta^\perp \\ x\cdot\omega = s}} \int_{-\infty}^{\infty} f(x+t\theta)\,dt\,dx$$

$$= \int_{\theta^\perp \cap \omega^\perp} \int_{-\infty}^{+\infty} f(s\omega + y + t\theta)\,dt\,dy$$

$$= \int_{\omega^\perp} f(s\omega + z)\,dz$$

$$= \mathbf{R}f(\omega, s).$$

Since $h = \mathbf{R}f$, the integrals coincide. This means that the Radon transforms of $g(\theta, \cdot)$, $\mathbf{P}f(\theta, \cdot)$ on $\theta^\perp$ coincide. But the Radon transform on $\mathscr{S}(\theta^\perp)$ is injective, hence $g = \mathbf{P}f$. □

Incidentally, Theorem 4.3 does not hold if the condition $g(\theta, x) = 0$ for $|x| \geq a$ (and the conclusion that $f(x) = 0$ for $|x| \geq a$) is dropped: let h be a non-trivial even function in $\mathscr{S}(\mathbb{R}^1)$ such that

$$\int_0^\infty s^m h(s)\,ds = 0, \qquad m = 0, 1, \ldots,$$

let $u \in C^\infty(S^{n-1})$ and let $g(\theta, x) = u(\theta)h(|x|)$. Then, $g \in \mathscr{S}(T)$, and

$$\int_{\theta^\perp} (x\cdot y)^m g(\theta, x)\,dx = u(\theta) \int_{\theta^\perp} (x\cdot y)^m h(|x|)\,dx$$

$$= u(\theta) \int_0^\infty s^{n-2+m} h(s)\,ds \int_{S^{n-1} \cap \theta^\perp} (\omega \cdot y)^m\,d\omega$$

$$= 0$$

where we have put $x = s\omega$ in $\theta^\perp$. Thus, g satisfies the consistency conditions of the theorem.

For $n > 3$, let $\omega \perp \theta$. Then,

$$\int_{x \perp \theta, x\cdot\omega = s} g(\theta, x)\,dx = u(\theta) \int_{x \perp \theta, x\cdot\omega = s} h(|x|)\,dx = u(\theta)\,\mathbf{R}h(\omega, s)$$

where h is considered as the radial function $x \to h(|x|)$ and **R** is the $(n-1)$-

dimensional Radon transform. On the other hand, if $g = \mathbf{P}f$ for some $f \in \mathscr{S}(\mathbb{R}^n)$, we have from (1.1)

$$\int_{x \perp \theta, x \cdot \omega = s} g(\theta, x) \, dx = \mathbf{R}f(\omega, s)$$

and it follows that

$$\mathbf{R}f(\omega, s) = u(\theta) \mathbf{R}h(\omega, s)$$

for $\omega \perp \theta$. This is a contradiction unless u is constant since $\mathbf{R}h$ is independent of ω and $\mathbf{R}h \neq 0$ because of the injectivity of $\mathbf{R}$.

II.5 Sobolev Space Estimates

In Theorem 1.6 we derived some simple continuity results in an L_2-setting. Since all the transforms considered in that theorem have a certain smoothing property, these results cannot be optimal. In particular, the inverses are not continuous as operators between L_2 spaces. However, they are continuous as operators between suitable Sobolev spaces. Sobolev space estimates are the basic tool for the treatment of our integral equations as ill-posed problems in IV.2.

The Sobolev spaces $H^\alpha(\Omega)$, $H_0^\alpha(\Omega)$ on $\Omega \subseteq \mathbb{R}^n$ are defined in VII.4. The Sobolev spaces on Z and T we are working with are defined by the norms

$$\|g\|_{H^\alpha(Z)}^2 = \int_{S^{n-1}} \int_{\mathbb{R}^1} (1+\sigma^2)^\alpha |\hat{g}(\theta, \sigma)|^2 \, d\sigma \, d\theta,$$

$$\|g\|_{H^\alpha(T)}^2 = \int_{S^{n-1}} \int_{\theta^\perp} (1+|\eta|^2)^\alpha |\hat{g}(\theta, \eta)|^2 \, d\eta \, d\theta.$$

The Fourier transforms are to be understood as in Section 1. Because of R3 from VII.1 an equivalent norm in $H^\alpha(Z)$ for $\alpha \geq 0$ an integer is

$$\|g\|_{\tilde{H}^\alpha(Z)}^2 = \int_{S^{n-1}} \int_{\mathbb{R}^1} \sum_{l \leq \alpha} |g^{(l)}(\theta, s)|^2 \, ds \, d\theta$$

where $g^{(l)}$ is the lth derivative with respect to s. For most of the results of this section it is essential that the functions have compact support. For simplicity we restrict everything to Ω^n.

THEOREM 5.1   For each α there exist positive constants $c(\alpha, n)$, $C(\alpha, n)$ such that for $f \in C_0^\infty(\Omega^n)$

$$c(\alpha, n) \|f\|_{H_0^\alpha(\Omega^n)} \leq \|\mathbf{R}f\|_{H^{\alpha+(n-1)/2}(Z)} \leq C(\alpha, n) \|f\|_{H_0^\alpha(\Omega^n)},$$

$$c(\alpha, n) \|f\|_{H_0^\alpha(\Omega^n)} \leq \|\mathbf{P}f\|_{H^{\alpha+1/2}(T)} \leq C(\alpha, n) \|f\|_{H_0^\alpha(\Omega^n)}.$$

Proof We start with the inequality for **R**. From Theorem 1.1 we have

$$(\mathbf{R}f)\hat{\,}(\theta, \sigma) = (2\pi)^{(n-1)/2}\hat{f}(\sigma\theta),$$

hence

$$\|\mathbf{R}f\|^2_{H^{\alpha+(n-1)/2}(Z)} = \int_{S^{n-1}}\int_{\mathbf{R}^1} (1+\sigma^2)^{\alpha+(n-1)/2} |(\mathbf{R}f)\hat{\,}(\sigma\theta)|^2 \, d\sigma \, d\theta$$

$$= (2\pi)^{n-1} \int_{S^{n-1}}\int_{\mathbf{R}^1} (1+\sigma^2)^{\alpha+(n-1)/2} |\hat{f}(\sigma\theta)|^2 \, d\sigma \, d\theta$$

$$= 2(2\pi)^{n-1} \int_{S^{n-1}}\int_0^\infty (1+\sigma^2)^{\alpha+(n-1)/2} |\hat{f}(\sigma\theta)|^2 \, d\sigma \, d\theta.$$

Substituting $\xi = \sigma\theta$ we get

$$\|\mathbf{R}f\|^2_{H^{\alpha+(n-1)/2}(Z)} = 2(2\pi)^{n-1} \int_{\mathbf{R}^n} |\xi|^{1-n} (1+|\xi|^2)^{\alpha+(n-1)/2} |\hat{f}(\xi)|^2 \, d\xi \quad (5.1)$$

$$\geq 2(2\pi)^{n-1} \int_{\mathbf{R}^n} (1+|\xi|^2)^\alpha |\hat{f}(\xi)|^2 \, d\xi$$

$$= 2(2\pi)^{n-1} \|f\|^2_{H_0^\alpha(\Omega^n)}.$$

This is the left-hand side of the inequality for **R**. For the right-hand side we start out from (5.1) and decompose the integral into an integral over $|\xi| \geq 1$ and an integral over $|\xi| \leq 1$. In the first one we have $|\xi|^2 \geq 2^{-1}(1+|\xi|^2)$, hence

$$\int_{|\xi|\geq 1} |\xi|^{1-n}(1+|\xi|^2)^{\alpha+(n-1)/2} |\hat{f}(\xi)|^2 \, d\xi \leq 2^{(n-1)/2} \int_{|\xi|\geq 1} (1+|\xi|^2)^\alpha |\hat{f}(\xi)|^2 \, d\xi$$

$$\leq 2^{(n-1)/2} \|f\|^2_{H_0^\alpha(\Omega^n)}. \quad (5.2)$$

The integral over $|\xi| \leq 1$ is estimated by

$$\int_{|\xi|\leq 1} |\xi|^{1-n}(1+|\xi|^2)^{\alpha+(n-1)/2} |\hat{f}(\xi)|^2 \, d\xi \leq \int_{|\xi|\leq 1} |\xi|^{1-n}(1+|\xi|^2)^{\alpha+(n-1)/2} \, d\xi$$

$$\times \sup_{|\xi|\leq 1} |\hat{f}(\xi)|^2$$

$$= c_1(\alpha, n) \sup_{|\xi|\leq 1} |\hat{f}(\xi)|^2. \quad (5.3)$$

In order to estimate the sup we choose a function $\chi \in C_0^\infty(\mathbb{R}^n)$ which is 1 on Ω'' and put $\chi_\xi(x) = e^{-ix\cdot\xi} \chi(x)$. Then, with R5 from VII.1, and with $\tilde{\chi}$ the inverse Fourier transform of χ,

$$|\hat{f}(\xi)| = (2\pi)^{-n/2} \left| \int_{\mathbb{R}^n} \chi_\xi(x) f(x) \, dx \right|$$

$$= (2\pi)^{-n/2} \left| \int_{\mathbb{R}^n} \tilde{\chi}_\xi(\eta) \hat{f}(\eta) \, d\eta \right|$$

$$= (2\pi)^{-n/2} \left| \int_{\mathbb{R}^n} \tilde{\chi}_\xi(\eta) (1+|\eta|^2)^{-\alpha/2} (1+|\eta|^2)^{\alpha/2} \hat{f}(\eta) \, d\eta \right|$$

$$\leq (2\pi)^{-n/2} \left(\int_{\mathbb{R}^n} (1+|\eta|^2)^{-\alpha} |\tilde{\chi}_\xi(\eta)|^2 \, d\eta \int_{\mathbb{R}^n} (1+|\eta|^2)^\alpha |\hat{f}(\eta)|^2 \, d\eta \right)^{1/2}$$

$$= (2\pi)^{-n/2} \|\chi_\xi\|_{H^{-\alpha}(\mathbb{R}^n)} \|f\|_{H_0^\alpha(\Omega')}. \tag{5.4}$$

The $H^{-\alpha}(\mathbb{R}^n)$ norm of χ_ξ is a continuous function of ξ, hence

$$\sup_{|\xi|\leq 1} \|\chi_\xi\|_{H^{-\alpha}(\mathbb{R}^n)} \leq c_2(\alpha, n) \tag{5.5}$$

with some constant $c_2(\alpha, n)$. Combining (5.1)–(5.5) we get

$$\|Rf\|^2_{H^{\alpha+(n-1)/2}(Z)} \leq 2(2\pi)^{n-1}(2^{(n-1)/2} + (2\pi)^{-n} c_2^2(\alpha, n) c_1(\alpha, n)) \|f\|^2_{H_0^\alpha(\Omega')}$$

and this is the right-hand side of the inequality for R.

For the inequality for P we also start out from Theorem 1.1, applying to the resulting integral formula (VII.2.8). We obtain

$$\|Pf\|^2_{H^{\alpha+1/2}(T)} = \int_{S^{n-1}} \int_{\theta^\perp} (1+|\eta|^2)^{\alpha+1/2} |(P_\theta f)^\wedge(\eta)|^2 \, d\eta \, d\theta$$

$$= 2\pi \int_{S^{n-1}} \int_{\theta^\perp} (1+|\eta|^2)^{\alpha+1/2} |\hat{f}(\eta)|^2 \, d\eta \, d\theta$$

$$= 2\pi |S^{n-2}| \int_{\mathbb{R}^n} |\xi|^{-1} (1+|\xi|^2)^{\alpha+1/2} |\hat{f}(\xi)|^2 \, d\xi.$$

This corresponds to (5.1) in the case of R. From here on we proceed exactly in the same way as above. □

In Theorem 5.1 we can put a stronger norm on Z which also includes derivatives with respect to θ. In order to do so we define the derivatives D_θ^k as in (1.5), i.e. we extend functions on Z to all of $(\mathbb{R}^n - \{0\}) \times \mathbb{R}^1$ by homogeneity of degree -1. Then we define for α an integer

$$\|g\|_{\bar{H}^\alpha(Z)}^2 = \int_{S^{n-1}} \int_{\mathbb{R}^1} \sum_{|k|+l \leq \alpha} \left| D_\theta^k \frac{\partial^l}{\partial s^l} g(\theta, s) \right|^2 ds\, d\theta.$$

For $\alpha \geq 0$ real we define $\bar{H}^\alpha(Z)$ by interpolation, i.e. we put for $0 \leq \vartheta \leq 1$ and α, β integers ≥ 0

$$\bar{H}^{\alpha(1-\vartheta)+\beta\vartheta}(Z) = (\bar{H}^\alpha(Z), \bar{H}^\beta(Z))_\vartheta.$$

As in (VII.4.6) this definition is independent of the choice of α, β because of the reiteration Lemma VII.4.3.

THEOREM 5.2 The norms $\|\cdot\|_{\bar{H}^\alpha(Z)}, \|\cdot\|_{H^\alpha(Z)}$ are equivalent on range (**R**) for $\alpha \geq 0$, **R** being considered as an operator on $C_0^\infty(\Omega^n)$

Proof We first show the equivalence for α an integer ≥ 0. From (1.5) we have

$$D_\theta^k \frac{\partial^l}{\partial s^l} \mathbf{R}f = (-1)^{|k|} \frac{\partial^{|k|+l}}{\partial s^{|k|+l}} \mathbf{R}(x^k f),$$

hence

$$\|\mathbf{R}f\|_{\bar{H}^\alpha(Z)}^2 = \sum_{|k|+l \leq \alpha} \int_{S^{n-1}} \int_{\mathbb{R}^1} \left| D_\theta^k \frac{\partial^l}{\partial s^l} \mathbf{R}f(\theta, s) \right|^2 ds\, d\theta$$

$$= \sum_{|k|+l \leq \alpha} \int_{S^{n-1}} \int_{\mathbb{R}^1} \left| \frac{\partial^{|k|+l}}{\partial s^{|k|+l}} \mathbf{R}(x^k f)(\theta, s) \right|^2 ds\, d\theta$$

$$\leq \sum_{|k| \leq \alpha} \|\mathbf{R}(x^k f)\|_{\bar{H}^\alpha(Z)}^2. \tag{5.6}$$

From Theorem 5.1 we get with some constant $c_1(\alpha, n)$

$$\|\mathbf{R}(x^k f)\|_{\bar{H}^\alpha(Z)} \leq c_1(\alpha, n) \|x^k f\|_{H_0^{\alpha-(n-1)/2}(\Omega^n)}.$$

Now choose $\chi \in C_0^\infty(\mathbb{R}^n)$ such that $\chi = 1$ on Ω^n. Then, $x^k f = x^k \chi f$, and since multiplication with the C_0^∞ function $x^k \chi$ is a continuous operation in Sobolev spaces (compare Lemma VII.4.5) we find that

$$\|\mathbf{R}(x^k f)\|_{\bar{H}^\alpha(Z)}^2 \leq c_2(\alpha, n) \|f\|_{H_0^{\alpha-(n-1)/2}(\Omega^n)}^2.$$

Combining this with (5.6) we get

$$\|\mathbf{R}f\|_{\bar{H}^\alpha(Z)} \leq c_3(\alpha, n) \|f\|_{H_0^{\alpha-(n-1)/2}(\Omega^n)}$$

where $c_3(\alpha, n)$ is an other constant. Now we use Theorem 5.1 again to estimate the $H_0^{\alpha-(n-1)/2}(\Omega^n)$-norm of f by the $H^\alpha(Z)$-norm of Rf, obtaining

$$\|Rf\|_{\bar{H}^\alpha(Z)} \leq c_4(\alpha, n) \|Rf\|_{H^\alpha(Z)}. \tag{5.7}$$

On the other hand we obviously have

$$\|Rf\|_{\bar{H}^\alpha(Z)} \geq \|Rf\|_{\bar{H}^\alpha(Z)} \geq c_5(\alpha, n) \|Rf\|_{H^\alpha(Z)} \tag{5.8}$$

with some positive constant $c_5(\alpha, n)$. (5.7), (5.8) show that the norms $\bar{H}^\alpha(Z)$, $H^\alpha(Z)$ are equivalent on range (R) for α an integer ≥ 0. In order to establish the equivalence for arbitrary real non-negative order we use an interpolation argument. Let $0 \leq \alpha < \beta$ be integers and let $\gamma = \alpha(1-\vartheta) + \beta\vartheta$ with some $\vartheta \in [0,1]$. From Theorems 5.1 and (5.7) we see that

$$\mathbf{R}: H_0^{\gamma-(n-1)/2}(\Omega^n) \to \bar{H}^\gamma(Z)$$

continuously for $\vartheta = 0, 1$. Hence, by Lemma VII.4.2, **R** is continuous for $0 < \vartheta < 1$, i.e.

$$\|Rf\|_{\bar{H}^\gamma(Z)} \leq c_6(\gamma, n) \|f\|_{H_0^{\gamma-(n-1)/2}(\Omega^n)}$$

with some constant $c_6(\gamma, n)$. Using Theorem 5.1 we can estimate the right-hand side by $\|Rf\|_{H^\gamma(Z)}$, obtaining

$$\|Rf\|_{\bar{H}^\gamma(Z)} \leq c_7(\gamma, n) \|Rf\|_{H^\gamma(Z)}.$$

The opposite inequality follows directly by interpolation since for α an integer ≥ 0,

$$\|g\|_{H^\alpha(Z)} \leq \|g\|_{\bar{H}^\alpha(Z)}$$

on all of $\bar{H}^\alpha(Z)$.

As a consequence the first half of Theorem 5.1 holds also for the stronger norm $\bar{H}^\alpha(Z)$:

THEOREM 5.3 For $\alpha \geq 0$ there exist positive constants $c(\alpha, n)$, $C(\alpha, n)$ such that for $f \in C_0^\infty(\Omega^n)$

$$c(\alpha, n) \|f\|_{H_0^\alpha(\Omega^n)} \leq \|Rf\|_{\bar{H}^{\alpha+(n-1)/2}(Z)} \leq C(\alpha, n) \|f\|_{H_0^\alpha(\Omega^n)}.$$

II.6 The Attenuated Radon Transform

In $\mathbb{R}^2$ we define for functions with compact support the attenuated Radon transform

$$\mathbf{R}_\mu f(\theta, s) = \int_{x \cdot \theta = s} e^{-D\mu(x, \theta^\perp)} f(x) \, dx.$$

Here we denote by $\theta^\perp$ the unit vector perpendicular to $\theta \in S^1$ for which $\det(\theta, \theta^\perp) = +1$. For $\theta = (\cos\varphi, \sin\varphi)^T$, $\theta^\perp = (-\sin\varphi, \cos\varphi)^T$. μ is a real function on $\mathbb{R}^2$ which plays the role of a parameter. $\mathbf{R}_\mu$ is the integral transform in emission tomography, see I.2. In this section we extend as far as possible the results about **R** in the previous sections to $\mathbf{R}_\mu$.

A special case occurs if the function μ has a constant value μ_0 in a convex domain Ω containing the support of f.

If $s\theta + \tau(\theta, s)\theta^\perp$ denotes that point in which the ray starting at $s\theta$ with direction $\theta^\perp$ hits the boundary of Ω, then

$$\mathbf{D}\mu(x, \theta^\perp) = (\tau(\theta, s) - x \cdot \theta^\perp)\mu_0 + a(\theta, s), \qquad a(\theta, s) = \int_{\tau(\theta, s)}^{\infty} \mu(s\theta + t\theta^\perp)\,dt$$

for $x \in \Omega$, $x \cdot \theta = s$. Therefore,

$$\mathbf{R}_\mu f(\theta, s) = \int_{x \cdot \theta = s} e^{-(\tau(\theta, s) - x \cdot \theta^\perp)\mu_0 - a(\theta, s)} f(x)\,dx$$

$$= e^{-\tau(\theta, s)\mu_0 - a(\theta, s)} \mathbf{T}_{\mu_0} f(\theta, s),$$

$$\mathbf{T}_{\mu_0} f(\theta, s) = \int_{x \cdot \theta = s} e^{\mu_0 x \cdot \theta^\perp} f(x)\,dx$$

$$= \int_{\mathbb{R}^1} e^{\mu_0 t} f(s\theta + t\theta^\perp)\,dt.$$

$\mathbf{T}_{\mu_0}$ is known as the exponential Radon transform.

In the following we extend some of the results for **R** to $\mathbf{R}_\mu$, $\mathbf{T}_\mu$. The proofs are omitted since they are obvious modifications of the proofs for **R**.

The projection theorem for $\mathbf{T}_\mu$ reads

$$(\mathbf{T}_\mu f)\hat{\,}(\theta, \sigma) = (2\pi)^{1/2} \hat{f}(\sigma\theta + i\mu\theta^\perp). \tag{6.1}$$

This formula is not as useful as Theorem 1.1 since it gives $\hat{f}$ on a two-dimensional surface in the space $\mathbb{C}^2$ of two complex variables while the Fourier inversion formula integrates over $\mathbb{R}^2$.

Theorems 1.2, 1.3 hold for $\mathbf{T}_\mu$ as well:

$$\mathbf{T}_\mu(f * g) = \mathbf{T}_\mu f * \mathbf{T}_\mu g \tag{6.2}$$

$$(\mathbf{T}^\#_{-\mu} g) * f = \mathbf{T}^\#_{-\mu}(g * \mathbf{T}_\mu f). \tag{6.3}$$

Here, the dual operators $\mathbf{T}^\#_\mu$, $\mathbf{R}^\#_\mu$ are

$$\mathbf{T}^\#_\mu g(x) = \int_{S^1} e^{\mu x \cdot \theta^\perp} g(\theta, x \cdot \theta)\,d\theta,$$

$$\mathbf{R}^\#_\mu g(x) = \int_{S^1} e^{-\mathbf{D}\mu(x, \theta^\perp)} g(\theta, x \cdot \theta)\,d\theta.$$

Theorem 1.5 extends even to R_μ in the form

$$\mathbf{R}^{\#}_{-\mu}\mathbf{R}_\mu f(x) = 2 \int_{\mathbb{R}^2} |x-y|^{-1} \cosh\left(\int_x^y \mu\, dt\right) f(y)\, dy. \tag{6.4}$$

For $\mathbf{T}_\mu$ this reduces to

$$\mathbf{T}^{\#}_{-\mu}\mathbf{T}_\mu f = k * f, \qquad k(x) = 2\frac{\cosh(\mu|x|)}{|x|}$$

This formula corresponds to Theorem 1.4 and is the starting point for a reconstruction method of the ρ-filtered layergram type, see V.6. A Radon type inversion formula for $\mathbf{T}_\mu$ is obtained in the next theorem.

THEOREM 6.1 Let $f \in C_0^\infty(\mathbb{R}^2)$. Then,

$$f = \frac{1}{4\pi} \mathbf{T}^{\#}_{-\mu} \mathbf{I}_\mu^{-1} g, \qquad g = Tf$$

where $\mathbf{I}_\mu^{-1}$ is the generalized Riesz potential

$$(\mathbf{I}_\mu^{-1} g)\hat{}(\sigma) = \begin{cases} |\sigma|\hat{g}(\sigma), & |\sigma| > |\mu|, \\ 0, & \text{otherwise}. \end{cases}$$

Proof We start out from (6.3), trying to determine the function g in that formula such that $\mathbf{T}^{\#}_\mu g$ is a constant multiple of the δ-function.

For some $b > |\mu|$ we put

$$\hat{w}_b(\theta, \sigma) = \begin{cases} |\sigma|, & |\mu| < |\sigma| < b, \\ 0, & \text{otherwise}. \end{cases}$$

and we compute

$$\mathbf{T}^{\#}_{-\mu} w_b(x) = \int_{S^1} e^{-\mu x \cdot \theta^\perp} w_b(\theta, x\cdot\theta)\, d\theta$$

$$= (2\pi)^{-1/2} \int_{S^1} e^{-\mu x \cdot \theta^\perp} \int_{\mathbb{R}^1} e^{i(x\cdot\theta)\sigma} \hat{w}_b(\theta, \sigma)\, d\sigma\, d\theta$$

$$= (2\pi)^{-1/2} \int_{|\mu|<|\sigma|<b} |\sigma| \int_{S^1} e^{-\mu x \cdot \theta^\perp + i(x\cdot\theta)\sigma}\, d\theta\, d\sigma.$$

In the inner integral we put $\theta = (\cos\varphi, \sin\varphi)^\mathsf{T}$, $x = r(\cos\psi, \sin\psi)$, obtaining

$$\int_{S^1} e^{-\mu x\cdot\theta^\perp + i(x\cdot\theta)\sigma}\, d\theta = \int_0^{2\pi} e^{\mu r \sin\varphi + i\sigma r \cos\varphi}\, d\varphi$$

$$= 2\pi J_0(r(\sigma^2 - \mu^2)^{1/2}),$$

see (VII.3.17). Hence

$$\mathbf{T}^{\#}_{-\mu}w_b(x) = (2\pi)^{1/2} \int_{|\mu|<|\sigma|<b} |\sigma| J_0(|x|(\sigma^2-\mu^2)^{1/2}) \, d\sigma$$

$$= 2(2\pi)^{1/2} \int_0^{\sqrt{(b^2-\mu^2)}} t J_0(|x|t) \, dt$$

$$= 2(2\pi)^{1/2}(b^2-\mu^2)^{1/2}|x|^{-1} J_1(|x|(b^2-\mu^2)^{1/2})$$

where we have used (VII.3.25). Comparing this with (VII.1.3) we see that

$$\tfrac{1}{2}(2\pi)^{-3/2}\mathbf{T}^{\#}_{-\mu}w_b = \delta^{\sqrt{(b^2-\mu^2)}}$$

is an approximate δ-function in the sense that $\delta^{\sqrt{(b^2-\mu^2)}} \to \delta$ pointwise in $\mathscr{S}'$ as $b \to \infty$. From (6.3) we have

$$\mathbf{T}^{\#}_{-\mu}w_b * f = \mathbf{T}^{\#}_{-\mu}(w_b * \mathbf{T}_\mu f). \tag{6.6}$$

It follows that

$$f = \tfrac{1}{2}(2\pi)^{-3/2} \lim_{b\to\infty} \mathbf{T}^{\#}_{-\mu}(w_b * \mathbf{T}_\mu f)$$

$$= \tfrac{1}{2}(2\pi)^{-1}\mathbf{T}^{\#}_{-\mu} I_\mu^{-1} \mathbf{T}_\mu f$$

where we have used R4 of VII.1. This is our inversion formula for $\mathbf{T}_\mu$. □

Theorem 6.1 is an extension of Theorem 2.1 to $\mathbf{T}_\mu$ for $\alpha = 0$. It is the basis for a filtered back-projection algorithm for the inversion of $\mathbf{T}_\mu$, see V.1. As for $\mathbf{R}$, the actual numerical implementation starts out from (6.6).

Next we consider the range of $\mathbf{R}_\mu$.

THEOREM 6.2   Let $f, \mu \in \mathscr{S}(\mathbb{R}^n)$. Then, for $k > m \geq 0$ integers, we have

$$\int_{\mathbb{R}^1} \int_0^{2\pi} s^m e^{\pm ik\varphi + 1/2(I \pm i\mathbf{H})\mathbf{R}\mu(\theta,s)} \mathbf{R}_\mu f(\theta,s) \, d\varphi \, ds = 0.$$

where $\theta = (\cos\varphi, \sin\varphi)^\mathsf{T}$.

Proof   The theorem follows essentially by considering the Fourier expansions

$$\mathbf{D}\mu(x,\theta) = \sum_l p_l(x) e^{-il\varphi}, \qquad \theta = (\cos\varphi, \sin\varphi)^\mathsf{T}$$

$$h(\theta, x\cdot\theta) = \sum_l q_l(x) e^{-il\varphi}$$

where h is a function on Z. We have

$$p_l(x) = \frac{1}{2\pi} \int_0^{2\pi} e^{il\varphi} \mathbf{D}\mu(x,\theta) \, d\varphi$$

$$= \frac{1}{2\pi} \int_0^{2\pi} e^{il\varphi} \int_0^\infty \mu(x+t\theta) \, dt \, d\varphi.$$

Putting $y = -t\theta$ we obtain

$$p_l(x) = \frac{1}{2\pi}(-1)^l \int_{\mathbb{R}^2} \mu(x-y) v_l(y) \, dy = \frac{1}{2\pi}(-1)^l (\mu * v_l)(x), \tag{6.7}$$

$$v_l(r\theta) = \frac{1}{r} e^{il\varphi}, \quad r > 0.$$

We compute the Fourier transform of v_l. With $\xi = \rho(\cos\Psi, \sin\Psi)^T$ we get

$$\hat{v}_l(\xi) = \frac{1}{2\pi} \int_{\mathbb{R}^2} e^{-ix\cdot\xi} v_l(x) \, dx$$

$$= \frac{1}{2\pi} \int_0^\infty \int_0^{2\pi} e^{-ir\rho\cos(\varphi-\Psi)+il\varphi} \, d\varphi \, dr$$

$$= \frac{1}{2\pi} \int_0^\infty e^{il\Psi} \int_0^{2\pi} e^{-ir\rho\cos\varphi+il\varphi} \, d\varphi \, dr$$

$$= i^l \frac{1}{\rho} \int_0^\infty J_l(-r\rho) \, dr \, e^{il\Psi}$$

where we have used (VII.3.16). From (VII.3.27) we get

$$\hat{v}_l(\xi) = \varepsilon_l i^{-l} \rho^{-1} e^{il\Psi} = \varepsilon_l i^{-l} v_l(\xi),$$

$$\varepsilon_l = \begin{cases} 1, & l \geq 0, \\ (-1)^l, & l < 0. \end{cases}$$

From (6.7) and R4 of VII.1 we get

$$\hat{p}_l = (-1)^l \hat{\mu} \hat{v}_l$$

$$= \varepsilon_l i^l \hat{\mu} v_l. \tag{6.8}$$

For q_l we have

$$q_l(x) = \frac{1}{2\pi} \int_0^{2\pi} e^{il\varphi} h(\theta, x \cdot \theta) d\theta$$

$$= \frac{1}{2\pi} \mathbf{R}^* (e^{il\varphi} h)(x).$$

From Theorem 1.4 we get

$$\hat{q}_l(\xi) = \frac{1}{2\pi} (\mathbf{R}^* (e^{il\varphi} h))^\wedge(\xi)$$

$$= (2\pi)^{-1/2} |\xi|^{-1} \left[e^{il\Psi} \hat{h}\left(\frac{\xi}{|\xi|}, |\xi|\right) + e^{il(\Psi + \pi)} \hat{h}\left(-\frac{\xi}{|\xi|}, -|\xi|\right) \right]$$

$$= (2\pi)^{-1/2} v_l(\xi) \left[\hat{h}\left(\frac{\xi}{|\xi|}, |\xi|\right) + (-1)^l \hat{h}\left(-\frac{\xi}{|\xi|}, -|\xi|\right) \right]. \tag{6.9}$$

The similarity between (6.8) and (6.9) is the core of the proof. We define two functions h_+, h_- on Z by

$$\hat{h}_\pm(\theta, \sigma) = (2\pi)^{1/2} \tfrac{1}{2}(1 \pm \text{sgn}(\sigma))\hat{\mu}(\sigma\theta)$$

and compute the Fourier coefficients $u_l(x)$ of the function

$$u_+(x, \theta) = h_+(\theta, x \cdot \theta) - D\mu(x, \theta^\perp).$$

From (6.9), (6.8) we get

$$\hat{u}_l = v_l \hat{\mu} - \varepsilon_l \hat{\mu} v_l$$

and this vanishes for $l \geq 0$. Hence the Fourier expansion of u_+ contains only terms with $l \leq 0$, and so does the Fourier expansion of $\exp\{u_+\}$. Since $(x \cdot \theta)^m$, $m \geq 0$ an integer, is a trigonometric polynomial of degree $\leq m$, the Fourier expansion of

$$(x \cdot \theta)^m e^{ik\varphi} e^{u_+(x, \theta)}$$

contains for $k > m$ only terms of positive order. Integrating over $[0, 2\pi]$ and inserting the explicit expression for u_+ we obtain for $k > m$

$$\int_0^{2\pi} (x \cdot \theta)^m e^{ik\varphi + h_+(\theta, x \cdot \theta)} e^{-D\mu(x, \theta^\perp)} d\varphi = 0.$$

But this can be written as

$$\mathbf{R}_\mu^\# w_+ = 0, \quad w_+(\theta, s) = s^m e^{ik\varphi + h_+(\theta, s)}.$$

In the same way we see that

$$\mathbf{R}_\mu^\# w_- = 0, \quad w_-(\theta, s) = s^m e^{-ik\varphi + h_-(\theta, x \cdot \theta)}.$$

for $k > m$. $\mathbf{R}_\mu^\#$ being the dual of $\mathbf{R}_\mu$ it follows that for $f \in \mathscr{S}(\mathbb{R}^2)$

$$(w_\pm, \mathbf{R}_\mu f)_{L_2(Z)} = (\mathbf{R}_\mu^\# w_\pm, f)_{L_2(\mathbb{R}^2)} = 0 \tag{6.10}$$

for $k > m$.

We give (6.10) a more explicit form. Making use of Theorem 1.1 we have

$$(\mathbf{R}\mu)\hat{\,}(\theta, \sigma) = (2\pi)^{1/2}\hat{\mu}(\sigma\theta).$$

For the Hilbert transform $\mathbf{H}$ we have

$$i(\mathbf{H}h)\hat{\,}(\sigma) = \text{sgn}(\sigma)\hat{h}(\sigma),$$

see (VII.1.11). Combining the last two formulas with the definition of $h_\pm$ yields

$$\hat{h}_\pm(\theta, \sigma) = \tfrac{1}{2}(1 \pm \text{sgn}(\sigma))(\mathbf{R}\mu)\hat{\,}(\theta\sigma)$$

or

$$h_\pm = \tfrac{1}{2}(I \pm i\mathbf{H})\mathbf{R}\mu.$$

Using this in (6.10) we obtain the theorem. □

Theorem 6.2 generalizes Theorem 4.1 to the attenuated Radon transform: if $\mu = 0$, then Theorem 6.2 states that

$$\int_0^{2\pi} e^{\pm ik\varphi} \int_{\mathbb{R}^1} s^m \mathbf{R}_\mu f(\theta, s) \, ds \, d\varphi = 0$$

for $k > m$. This means that the inner integral is a trigonometric polynomial of degree $\leq m$.

II.7 Bibliographical Notes

Most of the results for $\mathbf{R}$ and $\mathbf{P}$ extend to the general k-plane transform which integrates over k-dimensional subspaces, see Solmon (1976). In this way a unified treatment of $\mathbf{R}$ ($k = n - 1$) and $\mathbf{P}$ ($k = 1$) is possible.

The inversion formulas of Theorem 2.1 in the general form given here has first been obtained by Smith *et al.* (1977). Special cases have been known before, most notably Radon (1917) for $n = 2$, and also John (1934), Helgason (1965), Ludwig (1966). Theorem 2.2 has been obtained by Ludwig (1966), Theorem 2.3 by Deans (1979). The case $n = 2$ was been settled in 1963 by A. Cormack (1963, 1964) who received for this work the 1979 Nobel price for medicine, jointly with G. Hounsfield. However, it has also been used in a completely different context by Kershaw (1962, 1970) as early as 1962.

Theorem 3.1, with a completely different proof, is due to Helgason (1965). In two dimensions it is due to Cormack (1963). The other uniqueness theorems in Section 3 have been obtained, even for non-smooth functions, in Hamaker *et al.*, (1980), Smith *et al.* (1977); see also Leahy *et al.* (1979).

Theorem 4.2 is due to Helgason (1980). Different proofs have been given by Lax and Phillips (1970), Ludwig (1966), Smith, *et al.* (1977) and Droste (1983).

Theorem 4.3 has been obtained by Solmon (1976) in the L_2 case and by Helgason (1980) in the case given here. Solmon also observed that the condition of compact support in this theorem cannot be dropped (oral communication).

Sobolev space estimates such as given in Theorem 5.1 have been obtained in Natterer (1977, 1980) for $n = 2$ and by Smith et al. (1977), Louis (1981), Hertle (1983). That paper contains also the estimate of Theorem 5.3, see Natterer (1980) for the case $n = 2$.

The reduction of $\mathbf{R}_\mu$ to $\mathbf{T}_\mu$ for constant μ is due to Markoe (1986). The inversion formula for the exponential Radon transform has been given by Tretiak and Metz (1980). An inversion procedure based on (6.1) and Cauchy's theorem has been given in Natterer (1979). The consistency conditions for the range of the attenuated Radon transform given in Theorem 6.2 have been used to solve in simple cases the identification problem in ECT, see I.2: given $g = \mathbf{R}_\mu f$, find μ without knowing f. For this and similar problems see Natterer (1983a, b, 1984). Heike (1984) proved the analogue of Theorem 5.1 for $\mathbf{R}_\mu$, provided $\mathbf{R}_\mu$ is invertible. The invertibility of $\mathbf{R}_\mu$ has not yet been settled in general.

The attenuated Radon transform is a special case of the generalized Radon transform

$$\mathbf{R}_\Phi f(\theta, s) = \int_{x \cdot \theta = s} \Phi(x, \theta, s) f(x) \, dx$$

where the Lebesgue measure dx has been replaced by the smooth positive measure $\Phi(x, \theta, s) dx$. Quinto (1983) proved invertibility if $\mathbf{R}_\Phi$ is rotation invariant, Boman (1984b) if Φ is real analytic and positive, Markoe and Quinto (1985) obtained local invertibility. Hertle (1984) showed that $\mathbf{R}_\Phi$ is invertible if $\Phi(x, \theta, s) = \exp\{\varphi(x, \theta)\}$ with φ depending linearly on x. On the other hand, Boman (1984a) showed that $\mathbf{R}_\Phi$ is not invertible in general even if Φ is a C_0^∞ function.

Another type of generalized Radon transforms integrates over manifolds rather than over planes. As standard reference we mention Helgason (1980) and Gelfand et al. (1965). Funk (1913) derived a Radon type inversion formula for recovering a function on S^2 from integrals over great circles. John (1934), Romanov (1974), Cormack (1981), Cormack and Quinto (1980), Boman (1984b) and Bukhgeim and Lavrent'ev (1973) considered special families of manifolds.

III
Sampling and Resolution

In this chapter we want to find out how to properly sample $\mathbf{P}f$, $\mathbf{R}f$ for some function f. We have seen in Theorem II.3.7 that f is basically undetermined by $\mathbf{P}f(\theta_j, x)$ for finitely many directions θ_j even in the semi-discrete case in which x runs over all of $\theta_j^\perp$. Therefore we have to restrict f somehow. It turns out that positive and practically useful results are obtained for (essentially) band-limited functions f. These functions and their sampling properties are summarized in Section III.1. In Section III.2 we study the possible resolution if the Radon transform is available for finitely many directions. In Section III.3. we find the resolution of some fully discrete sampling schemes in the plane.

III.1 The Sampling Theorem

One of the basic problems in digital image processing is the sampling of images and the reconstruction of images from samples, see e.g. Pratt (1978). Since an image is described by its density function f the mathematical problem is to discretize f and to compute f from the discrete values.

The fundamental theorem in sampling is Shannon's sampling theorem, see Jerry (1977) for a survey. It deals with band-limited functions. We give a very brief account of band-limited functions which play an important role in communication theory.

A function in $\mathbb{R}^n$ is called band-limited with bandwidth b (or b-band-limited) if its Fourier transform is locally integrable and vanishes a.e. outside the ball of radius b. The simplest example of a band-limited function in $\mathbb{R}^1$ is the sinc-function

$$\text{sinc}(x) = \frac{1}{2} \int_{-1}^{+1} e^{ix\xi} d\xi$$

$$= \begin{cases} \dfrac{\sin x}{x}, & x \neq 0, \\ 1, & x = 0. \end{cases}$$

Since it is the inverse Fourier transform of a function vanishing outside $[-1, +1]$ its bandwidth is 1. In $\mathbb{R}^n$ we define the sinc-function by

$$\mathrm{sinc}(x) = \mathrm{sinc}(x_1) \ldots \mathrm{sinc}(x_n)$$

where $x = (x_1, \ldots, x_n)^\mathsf{T}$. The function $\mathrm{sinc}_b(x) = \mathrm{sinc}(bx)$ is another example of a band-limited function, and we have with χ the characteristic function of $[-1, +1]^n$

$$\widehat{\mathrm{sinc}_b} = \left(\frac{\pi}{2}\right)^{n/2} b^{-n} \chi_{1/b}, \quad \chi_a(\xi) = \chi(a\xi).$$

In Fig. III.1 we show the graph of sinc_b. It is positive in $|x| < \pi/b$ and decays in an oscillating way outside of that interval. In the jargon of digital image processing, sinc_b represents a detail of size $2\pi/b$. Hence, a b-band-limited function contains no details smaller than $2\pi/b$, and for representing details of this size one needs functions of bandwidth at least b. We also say that details of size $2\pi/b$ or less in an image with density f are described by the values of $\hat{f}(\xi)$ for $|\xi| > b$ while the values of $\hat{f}(\xi)$ for $|\xi| < b$ are responsible for the coarser features. Therefore the variable ξ is sometimes called spacial frequency.

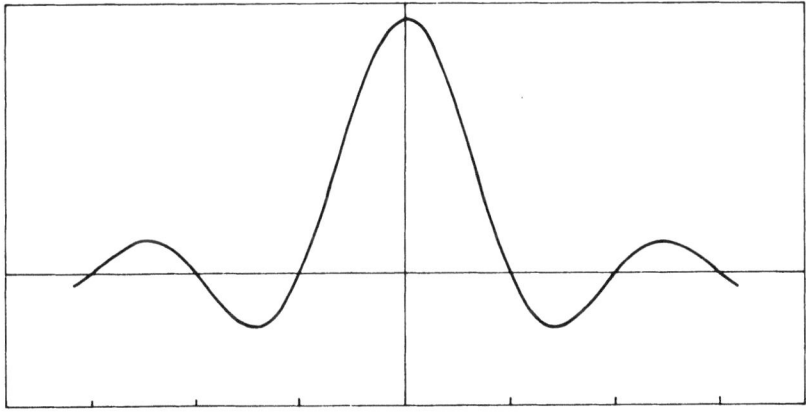

FIG. III.1 Graph of sinc_b

Since images are usually of finite extent, the density functions we have to deal with have compact support. The Fourier transform of such a function is analytic and cannot vanish outside a ball unless it is identically 0. Thus, image densities are usually not band-limited in the strict sense. Therefore we call a function f essentially b-band-limited if $\hat{f}(\xi)$ is negligible for $|\xi| > b$ in some sense. Essentially band-limited functions admit a similar interpretation as (strictly) band-limited functions.

The Shannon sampling theorem, in its simplest form, reads as follows.

THEOREM 1.1 Let f be b-band-limited, and let $h \leq \pi/b$. Then, f is uniquely determined by the values $f(hk)$, $k \in \mathbb{Z}^n$, and, in $L_2(\mathbb{R}^n)$,

$$f(x) = \sum_k f(hk) \operatorname{sinc} \frac{\pi}{h}(x - hk). \tag{1.1}$$

Moreover, we have

$$\hat{f}(\xi) = (2\pi)^{-n/2} h^n \sum_k f(hk) e^{-ih\xi \cdot k} \tag{1.2}$$

in $L_2([-(\pi/h), \pi/h]^n)$. If g is another b-band-limited function, we have

$$\int_{\mathbb{R}^n} f(x) \bar{g}(x) \, dx = h^n \sum_k f(hk) \bar{g}(hk). \tag{1.3}$$

Proof Since $\hat{f}$ vanishes outside $[-(\pi/h), \pi/h]^n$, (1.2) is simply the Fourier expansion of $\hat{f}$ in $[-(\pi/h), \pi/h]^n$, see VII.1, and (1.3) is Parseval's relation. Multiplying (1.2) with the characteristic function $\chi_{h/\pi}$ of $[-(\pi/h), \pi/h]^n$ yields

$$\hat{f}(\xi) = (2\pi)^{-n/2} h^n \sum_k f(hk) \chi_{h/\pi}(\xi) e^{-ih\xi \cdot k}$$

in all of $\mathbb{R}^n$. Since this series converges in $L_2(\mathbb{R}^n)$ we can take the inverse Fourier transform term by term. The result is (1.1). □

A few remarks are in order. The condition $h \leq \pi/b$ is called the Nyquist condition. It requires that f be sampled with a sampling distance at most half of the smallest detail contained in f. If it is satisfied, f can be reconstructed from its samples by means of the sinc series (1.1), and this reconstruction process is stable in the sense that

$$\|f\|_{L_2(\mathbb{R}^n)} = (h^n \sum_k |f(hk)|^2)^{1/2},$$

see (1.3) for $f = g$. From (1.2), (1.3) we see that under the Nyquist condition, Fourier transforms and inner products can be computed exactly by the trapezoidal rule.

If the Nyquist condition is over-satisfied, i.e. if $h < \pi/b$, then f is called over-sampled. The next theorem deals with that case.

THEOREM 1.2 Let f be b-band-limited, and let $h < \pi/b$. Let $\gamma \in C^\infty(\mathbb{R}^n)$ vanish for $|x| \geq 1$ and

$$\int_{\mathbb{R}^n} \gamma(x) \, dx = (2\pi)^{-n/2}.$$

Then,
$$f(x) = \sum_k f(hk)\tilde{\gamma}\left[\left(\frac{\pi}{h} - b\right)(x - hk)\right] \operatorname{sinc} \frac{\pi}{h}(x - hk). \tag{1.4}$$

Proof Again we start out from (1.2) which holds in $[-(\pi/h), \pi/h]^n$. The right-hand side of (1.2) is the periodic extension of $\hat{f}$ with period $2\pi/h$, whose support is

$$\bigcup_{k \in \mathbb{Z}}\left(\frac{2\pi}{h}k + \operatorname{supp}(\hat{f})\right).$$

Since $\operatorname{supp}(\hat{f}) \subseteq [-b, b]^n$, (1.2) holds in $[-a, a]^n$ where $a = 2\pi/h - b > \pi/h$. Thus, if $\psi \in C^\infty$ is 1 on $[-b, b]^n$ and 0 outside $[-a, a]^n$ we have

$$\hat{f}(\xi) = (2\pi)^{-n/2} h^n \sum_k f(hk)\psi(\xi) e^{-ih\xi \cdot k}$$

in all of $\mathbb{R}^n$. If γ is as in the theorem, then

$$\psi = \left(\frac{\pi}{h} - b\right)^{-n}(2\pi)^{n/2}\gamma_{1/(\pi/h-b)} * \chi_{h/\pi}$$

with $\gamma_a(\xi) = \gamma(a\xi)$ satisfies the above conditions, and the theorem follows by an inverse Fourier transform. □

The significance of Theorem 1.3 lies in the fact that (1.4) converges much faster than the sinc series (1.1). The reason is that the function $\tilde{\gamma}$, being the inverse Fourier transform of a C_0^∞-function, decays at infinity faster than any power of $|x|$. This means that for the computation of f from (1.4) one needs to evaluate only a few terms of the series, i.e. an over-sampled function can be evaluated very efficiently. For a more explicit version of Theorem 1.2 see Natterer (1986).

If, on the other hand, the Nyquist condition is not satisfied, i.e. if $h > \pi/b$, then f is called under-sampled. This is always the case if f is not band-limited at all, i.e. if $b = \infty$. If f is nevertheless computed from its sinc series

$$S_h f(x) = \sum_k f(hk) \operatorname{sinc} \frac{\pi}{h}(x - hk)$$

we commit an error which we will now consider.

THEOREM 1.3 Let $f \in \mathcal{S}$. Then, there is a L_∞-function χ_x with $|\chi_x| \le 1$ such that

$$(S_h f - f)(x) = 2(2\pi)^{-n/2} \int_{\mathbb{R}^n - [-(\pi/h), \pi/h]^n} \chi_x(\xi)\hat{f}(\xi) d\xi. \tag{1.5}$$

We also have

$$\hat{f}(\xi) - (2\pi)^{-n/2} h^n \sum_k f(hk) e^{-ih\xi \cdot k} = -\sum_{l \ne 0} \hat{f}\left(\xi - \frac{2\pi}{h}l\right). \tag{1.6}$$

If $f, g \in \mathscr{S}$ then

$$(f \overset{h}{*} g)\hat{}(\xi) - (f * g)\hat{}(\xi) = (2\pi)^{n/2} \hat{f}(\xi) \sum_{l \neq 0} \hat{g}\left(\xi - \frac{2\pi}{h} l\right) \tag{1.7}$$

where the discrete convolution is defined by

$$f \overset{h}{*} g(x) = h^n \sum_l f(x - h l) g(h l).$$

Proof (1.6) is simply (VII.1.4). To prove (1.7) we use R2 from VII.1 to compute

$$(f \overset{h}{*} g)\hat{}(\xi) = h^n \sum_l e^{-ihl \cdot \xi} \hat{f}(\xi) g(h l)$$

$$= (2\pi)^{n/2} \hat{f}(\xi) \sum_l \hat{g}\left(\xi - \frac{2\pi}{h} l\right)$$

where we have applied (VII.1.4) to g. Hence

$$(f \overset{h}{*} g)\hat{}(\xi) - (2\pi)^{n/2} \hat{f}(\xi) \hat{g}(\xi) = (2\pi)^{n/2} \hat{f}(\xi) \sum_{l \neq 0} \hat{g}\left(\xi - \frac{2\pi}{h} l\right)$$

and (1.7) follows by R4 of VII.1.

Putting

$$g(\xi) = \sum_l \hat{f}\left(\xi - \frac{2\pi}{h} l\right)$$

we have from (VII.1.4)

$$g(\xi) = (2\pi)^{-n/2} h^n \sum_k f(h k) e^{-ih\xi \cdot k}$$

in $[-(\pi/h), \pi/h]^n$. Comparing this with the Fourier transform of $S_h f$ we find that

$$(S_h f)\hat{} = \chi_{h/\pi} g$$

with $\chi_{h/\pi}$ the characteristic function of $[-(\pi/h), \pi/h]^n$. Now we decompose g into $\hat{f} + \hat{a}$ with

$$\hat{a}(\xi) = \sum_{l \neq 0} \hat{f}\left(\xi - \frac{2\pi}{h} l\right)$$

hence

$$(S_h f)\hat{} - \hat{f} = \chi_{h/\pi} g - \hat{f} = \chi_{h/\pi} (\hat{f} + \hat{a}) - \hat{f}$$

$$= (\chi_{h/\pi} - 1) \hat{f} + \chi_{h/\pi} \hat{a}. \tag{1.8}$$

Taking the inverse Fourier transform we obtain

$$(S_h f - f)(x) = (2\pi)^{-n/2} \int (S_h f - f)\hat{}(\xi) e^{ix \cdot \xi} d\xi$$

$$= (2\pi)^{-n/2} \int ((\chi_{h/\pi} - 1) \hat{f} + \chi_{h/\pi} \hat{a})(\xi) e^{ix \cdot \xi} d\xi$$

$$= (2\pi)^{-n/2} \int_{\mathbb{R}^n - [-(\pi/h), \pi/h]^n} (-1)\hat{f}(\xi) e^{ix\cdot\xi} d\xi$$

$$+ (2\pi)^{-n/2} \int_{[-(\pi/h), \pi/h]^n} \hat{a}(\xi) e^{ix\cdot\xi} d\xi.$$

Inserting $\hat{a}$ and putting $\eta = \xi - (2\pi/h)l$ the second integral becomes

$$\int_{[-(\pi/h), \pi/h]^n} \hat{a}(\xi) d\xi = \sum_{l \neq 0} \int_{[-(\pi/h), \pi/h]^n} \hat{f}\left(\xi - \frac{2\pi}{h}l\right) e^{ix\cdot\xi} d\xi$$

$$= \sum_{l \neq 0} \int_{[-(\pi/h), \pi/h]^n + (2\pi/h)l} \hat{f}(\eta) e^{ix\cdot[\eta + (2\pi/h)l]} d\eta$$

$$= \int_{\mathbb{R}^n - [-(\pi/h), \pi/h]^n} \chi_x^*(\eta) \hat{f}(\eta) d\eta$$

where

$$\chi_x^*(\eta) = e^{ix\cdot[\eta + (2\pi/h)l]}, \qquad \eta \in \left[-\frac{\pi}{h}, \frac{\pi}{h}\right]^n + \frac{2\pi}{h}l.$$

The theorem follows with $\chi_x(\eta) = (e^{ix\cdot\eta} + \chi_x^*(\eta))/2$. □

We want to make some remarks.

(1) If f is b-band-limited and $h \leq \pi/b$, then $\hat{f}$ vanishes outside $[-(\pi/h), \pi/h]^n$ and we obtain $S_h f = f$, i.e. (1.1). If f is essentially b-band-limited in the sense that

$$\int_{|\xi| \geq b} |\hat{f}(\xi)| d\xi \leq \varepsilon$$

and $h \leq \pi/b$, then

$$|S_h f - f| \leq 2 (2\pi)^{-n/2} \varepsilon$$

i.e. we have an error estimate for the reconstruction of an essentially b-band-limited function by its sinc series.

(2) The spectral composition of the error $S_h f - f$ is more interesting than the above estimate. According to (1.8) it consists of two functions.

The Fourier transform of the first function is $(\chi_{h/\pi} - 1)\hat{f}$ which vanishes in $[-(\pi/h), \pi/h]^n$, i.e. this function describes only details of size less than $2h$. According to our interpretation of Shannon's sampling theorem, this part of the error is to be expected since for the proper sampling of such details a sampling distance less than h is required.

The Fourier transform of the second function is $\chi_{h/\pi} \hat{a}$ which vanishes outside $[-(\pi/h), \pi/h]^n$, i.e. this function describes only features of size $2h$ and larger.

Thus we see that under-sampling not only produces spurious details twice as big or smaller than the sampling distance but also global artefacts perturbing, or aliasing, the image.

In order to prevent aliasing one has to band-limit the function prior to sampling. This can be done by filtering.

Let F be a b-band-limited function and put

$$f_F = F * f.$$

Then f_F is also b-band-limited and can be properly sampled with step-size $h \leq \pi/b$. In this context, F is called a low-pass filter with cut-off frequency b. An example is the ideal low-pass filter which is defined by

$$\hat{F}(\xi) = \begin{cases} 1, & |\xi| \leq b, \\ 0, & |\xi| > b. \end{cases}$$

F has been computed in (VII.1.3).

The sinc series renders possible error-free evaluation of properly sampled functions. However, the sinc series—even in the generalized form of Theorem 1.3—is rather difficult to compute. Therefore we shall make use occasionally of simple B-spline interpolation.

Let χ be the characteristic function of $[-\frac{1}{2}, \frac{1}{2}]$, i.e. χ is 1 in that interval and 0 outside. Let

$$B = \chi * \ldots * \chi \quad (k \text{ factors}).$$

B is called a B-spline of order k. Obviously, B is $(k-2)$ times continuously differentiable, vanishes outside $[-(k/2), k/2]$ and reduces to a polynomial of degree $k-1$ in each of the intervals $[l, l+1]$ for k even and $[l-\frac{1}{2}, l+\frac{1}{2}]$ for k odd, l being an integer.

Let $g \in \mathscr{S}(\mathbb{R}^1)$ and $h > 0$. With $B_{1/h}(s) = B(s/h)$ we define

$$I_h g(s) = \sum_l g(hl) B_{1/h}(s - hl) \tag{1.9}$$

and consider $I_h g$ as an approximation to g. For $k = 1(2)$, $I_h g$ is the piecewise constant (linear) function interpolating g.

In the following theorem we shall see that the effect of approximating a band-limited function g by $I_h g$ is equivalent to applying a low-pass filter and adding a high frequency function.

THEOREM 1.4 Let g be band-limited with bandwidth π/h. Then,

$$I_h g = F_h * g + a_h, \quad \hat{F}_h(\sigma) = \begin{cases} (2\pi)^{-1/2} \left(\operatorname{sinc}\frac{\sigma h}{2}\right)^k, & |\sigma| \leq \frac{\pi}{h}, \\ 0 & \text{otherwise} \end{cases}$$

where $\hat{a}_h(\sigma) = 0$ for $|\sigma| \leq \pi/h$, and for $\alpha, \beta \geq 0$

$$|a_h|_{H^{-\alpha}(\mathbb{R}^1)} \leq \left(\frac{2}{\pi}\right)^{k-1} \left(\frac{h}{\pi}\right)^{\beta - \alpha} |g|_{H^{-\alpha}(\mathbb{R}^1)}.$$

The semi-norm $|\cdot|_{H^s(\mathbf{R}^1)}$ is defined by

$$|g|^2_{H^s(\mathbf{R}^1)} = \int |\sigma|^{2\alpha} |\hat{g}(\sigma)|^2 \, d\sigma.$$

Proof With R2 from VII.1 we compute

$$(I_h g)\,\hat{}\,(\sigma) = \hat{B}_{1/h}(\sigma) \sum_l g(h\,l) e^{-ihl\sigma}$$

$$= \hat{B}_{1/h}(\sigma)(2\pi)^{1/2} h^{-1} \sum_l \hat{g}\left(\sigma - \frac{2\pi}{h} l\right) \quad (1.10)$$

where we have used (VII.1.4). With R1, R4 from VII.1 we obtain

$$\hat{B}_{1/h}(\sigma) = h\hat{B}(h\sigma) = h(2\pi)^{(k-1)/2} (\hat{\chi}(h\sigma))^k$$

$$= h(2\pi)^{-1/2} \left(\mathrm{sinc}\left(\frac{\sigma h}{2}\right)\right)^k.$$

Hence, from (1.10),

$$(I_h g)\,\hat{}\,(\sigma) = \left(\mathrm{sinc}\left(\frac{\sigma h}{2}\right)\right)^k \sum_l \hat{g}\left(\sigma - \frac{2\pi}{h} l\right)$$

$$= \left(\mathrm{sinc}\left(\frac{\sigma h}{2}\right)\right)^k \hat{g}(\sigma) + \hat{a}_h(\sigma),$$

$$\hat{a}_h(\sigma) = \left(\mathrm{sinc}\left(\frac{\sigma h}{2}\right)\right)^k \sum_{l \neq 0} \hat{g}\left(\sigma - \frac{2\pi}{h} l\right).$$

Since g has bandwidth π/h, $\hat{a}_h(\sigma) = 0$ for $|\sigma| \leq \pi/h$. The estimate on a_h is obtained as follows. We have

$$|a_h|^2_{H^{-s}(\mathbf{R}^1)} = \int_{|\sigma| \geq \pi/h} |\sigma|^{-2\beta} |\hat{a}_h(\sigma)|^2 \, d\sigma$$

$$\leq \int_{|\sigma| \geq \pi/h} |\sigma|^{-2\beta} \left(\mathrm{sinc}\,\frac{\sigma h}{2}\right)^{2k} \left(\sum_{l \neq 0} \left|\hat{g}\left(\sigma - \frac{2\pi}{h} l\right)\right|\right)^2 d\sigma.$$

Since the support of the functions in the sum do not overlap we can continue

$$\leq \sum_{l \neq 0} \int_{|\sigma| \leq \pi/h} \left|\sigma - \frac{2\pi}{h} l\right|^{-2\beta} \left(\mathrm{sinc}\left(\sigma - \frac{2\pi}{h} l\right)\frac{h}{2}\right)^{2k} |\hat{g}(\sigma)|^2 \, d\sigma$$

$$\leq \sum_{l \neq 0} \left(\frac{\pi}{2}(2|l|-1)\right)^{-2k} \int_{|\sigma| \leq \pi/h} \left|\sigma - \frac{2\pi}{h}\right|^{-2\beta} |\hat{g}(\sigma)|^2 \, d\sigma.$$

The sum is
$$2\left(\frac{2}{\pi}\right)^{2k} \sum_{l=1}^{\infty} (2l-1)^{-2k} \le \left(\frac{2}{\pi}\right)^{2k-2}$$
where we have used that $1 + 3^{-2} + 5^{-2} + \ldots = \pi^2/8$, hence

$$\begin{aligned}
|a_h|^2_{H^{-\beta}(\mathbb{R}^1)} &\le \left(\frac{2}{\pi}\right)^{2k-2} \int_{|\sigma| \le \pi/h} \left|\sigma - \frac{2\pi}{h}\right|^{-2\beta} |\sigma|^{2\alpha} |\sigma|^{-2\alpha} |\hat{g}(\sigma)|^2 \, d\sigma \\
&\le \left(\frac{2}{\pi}\right)^{2k-2} \sup_{|\sigma| \le \pi/h} \left(\left|\sigma - \frac{2\pi}{h}\right|^{-2\beta} |\sigma|^{2\alpha}\right) |g|^2_{H^{-\alpha}(\mathbb{R}^1)} \\
&\le \left(\frac{2}{\pi}\right)^{2k-2} \left(\frac{h}{\pi}\right)^{2(\beta-\alpha)} |g|^2_{H^{-\alpha}(\mathbb{R}^1)}.
\end{aligned}$$

The theorem now follows from R4 of VII.1. □

So far the Cartesian grid $h\mathbb{Z}^n$ and the cube $[-(\pi/h), \pi/h]^n$ played a special role: if $\hat{f}$ vanishes outside that cube, reconstruction of f from its values on the grid is possible. Below we will prove a sampling theorem for arbitrary grids, replacing the cube by a suitable set. We need a fairly general version of that theorem which goes back to Peterson and Middleton (1962). Here, a function f on $\mathbb{R}^n$ is sampled on the grid
$$\{Wl = l \in \mathbb{Z}^n\}$$
where W is a real non-singular $n \times n$ matrix, and the reconstruction is done by the formula
$$S_W f(x) = \det(W)(2\pi)^{-n/2} \sum_l f(Wl) \hat{\chi}_K (x - Wl)$$
where χ_K is the characteristic function of some open set $K \subseteq \mathbb{R}^n$.

THEOREM 1.5 Assume that the sets $K + 2\pi(W^{-1})^\mathsf{T} k$, $k \in \mathbb{Z}^n$ are mutually disjoint, and let $g \in \mathscr{S}$. Then, there is a L_∞ function χ_x vanishing on K with $|\chi_x| \le 1$ such that

$$(S_W g - g)(x) = 2(2\pi)^{-n/2} \int_{\mathbb{R}^n} \chi_x(\xi) \hat{g}(\xi) \, d\xi.$$

Proof we repeat the proof of Theorem 1.3 for the function
$$f(x) = g(Wx)$$
and replace the cube $(-(\pi/h), \pi/h)^n$ by K. □

We shall apply Theorem 1.5 to functions g which vanish on the grid

$\{Wl: l \in \mathbb{Z}^n\}$. Then,

$$|g(x)| \leq 2(2\pi)^{-n/2} \int_{\mathbb{R}^n - K} |\hat{g}(\xi)| \, d\xi. \qquad (1.11)$$

If g is a $2a$-periodic C^∞ function, we get from (VII.1.7)

$$\hat{g} = (2\pi)^{n/2} \sum_k \hat{g}_k \, \delta_{\pi k/a}$$

and we expect from (1.11)

$$|g(x)| \leq 2 \sum_{\pi k/a \notin K} |\hat{g}_k| \qquad (1.12)$$

to hold. This is in fact the case. To prove (1.12) we choose a real valued function $w \in \mathscr{S}$ and apply Theorem 1.5 to the function $wg \in \mathscr{S}$, obtaining

$$(wg)(x) = 2(2\pi)^{-n/2} \int_{\mathbb{R}^n} \chi_x(\xi)(wg)\hat{}(\xi) \, d\xi$$

where χ_x is a L_∞ function which vanishes on K and $|\chi_x| \leq 1$. Proceeding formally we obtain

$$\int_{\mathbb{R}^n} \chi_x(\xi)(wg)\hat{}(\xi) \, d\xi = (2\pi)^{-n/2} \int_{\mathbb{R}^n} \chi_x(\xi)(\hat{w} * \hat{g})(\xi) \, d\xi \qquad (1.13)$$

$$= (2\pi)^{-n/2} \int_{\mathbb{R}^n} (\tilde{w} * \chi_x)(\xi) \hat{g}(\xi) \, d\xi$$

$$= (2\pi)^{-n/2} \hat{g}(\tilde{w} * \chi_x)$$

where $\hat{g}$ is to be understood as the extension of $\hat{g}$ from $\mathscr{S}$ to the bounded C^∞ functions, i.e.

$$\hat{g}(\tilde{w} * \chi_x) = (2\pi)^{n/2} \sum_k \hat{g}_k (\tilde{w} * \chi_x)(\pi k/a).$$

(1.13) is easily justified by explicit computation. It follows that

$$|(wg)(x)| \leq 2(2\pi)^{-n/2} \sum_k |\hat{g}_k| \, |(\tilde{w} * \chi_x)(\pi k/a)|$$

and (1.12) follows by letting $w \to 1$ in a suitable way: for $\psi \in C_0^\infty(\Omega^n)$ a radial function with mean value 1 we put $\tilde{w}(\xi) = (2\pi)^{n/2} \varepsilon^{-n} \psi(\xi/\varepsilon)$, i.e. $w(0) = 1$. We obtain for each $\varepsilon > 0$

$$|(wg)(x)| \leq 2 \sum_k |\hat{g}_k| \sup_{|\pi k/a - \xi| \leq \varepsilon} |\chi_x(\xi)|$$

and (1.12) follows by letting $\varepsilon \to 0$.

If $g \in C^\infty(\mathbb{R}^2)$ has period 2π in its first variable only and is in $\mathscr{S}(\mathbb{R}^1)$ as a function of the second variable, then

$$|g(x)| \leq 2(2\pi)^{-1/2} \sum_k \int_{(k,\sigma) \notin K} |\hat{g}_k(\sigma)| d\sigma. \quad (1.14)$$

This can be established in the same way as (1.12).

III.2 Resolution

In this section we consider the Radon transform Rf of a function f which is supported in the unit ball Ω^n of $\mathbb{R}^n$ and which is essentially b-band-limited in a sense to be made precise later. We want to find out for which discrete directions $\theta \in S^{n-1}$ the function $R_\theta f$ must be given if f is to be recovered reliably, i.e. if details of size $2\pi/b$ are to be resolved. Since sampling conditions for $\mathbf{P}$ in three dimensions can be obtained by applying the sampling conditions for $\mathbf{R}$ to planes we consider only $\mathbf{R}$.

Let H'_m be the set of spherical harmonics of degree $\leq m$ which are even for m even and odd for m odd. We show that

$$\dim H'_m = \binom{m+n-1}{n-1}. \quad (2.1)$$

We proceed by induction. For $m = 0, 1$, we have $H'_0 = \langle 1 \rangle$, $H'_1 = \langle x_1, \ldots, x_n \rangle$, hence

$$\dim H'_0 = 1 = \binom{n-1}{n-1}, \qquad \dim H'_1 = n = \binom{n}{n-1},$$

i.e. (2.1) is correct for $m = 0, 1$. Assume that it is correct for some $m \geq 1$. Then, from (VII.3.11),

$$\dim H'_{m+2} = \dim H'_m + N(n, m+2)$$

$$= \binom{m+n-1}{n-1} + \frac{(2m+n+2)(n+m-1)!}{(m+2)!(n-2)!}$$

$$= \frac{(m+n-1)!}{(m+2)!(n-1)!}((m+1)(m+2) + (2m+n+2)(n-1))$$

$$= \frac{(m+n-1)!}{(m+2)!(n-1)!}(m+n)(m+n+1)$$

$$= \frac{(m+n+1)!}{(m+2)!(n-1)!} = \binom{m+n+1}{n-1}.$$

This is (2.1) with m replaced by $m+2$, hence (2.1) is established.

Now we make a definition which is crucial for questions of resolution. A set $A \subseteq S^{n-1}$ is called m-resolving if no non-trivial $h \in H'_m$ vanishes on A.

If A is m-resolving then the number $|A|$ of elements of A satisfies

$$|A| \geq \dim H'_m = \binom{m+n-1}{n-1}. \tag{2.2}$$

Conversely, if $|A|$ satisfies (2.2) it usually will be m-resolving, except if A lies on a certain algebraic manifold of degree m on S^{n-1}.

THEOREM 2.1 Let A be m-resolving, let $f \in C_0^\infty(\Omega^n)$, and let $\lambda > -1/2$. If $\mathbf{R}_\theta f$ vanishes for $\theta \in A$, then

$$\mathbf{R}_\theta f(s) = (1-s^2)^{\lambda - 1/2} \sum_{l > m} C_l^\lambda(s) h_l(\theta) \tag{2.3}$$

with C_l^λ the Gegenbauer polynomials (see VII.3) and $h_l \in H'_l$.

Proof According to (II.4.2) we have the expansion

$$\mathbf{R}_\theta f(s) = (1-s^2)^{\lambda - 1/2} \sum_{l=0}^\infty C_l^\lambda(s) h_l(\theta)$$

with $h_l \in H'_l$. If $\mathbf{R}_\theta f = 0$ for some θ it follows that $h_l(\theta) = 0$ for each l. Since A is m-resolving it follows that $h_l = 0$ for $l \leq m$, hence the theorem. □

Theorem 2.1 tells us that the expansion of $\mathbf{R}_\theta f$ in Gegenbauer polynomials starts with the $(m+1)$st term. For m large, $\mathbf{R}_\theta f$ is therefore a highly oscillating function. In fact, we shall see in the next theorem that $|(\mathbf{R}_\theta f)^\wedge|$ is negligible in an interval only slightly smaller than $[-m, +m]$ for m large. In order to formulate statements like this we introduce the following notation. For $0 < \vartheta < 1$ and $b \geq 0$ we denote by $\eta(\vartheta, b)$ any quantity which admits an estimate of the form

$$0 \leq \eta(\vartheta, b) \leq C(\vartheta) e^{-\lambda(\vartheta) b} \tag{2.4}$$

provided $b \geq B(\vartheta)$, where $\lambda(\vartheta), C(\vartheta), B(\vartheta)$ are positive numbers. Thus, for $\vartheta < 1$ fixed, $\eta(\vartheta, b)$ decays exponentially as b tends to infinity. We shall use the notation η in a generic way, i.e. different quantities are denoted by the same symbol η if they only satisfy (2.4). Specific examples of functions η are

$$\eta_1(\vartheta, m) = \sup_{|r| \leq 1} \int_{-\vartheta m}^{\vartheta m} |J_m(r\sigma)| d\sigma \tag{2.5}$$

as can be seen from (VII.3.20). In fact, a short calculation shows that

$$\eta_1(\vartheta, m) \leq C(\vartheta) m^{1/2} e^{-(1-\vartheta^2)^{3/2} m/3}.$$

Since for $\lambda > 0$, $d > 0$ and $\lambda - d/m > 0$

$$\sum_{l > m} l^d e^{-\lambda l} \leq \frac{1}{\lambda - d/m} m^d e^{-\lambda m} \tag{2.6}$$

as can be as seen from the inequality

$$\sum_{l>m} l^d e^{-\lambda l} \le \int_m^\infty x^d e^{-\lambda x}\, dx,$$

the functions

$$\eta_2(\vartheta, b) = \sum_{m \ge b} \eta_1(\vartheta, m)$$

$$\eta_3(\vartheta, b) = \sum_{m \ge b} \eta_2(\vartheta, m) \tag{2.7}$$

$$\eta_{4,d}(\vartheta, b) = \sum_{m \ge b} m^d \eta_1(\vartheta, m)$$

also satisfy (2.4). Of course, the functions

$$b^d \eta(\vartheta, b), \quad \eta\left(\vartheta, \left(\frac{1}{\vartheta} - 1\right)b\right) \tag{2.8}$$

fulfil (2.4) if η does.

In order to express what we mean by an essentially band-limited function we introduce the notation

$$\varepsilon_d(f, b) = \int_{|\xi| > b} |\xi|^d |f(\xi)|\, d\xi.$$

For $0 < \vartheta$ and $b \ge 1$ we have

$$\sum_{k \ge b/\vartheta} \varepsilon_d(f, \vartheta k) \le \frac{1}{\vartheta} \varepsilon_{d+1}(f, b). \tag{2.9}$$

This can be seen as follows. If h is a non-negative function, then

$$\sum_{k \ge b} \int_{\vartheta k}^\infty h(\sigma)\, d\sigma \le \frac{1}{\vartheta} \int_{\vartheta b}^\infty \sigma h(\sigma)\, d\sigma \tag{2.10}$$

whenever the integrals make sense. To establish (2.10) we write

$$\sum_{k \ge b} \int_{\vartheta k}^\infty h(\sigma)\, d\sigma \le \int_{\vartheta b}^\infty h(\sigma)\, d\sigma + \int_{\vartheta(b+1)}^\infty h(\sigma)\, d\sigma + \ldots$$

$$= \int_{\vartheta b}^{\vartheta(b+1)} h(\sigma)\, d\sigma + 2 \int_{\vartheta(b+1)}^{\vartheta(b+2)} h(\sigma)\, d\sigma + \ldots$$

$$\le \int_{\vartheta b}^{\vartheta(b+1)} \frac{\sigma}{\vartheta} h(\sigma)\, d\sigma + \int_{\vartheta(b+1)}^{\vartheta(b+2)} \frac{\sigma}{\vartheta} h(\sigma)\, d\sigma + \ldots$$

which holds for $b \geq 1$. This proves (2.10). Applying (2.10) with
$$h(\sigma) = |\sigma|^{d+n-1} |\hat{f}(\sigma\theta)|$$
and integrating over S^{n-1} yields (2.9).

THEOREM 2.2 Let A be m-resolving and let $f \in C_0^\infty(\Omega^n)$. If $\mathbf{R}_\theta f$ vanishes for $\theta \in A$, then
$$\int_{|\sigma| \leq \vartheta m} |(\mathbf{R}_\theta f)\hat{\,}(\sigma)|\, d\sigma \leq \eta(\vartheta, m) \|\mathbf{R}_\theta f\|_{L_1(\mathbf{R}^1)}$$
for $\theta \in S^{n-1}$.

Proof We use Theorem 2.1 with $\lambda = 0$, obtaining
$$\mathbf{R}_\theta f(s) = (1-s^2)^{-1/2} \sum_{l > m} T_l(s) h_l(\theta),$$
$$|h_l(\theta)| = \frac{2}{\pi} \left| \int_{-1}^{+1} \mathbf{R}_\theta f(s) T_l(s)\, ds \right| \leq \frac{2}{\pi} \|\mathbf{R}_\theta f\|_{L_1(\mathbf{R}^1)}. \tag{2.11}$$

Taking the Fourier transform term by term we obtain from (VII.3.18)
$$(\mathbf{R}_\theta f)\hat{\,}(\sigma) = (\pi/2)^{1/2} \sum_{l > m} i^{-l} J_l(\sigma) h_l(\theta).$$

Integrating it follows from (2.11) that
$$\int_{|\sigma| < \vartheta m} |(\mathbf{R}_\theta f)\hat{\,}(\sigma)|\, d\sigma \leq 2(\pi/2)^{1/2} \frac{2}{\pi} \|\mathbf{R}_\theta f\|_{L_1(\mathbf{R}^1)} \sum_{l > m} \int_0^{\vartheta m} |J_l(\sigma)|\, d\sigma$$
$$\leq (2/\pi)^{1/2} \|\mathbf{R}_\theta f\|_{L_1(\mathbf{R}^1)} \sum_{l > m} \eta_1(\vartheta, l)$$
$$\leq (2/\pi)^{1/2} \|\mathbf{R}_\theta f\|_{L_1(\mathbf{R}^1)} \eta_2(\vartheta, m)$$

where we have used (2.5) and (2.7). This is the theorem with $\eta(\vartheta, m) = (2/\pi)^{1/2} \eta_2(\vartheta, m)$.

By means of Theorem II.1.1, Theorem 2.2 translates into the corresponding theorem for f.

THEOREM 2.3 Let A be m-resolving, and let $f \in C_0^\infty(\Omega^n)$. If $\mathbf{R}_\theta f$ vanishes for $\theta \in A$, then
$$\int_{|\xi| \leq \vartheta m} |\hat{f}(\xi)|\, d\xi \leq \eta(\vartheta, m) \|f\|_{L_1(\Omega)}.$$

Proof From Theorem II.1.1 and Theorem 2.2,

$$\int_{|\xi| \le \vartheta m} |\hat{f}(\xi)| d\xi = \int_{S^{n-1}} \int_0^{\vartheta m} |\hat{f}(\sigma\theta)| \sigma^{n-1} d\sigma d\theta$$

$$= (2\pi)^{(1-n)/2} \int_{S^{n-1}} \int_0^{\vartheta m} |(R_\theta f)^\wedge(\sigma)| \sigma^{n-1} d\sigma d\theta$$

$$\le (2\pi)^{(1-n)/2} m^{n-1} \frac{1}{2} \eta(\vartheta, m) \int_{S^{n-1}} \|R_\theta f\|_{L_1(R^1)} d\theta$$

with η from Theorem 2.2. Since $m^{n-1} \eta(\vartheta, m)$ satisfies (2.4) if η does, the theorem follows. □

An easy consequence is

THEOREM 2.4 Let A be m-resolving and let $f \in C_0^\infty(\Omega^n)$. If $R_\theta f$ vanishes for $\theta \in A$, then

$$\|f\|_{L_\infty(\Omega^n)} \le \frac{(2\pi)^{-n/2}}{1 - \eta(\vartheta, m)} \varepsilon_0(f, \vartheta m).$$

Proof We have
$$|f(x)| = (2\pi)^{-n/2} |\int e^{ix \cdot \xi} \hat{f}(\xi) d\xi|$$

$$\le (2\pi)^{-n/2} \left\{ \int_{|\xi| \le \vartheta m} |\hat{f}(\xi)| d\xi + \int_{|\xi| \ge \vartheta m} |\hat{f}(\xi)| d\xi \right\}$$

$$\le (2\pi)^{-n/2} \{ \eta(\vartheta, m) \|f\|_{L_1(\Omega)} + \varepsilon_0(f, \vartheta m) \}$$

where we have used Theorem 2.3. It follows that

$$\|f\|_{L_\infty(\Omega^n)} \le (2\pi)^{-n/2} \{ \eta(\vartheta, m) |\Omega^n| \|f\|_{L_\infty(\Omega^n)} + \varepsilon_0(f, \vartheta m) \}$$

and the theorem follows by solving for $\|f\|_{L_\infty(\Omega^n)}$. □

The last two theorems clearly give an answer to the question of resolution. Theorem 2.3 says that the Fourier transform of a function on Ω^n whose Radon transform vanishes on a m-resolving set is almost entirely concentrated outside the ball of radius ϑm around the origin, provided m is large. In the light of Section III.1 this can be rephrased for ϑ close to 1 somewhat loosely as a statement on resolution:

A function on Ω^n whose Radon transform vanishes on a m-resolving set does not contain details of size $2\pi/m$ or larger.

Similarly, Theorem 2.4 admits the following interpretation. If a function f on

Ω^n is essentially b-band-limited in the sense that ε_0 (f, b) is negligible, then f can be recovered reliably from the values of Rf on a m-resolving set, provided $b \le \vartheta m$ and b large. Or, in a less exact but more practical fashion: a function on Ω^n which does not contain details of size $2\pi/b$ or smaller can be recovered reliably from the values of its Radon transform on an m-resolving set, provided that $m > b$.

To conclude this section we want to find out which sets A are m-resolving. We have found in (2.2) that, apart from exceptional cases, a set is m-resolving if and only if it contains

$$\binom{m+n-1}{n-1} = \frac{1}{(n-1)!} m^{n-1} (1 + 0(m)) \tag{2.12}$$

directions. So, for m large, we may think of an m-resolving set as a collection of $m^{n-1}/(n-1)!$ directions. For $n = 2$, this is in fact correct. For, let $A = \{\theta_1, \ldots, \theta_p\} \subseteq S^1$, $\theta_j = \begin{pmatrix} \cos \varphi_j \\ \sin \varphi_j \end{pmatrix}$, $0 \le \varphi_j < \pi$. In order that A be m-resolving we must have $p \ge \dim H'_m = \binom{m+1}{1} = m+1$, and $\theta_1, \ldots, \theta_p$ must not be the zeros of a function $h_m \in H'_m$. From (VII.3.14) we know that such a function h_m is a trigonometric polynomial of the form

$$h_m(\theta) = \sum_{k=0}^{m}{}' \{a_k \cos k\varphi + b_k \sin k\varphi\}$$

where $\theta = \begin{pmatrix} \cos \varphi \\ \sin \varphi \end{pmatrix}$, and Σ' denotes summation over $k+m$ even only. If h_m vanishes for $p > m$ mutually different angles $\varphi_j \in [0, \pi]$, then $h_m = 0$. Hence, for $n = 2$, A is m-resolving if and only if it contains $p > m$ mutually different directions in the angular interval $[0, \pi]$. This means that we can reconstruct reliably functions of essential bandwidth $b < \vartheta p$ from p mutually different directions in $[0, \pi]$. No assumption on the distribution of these directions is needed. For instance, the directions could be concentrated in a small angular interval. This is the discrete analogue to the uniqueness result of Theorem II.3.4.

Now let $n = 3$. Here, the condition that A be m-resolving means that $p \ge \dim H'_m = \binom{m+2}{2} = \frac{1}{2}(m+2)(m+1)$ and that no non-trivial function h_m of the form (see (VII.3.15))

$$h_m(\theta) = \sum_{l=0}^{m}{}' \left\{ a_l P_l(\cos \psi) + \sum_{k=1}^{l} (a_{lk} \cos k\varphi + b_{lk} \sin k\varphi) P_l^k(\cos \psi) \right\}$$

vanishes on A, where ψ, φ are the spherical coordinates of θ. We show that the $(m+1)^2$ directions θ_{jl} with spherical coordinates (see VII.2)

$$\begin{aligned} 0 \le \psi_0 < \psi_1 < \ldots < \psi_m < \pi, \\ 0 \le \varphi_0 < \varphi_1 < \ldots < \varphi_m < \pi \end{aligned} \tag{2.13}$$

form a m-resolving set. The proof depends on the fact that a function in H'_m, being a trigonometric polynomial of degree m on a circle on S^2, can have only $2m$ zeros on a circle, unless being there identically zero. For each $i = 0, \ldots, m$ consider the great circle C_i on which $\varphi = \varphi_i$ or $\varphi = \varphi_i + \pi$. If $h_m \in H'_m$ vanishes on (2.13) it has $2m + 2$ zeros on each C_i, namely those with spherical coordinates ψ_j, φ_i, $j = 0, \ldots, m$, and its antipodals. Hence $h_m = 0$ on each of the great circles C_i. It follows that h_m has $2m + 2$ zeros on each horizontal circle on S^2, i.e. $h_m = 0$ on S^2. This proves that (2.13) is m-resolving. Since, for $\varphi_j = \pi j/(m+1), j = 0, \ldots, m$, the function

$$P_{m+1}^{m+1}(\cos\psi)\sin(m+1)\varphi$$

which is in H'_{m+1} vanishes on (2.13), (2.13) is certainly not $(m+1)$-resolving in general.

We conclude that f can be recovered reliably from the directions (2.13), provided f is essentially b-band-limited with $b \leq 9m$.

From (2.12) we expect m-resolving sets with $(m+2)(m+1)/2$ directions to exist. A possible candidate for such a set, for m even, is

$$0 < \psi_0 < \psi_1 < \ldots < \psi_{m/2} < \pi/2$$
$$\varphi_i = 2\pi i/(m+1), \quad i = 0, \ldots, m. \tag{2.14}$$

For $m = 2$ we can show that (2.14) is m-resolving: if h vanishes on (2.14) it has four zeros on each great circle C_i on which $\varphi = \varphi_i$ or $\varphi = \varphi_i \pm \pi$, namely those with spherical coordinates $\psi_j, \varphi_i, j = 0, 1$ and its antipodals. If $h \neq 0$ at the North Pole these are the only zeros of h on $C_i, i = 0, 1, 2$. Thus h has six sign changes along each circle with ψ fixed in (ψ_0, ψ_1) what is impossible. If $h = 0$ at the North Pole, then h has six zeros on C_i, hence $h = 0$ on C_i, hence $h = 0$ on S^2.

So far we have assumed that $\mathbf{R}_\theta f(s)$ is known for $\theta \in A$ and for all values of s. In practice we know $\mathbf{R}_\theta f(s)$ for finitely many values of s only. In view of Theorem II.1.1, $\mathbf{R}_\theta f$ is essentially b-band-limited if f is. This suggests to apply Theorem 1.3 to $\mathbf{R}_\theta f$, with the result that the sampling is correct if the Nyquist condition is satisfied, i.e. if $\mathbf{R}_\theta f(s_l)$ is known for

$$s_l = l/q, \quad l = -q, \ldots, q, \quad q \geq b/\pi.$$

From (2.12) we know that the number p of directions we need to recover such a function f is essentially $p \geq b^{n-1}/(n-1)!$ Thus for the minimal numbers p, q we have approximately

$$p = cq^{n-1}, \quad c = \pi^{n-1}/(n-1)! \tag{2.15}$$

But we have to be cautious: $\mathbf{R}_\theta f(s_l) = 0$ implies only that $\mathbf{R}_\theta f$ is small, but we do not know how large $\mathbf{R}f$ can be if $\mathbf{R}_\theta f$ is small for $\theta \in A$. In fact, we shall see in VI.2 that there is no reasonable estimate of $\mathbf{R}f$ in terms of $\mathbf{R}_\theta f, \theta \in A$ if A is a proper subset of the half-sphere, even if A is infinite.

In order to obtain a positive statement we would have to put a stability requirement on A which guarantees that $h \in H'_m$ is small on all of S^{n-1} if it is small on A. However, we will not pursue this approach further. Rather we shall consider in the next section some specific fully discrete sampling schemes.

III.3 Some Two-Dimensional Sampling Schemes

In this section we study the resolution of some sampling schemes—or, in the jargon of CT, scanning geometries—in the plane which are fully discrete and which are actually used in practice. We assume f to be supported in the unit disk Ω^2 and to be essentially b-band-limited in an appropriate sense.

We start with the (standard) parallel scanning geometry. Here, for each of the directions $\theta_1, \ldots, \theta_p$ uniformly distributed over the half-circle, $\mathbf{R}_{\theta_j} f$ is sampled at $2q+1$ equally spaced points s_l. We have

$$\theta_j = \begin{pmatrix} \cos \varphi_j \\ \sin \varphi_j \end{pmatrix}, \quad \varphi_j = \pi(j-1)/p, j = 1, \ldots, p,$$

$$s_l = hl, l = -q, \ldots, q, h = \frac{1}{q}.$$

From the discussion at the end of Section III.2 we guess that the correct sampling conditions are $p \geq b$ and $q \geq b/\pi$. Below we shall see that this is in fact the case. Surprisingly enough, this scanning geometry is by no means optimal. We shall see that the interlaced parallel geometry which samples the functions $\mathbf{R}_{\theta_j} f$ only at points s_l with $l+j$ even has the same resolution as the standard parallel geometry with only one-half of the data.

Our approach will be based on Theorem 1.5 applied to $\mathbf{R}f$ considered as a function on $\mathbb{R}^2$, the crucial point being the shape of the (essential) support of the Fourier transform of that function viewed as a periodic distribution.

THEOREM 3.1 Let $f \in C_0^\infty(\Omega^2)$, and let

$$g(\varphi, s) = \mathbf{R}f(\theta, s), \quad \theta = \begin{pmatrix} \cos \varphi \\ \sin \varphi \end{pmatrix}.$$

For $0 < \vartheta < 1$ and $b \geq 1$, define the set

$$K = \{(k, \sigma): |\sigma| < b, |k| < \max(|\sigma|/\vartheta, (1/\vartheta - 1)b)\} \quad (3.1)$$

in $\mathbb{R}^2$, see Fig. III.2. Let W be a real non-singular 2×2 matrix such that the sets $K + 2\pi(W^{-1})^T l$, $l \in \mathbb{Z}^2$, are mutually disjoint. If $g(Wl) = 0$ for $l \in \mathbb{Z}^2$, then

$$\|\mathbf{R}f\|_{L_\infty(Z)} \leq \eta(\vartheta, b) \|f\|_{L_1(\Omega^2)} + \frac{8}{\pi \vartheta} \varepsilon_0(f, b). \quad (3.2)$$

Proof Let $\hat{g}$ be the one-dimensional Fourier transform of g with respect to s and $\hat{g}_k$ the kth Fourier coefficient of $\hat{g}$, i.e.

$$\hat{g}_k(\sigma) = \frac{1}{2\pi} \int_0^{2\pi} \hat{g}(\varphi, \sigma) e^{-ik\varphi} d\varphi.$$

$\hat{g}_k$ can be computed by Theorem II.1.1 and the integral representation (VII.3.16) for the Bessel functions. We obtain

$$\hat{g}_k(\sigma) = (2\pi)^{-1/2} \int_0^{2\pi} \hat{f}(\sigma\theta) e^{-ik\varphi} d\varphi$$

$$= (2\pi)^{-3/2} \int_0^{2\pi} \int_{\Omega^2} e^{-i\sigma\theta \cdot x} f(x) dx\, e^{-ik\varphi} d\varphi$$

$$= (2\pi)^{-3/2} \int_{\Omega^2} f(x) \int_0^{2\pi} e^{-i\sigma\theta \cdot x - ik\varphi} d\varphi\, dx$$

$$= (2\pi)^{-3/2} \int_{\Omega^2} f(x) \int_0^{2\pi} e^{-i\sigma|x|\cos(\varphi-\psi) - ik\varphi} d\varphi\, dx$$

where we have put $x = |x| \begin{pmatrix} \cos\psi \\ \sin\psi \end{pmatrix}$,

$$= (2\pi)^{-3/2} \int_{\Omega^2} f(x) e^{-ik\psi} \int_0^{2\pi} e^{-i\sigma|x|\cos\varphi - ik\varphi} d\varphi\, dx$$

$$= (2\pi)^{-1/2} i^k \int_{\Omega^2} f(x) e^{-ik\psi} J_k(-\sigma|x|)\, dx.$$

We deduce the estimates

$$\int_{|\sigma|>b} |\hat{g}_k(\sigma)| d\sigma \leq 2(2\pi)^{-1/2} \varepsilon_{-1}(f, b) \tag{3.3}$$

$$\int_{|\sigma|<\vartheta|k|} |\hat{g}_k(\sigma)| d\sigma \leq (2\pi)^{-1/2} \eta_1(\vartheta, |k|) \tag{3.4}$$

where we have assumed for convenience that $\|f\|_{L_1(\Omega^2)} = 1$.

From Fig. III.2 we see that

$$\sum_k \int_{(k,\sigma)\notin K} |\hat{g}_k(\sigma)| d\sigma = \Sigma_1 + \Sigma_2 + \Sigma_3,$$

$$\Sigma_1 = \sum_{|k| \geq (1/\vartheta - 1)b} \int_{|\sigma|<\vartheta|k|} |\hat{g}_k(\sigma)| d\sigma,$$

$$\Sigma_2 = \sum_{|k| < b/\vartheta} \int_{|\sigma| > b} |\hat{g}_k(\sigma)| \, d\sigma,$$

$$\Sigma_3 = \sum_{|k| \geq b/\vartheta} \int_{|\sigma| > \vartheta|k|} |\hat{g}_k(\sigma)| \, d\sigma.$$

For Σ_1 we get from (3.4) and (2.7) immediately

$$\Sigma_1 \leq \sum_{|k| \geq (1/\vartheta - 1)b} (2\pi)^{-1/2} \eta_1(\vartheta, |k|)$$

$$= 2(2\pi)^{-1/2} \eta_2(\vartheta, (1/\vartheta - 1)b).$$

In Σ_2 we have no more than $2b/\vartheta$ terms. From (3.3) we get

$$\Sigma_2 \leq \frac{4b}{\vartheta} (2\pi)^{-1/2} \varepsilon_{-1}(f, b)$$

$$\leq \frac{4}{\vartheta} (2\pi)^{-1/2} \varepsilon_0(f, b).$$

In Σ_3 we use (3.3) with b replaced by $\vartheta|k|$ to obtain

$$\Sigma_3 \leq 2 \sum_{|k| \geq b/\vartheta} (2\pi)^{-1/2} \varepsilon_{-1}(f, \vartheta|k|)$$

$$\leq \frac{4}{\vartheta} (2\pi)^{-1/2} \varepsilon_0(f, b)$$

where we have used (2.9). Combining the estimates for $\Sigma_1 - \Sigma_3$ we obtain

$$\sum_k \int_{(k,\sigma) \notin K} |\hat{g}_k(\sigma)| \, d\sigma \leq \eta(\vartheta, b) + \frac{8}{\vartheta} (2\pi)^{-1/2} \varepsilon_0(f, b),$$

$$\eta(\vartheta, b) = 2(2\pi)^{-1/2} \eta_2(\vartheta, (1/\vartheta - 1)b).$$

According to our hypothesis we can apply Theorem 1.5 in the form of (1.14) to g, K and W, obtaining

$$\|g\|_{L_\infty(\mathbb{R}^2)} \leq 2(2\pi)^{-1/2} \sum_k \int_{(k,\sigma) \notin K} |\hat{g}_k(\sigma)| \, d\sigma$$

$$\leq 2(2\pi)^{-1/2} \left\{ \eta(\vartheta, b) + \frac{8}{\vartheta} (2\pi)^{-1/2} \varepsilon_0(f, b) \right\}$$

and this is (3.2). □

Theorem 3.1 tells us that a function f which is essentially b-band-limited in the sense that $\varepsilon_0(f, b)$ is negligible can be recovered reliably from the values of $g = \mathbf{R}f$

on the grid $Wl, l \in \mathbb{Z}^2$ if the sets $K + 2\pi(W^{-1})^\mathsf{T}l, l \in \mathbb{Z}^2$ are mutually disjoint. This holds for ϑ arbitrarily close to 1 and b large.

For the standard parallel geometry we have

$$W = \begin{pmatrix} \pi/p & 0 \\ 0 & 1/q \end{pmatrix}, \quad 2\pi(W^{-1})^\mathsf{T} = \begin{pmatrix} 2p & 0 \\ 0 & 2\pi q \end{pmatrix}$$

and from Fig. III.2 we see that the sets $K + 2\pi(W^{-1})^\mathsf{T}l, l \in \mathbb{Z}^2$ are mutually disjoint if

$$b \leq p\vartheta, \quad b \leq \pi q. \tag{3.5}$$

These are the sampling requirements for the standard parallel geometry. There is no point in over-satisfying either of these inequalities. Therefore it is reasonable to tie p to q by the relation $p = \pi q/\vartheta$.

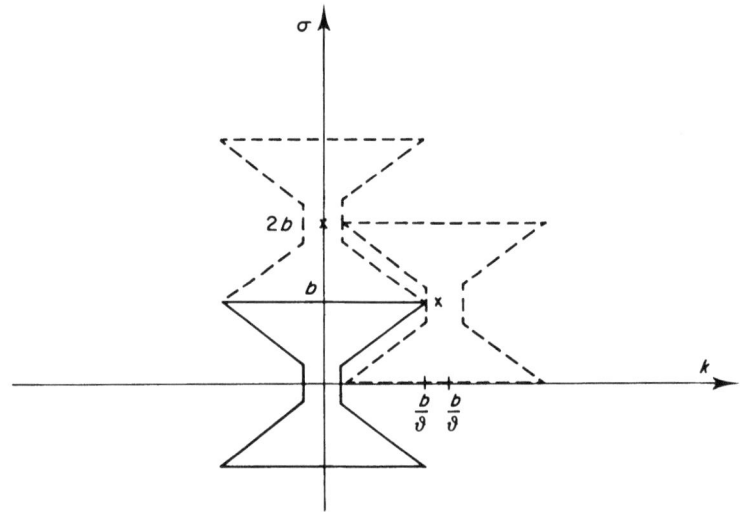

FIG. III.2 The set K defined in (3.1) and some of its translates (dashed) for the interlaced parallel geometry. Crosses indicate the columns of $2\pi(W^{-1})^\mathsf{T}$ ($\vartheta = 4/5$, $\vartheta' = \vartheta/(2-\vartheta) = 2/3$).

In order to obtain the interlaced parallel geometry we choose

$$2\pi(W^{-1})^\mathsf{T} = b\begin{pmatrix} 1/\vartheta' & 0 \\ 1 & 2 \end{pmatrix}, \quad 0 < \vartheta' \leq \frac{\vartheta}{2-\vartheta}$$

In Fig. III.2 we have drawn some of the sets $K + 2\pi(W^{-1})^\mathsf{T}l$. We see that these sets are also mutually disjoint and they cover the plane more densely than the corresponding sets for the standard parallel geometry. The grid generated by

$$W = \frac{\pi}{b}\begin{pmatrix} 2\vartheta' & -\vartheta' \\ 0 & 1 \end{pmatrix}$$

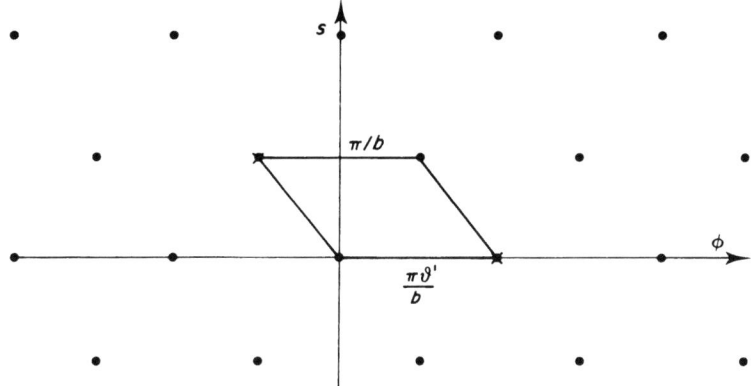

FIG. III.3 The sampling points of the interlaced parallel geometry in the $\varphi - s$ plane. The crosses indicate the columns of W ($\vartheta' = 4/5$).

is shown in Fig. III.3. It is identical to the interlaced parallel geometry with

$$q = b/\pi, \qquad p = b/\vartheta'$$

provided b/ϑ' is an even integer. The sampling conditions for the interlaced parallel geometry are therefore

$$p = \pi q/\vartheta', \qquad b \leq \pi q. \tag{3.6}$$

Note that ϑ' is an arbitrary number in $(0, 1)$ as is ϑ since for any $\vartheta' \in (0, 1)$ we can find $\vartheta \in (0, 1)$ with $\vartheta' \leq \vartheta/(2 - \vartheta)$.

We remark that the first of these conditions which we stipulated for the standard parallel geometry simply to avoid redundancy is mandatory here since it prevents the sets $K + 2\pi (W^{-1})^T l$, $l \in \mathbb{Z}^2$ from overlapping.

Now we turn to fan-beam scanning geometries. Let $r > 1$ and let $a = r \begin{pmatrix} \cos \beta \\ \sin \beta \end{pmatrix}$, $0 \leq \beta < 2\pi$ be a point (the source) on the circle with radius r around the origin. With $L(\beta, \alpha)$ we denote the straight line through a which makes an angle α with the line joining a with the origin. $L(\beta, \alpha)$, which is the dashed line in Fig. III.4, is given by $x \cdot \theta = s$, $\theta = \begin{pmatrix} \cos \varphi \\ \sin \varphi \end{pmatrix}$, where s, φ satisfy

$$\begin{aligned} s &= r \sin \alpha, \\ \varphi &= \beta + \alpha - \pi/2. \end{aligned} \tag{3.7}$$

The first relation is obvious since $s\theta$ is the orthogonal projection of a onto $\langle \theta \rangle$. For the second one it suffices to remark that the angle $\beta - \varphi$ between a and θ is $\pi/2 - \alpha$. Note that for each line L meeting Ω^2 there are precisely two representations in terms of the coordinates α, β as well as in the coordinates s, φ, but the relation (3.7) between these coordinate systems is nevertheless one-to-one.

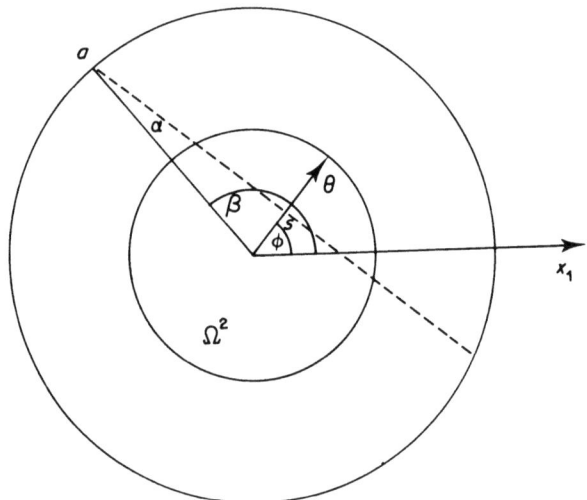

FIG. III.4 Fan-beam scanning. The reconstruction region Ω^2 is the disk with radius 1, while the sources are on the circle with radius $r > 1$ ($r = 2$ in the figure). Compare Figure I.1.

In fan-beam scanning, $D_{a_j} f$ is sampled for $2q + 1$ equally spaced directions for p sources $a_1, \ldots, a_p$ uniformly distributed over the circle of radius $r > 1$ around the origin. This amounts to sampling the function g in (3.8) below at (β_j, α_l), $j = 1, \ldots, p, l = -q, \ldots, q$ where

$$\beta_j = 2\pi(j-1)/p, \quad \alpha_l = \pi l/(2q).$$

Of course only the lines $L(\beta_j, \alpha_l)$ meeting Ω^2 need to be measured, i.e. those for which $|\alpha_l| \leq \bar{\alpha}(r) = \arcsin(1/r)$. Thus the number of data is practically

$$p \frac{\bar{\alpha}(r)}{\pi/2} 2q = 4 \frac{\bar{\alpha}(r)}{\pi} pq.$$

A special case arises for $p = 2q$. In this case, the scanning geometry is made up of the $p(p-1)/2$ lines joining the p sources, see Fig. III.5. Since this geometry arises, at least in principle, in positron emission tomography (PET), see I.2, we speak of the PET geometry. It can be rearranged to become a parallel geometry with non-uniform interlaced lateral sampling, see Fig. III.5. The directions θ_j for this parallel geometry are, for p even,

$$\theta_j = \begin{pmatrix} \cos \varphi_j \\ \sin \varphi_j \end{pmatrix}, \quad \varphi_j = \pi j/p, \quad j = 0, \ldots, p-1$$

and, for each j, the lateral sampling points s_l^j are

$$s_l^j = r \cos l\pi/p, \quad l = 0, \ldots, p, j+l \text{ even.}$$

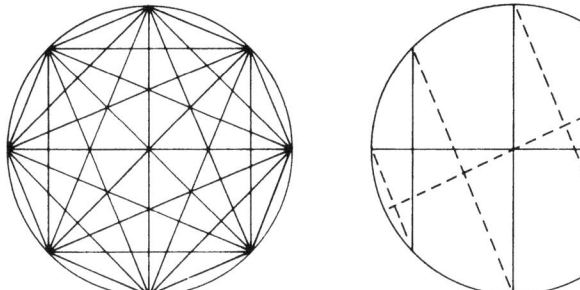

FIG. III.5 PET geometry with $p = 8$. *Left*: Measured lines. *Right*: Rearrangement into a parallel geometry. Solid line: j even. Dashed line: j odd.

Our analysis of fan-beam scanning is analogous to our treatment of the parallel case but technically more complicated.

THEOREM 3.2 Let $f \in C_0^\infty(\Omega^2)$, and let

$$g(\beta, \alpha) = \mathbf{R}f(\theta, r \sin \alpha), \quad \theta = \begin{pmatrix} \cos(\beta + \alpha - \pi/2) \\ \sin(\beta + \alpha - \pi/2) \end{pmatrix}. \quad (3.8)$$

For $0 < \vartheta < 1$ and $b \geq 1$ define the set

$$K = \{(k, 2m) : |k| < b/\vartheta, |k - 2m| < rb/\vartheta, |k| \leq \max(|k - 2m|, (1/\vartheta - 1)rb)\} \quad (3.9)$$

in $\mathbb{R}^2$, see Fig. III.6. Let W be a real non-singular 2×2 matrix such that the sets $K + 2\pi(W^{-1})^\mathsf{T} l, l \in \mathbb{Z}^2$ are mutually disjoint. Then, if $g(Wl) = 0$ for $l \in \mathbb{Z}^2$, we have

$$\|\mathbf{R}f\|_{L_\infty(Z)} \leq \eta(\vartheta, b') \|f\|_{L_1(\Omega^2)} + \frac{20r}{\pi \vartheta^2} \varepsilon_1(f, b) \quad (3.10)$$

where $b' = b \min\{1, \ln r\}$.

Proof We consider g as a function on $\mathbb{R}^2$ with period 2π in β and π in α. Its Fourier coefficients are

$$\hat{g}_{km} = (2\pi^2)^{-1} \int_0^{2\pi} \int_{-\pi/2}^{\pi/2} g(\beta, \alpha) e^{-i(k\beta + 2m\alpha)} \, d\alpha \, d\beta.$$

The $\hat{g}_{km}$ will be computed by transforming the integral to the coordinates φ, s. In

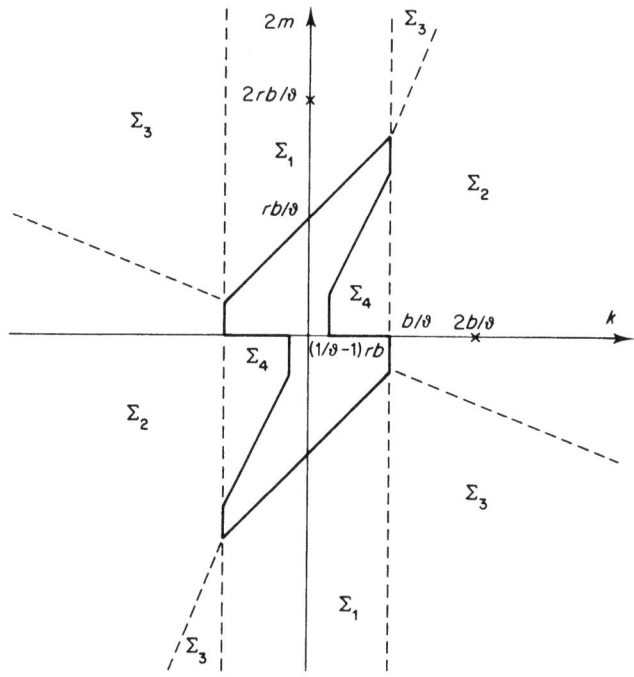

FIG. III.6 The set K of (3.9) for $r = 7/5$ and $\vartheta = 4/5$. The crosses indicate the columns of $2\pi (W^{-1})^T$ for the fan-beam geometry. Dashed lines separate the ranges of the sums in (3.16).

the inner integral we substitute $\varphi = \beta + \alpha - \pi/2$ for α. This yields with $\theta = \begin{pmatrix} \cos\varphi \\ \sin\varphi \end{pmatrix}$

$$\int_{-\pi/2}^{\pi/2} g(\beta, \alpha) e^{-2im\alpha} d\alpha = (-1)^m e^{2im\beta} \int_{\beta-\pi}^{\beta} Rf(\theta, \theta \cdot a) e^{-2im\varphi} d\varphi$$

$$= (-1)^m e^{2im\beta} \frac{1}{2} \int_0^{2\pi} Rf(\theta, \theta \cdot a) e^{-2im\varphi} d\varphi$$

where we have used that, due to the evenness of Rf, the integrand has period π. Here we use Theorem II.1.1 to obtain

$$Rf(\theta, \theta \cdot a) = (2\pi)^{-1/2} \int_{R^1} (Rf)^\wedge(\theta, \sigma) e^{i\sigma\theta \cdot a} d\sigma$$

$$= \int_{R^1} \hat{f}(\sigma \theta) e^{i\sigma\theta \cdot a} d\sigma.$$

Inserting this and interchanging integrations we get

$$\hat{g}_{km} = (2\pi^2)^{-1}(-1)^m \frac{1}{2} \int_{R^1} \hat{f}(\sigma\,\theta) \int_0^{2\pi} e^{-2im\varphi} \int_0^{2\pi} e^{i(2m-k)\beta + i\sigma\theta \cdot a}\,d\beta\,d\varphi\,d\sigma.$$

According to (VII.3.16) the inner integral is

$$\int_0^{2\pi} e^{i(2m-k)\beta + i\sigma\theta \cdot a}\,d\beta = \int_0^{2\pi} e^{i(2m-k)\beta + i\sigma r \cos(\beta-\varphi)}\,d\beta$$

$$= 2\pi(-1)^m i^k e^{(2m-k)i\varphi} J_{k-2m}(\sigma r)$$

hence

$$\hat{g}_{km} = \pi^{-1} i^k \frac{1}{2} \int_{R^1} \int_0^{2\pi} \hat{f}(\sigma\,\theta) e^{-ik\varphi}\,d\varphi\,J_{k-2m}(\sigma r)\,d\sigma.$$

The integral is broken into an integral over $|\sigma| \leq \sigma_0$ with σ_0 chosen suitably later on, and the rest whose absolute value can be estimated by $2\varepsilon_{-1}(f,\sigma_0)$. Hence

$$|\hat{g}_{km}| \leq \frac{1}{2\pi} \left| \int_{-\sigma_0}^{\sigma_0} \int_0^{2\pi} \hat{f}(\sigma\,\theta) e^{-ik\varphi}\,d\varphi\,J_{k-2m}(\sigma r)\,d\sigma \right| + \frac{1}{\pi}\varepsilon_{-1}(f,\sigma_0). \quad (3.11)$$

In the inner integral we express f by the Fourier integral, obtaining

$$\int_0^{2\pi} \hat{f}(\sigma\,\theta) e^{-ik\varphi}\,d\varphi = \frac{1}{2\pi} \int_{\Omega^2} f(x) \int_0^{2\pi} e^{-i\sigma\theta \cdot x - ik\varphi}\,d\varphi\,dx$$

$$= \frac{1}{2\pi} \int_{\Omega^2} f(x) \int_0^{2\pi} e^{-i\sigma|x|\cos(\varphi-\psi) - ik\varphi}\,d\varphi\,dx$$

where $x = |x|\begin{pmatrix} \cos\psi \\ \sin\psi \end{pmatrix}$. Again with (VII.3.16) we get

$$\int_0^{2\pi} \hat{f}(\sigma\,\theta) e^{-ik\varphi}\,d\varphi = i^k \int_{\Omega^2} f(x) e^{-ik\psi} J_k(-\sigma|x|)\,dx.$$

Inserting this in (3.11) yields

$$|\hat{g}_{km}| \leq \frac{1}{2\pi} \int_{\Omega^2} |f(x)| \left| \int_{-\sigma_0}^{\sigma_0} J_k(\sigma|x|) J_{k-2m}(\sigma r)\,d\sigma \right| dx + \frac{1}{\pi}\varepsilon_{-1}(f,\sigma_0). \quad (3.12)$$

We use (3.12) to estimate $\hat{g}_{km}$ for $(k,2m) \notin K$. For convenience we assume that $\|f\|_{L_1(\Omega^2)} = 1$. The estimates depend on a judicious choice of σ_0.

If $r|k| \geq |k-2m|$ we put $\sigma_0 = \vartheta |k|$, obtaining from (2.5)

$$|\hat{g}_{km}| \leq \frac{1}{2\pi} \eta_1(\vartheta, |k|) + \frac{1}{\pi} \varepsilon_{-1}(f, \vartheta|k|). \tag{3.13}$$

On the other hand, if $r|k| < |k-2m|$ we choose $\sigma_0 = \vartheta|k-2m|/r$ to obtain, again from (2.5),

$$|\hat{g}_{km}| \leq \frac{1}{2\pi} \int_{|\sigma| \leq \vartheta|k-2m|/r} |J_{k-2m}(\sigma r)| \, d\sigma + \frac{1}{\pi} \varepsilon_{-1}(f, \vartheta|k-2m|/r)$$

$$= \frac{1}{2\pi r} \int_{|\sigma| \leq \vartheta|k-2m|} |J_{k-2m}(\sigma)| \, d\sigma + \frac{1}{\pi} \varepsilon_{-1}(f, \vartheta|k-2m|/r)$$

$$\leq \frac{1}{2\pi r} \eta_1(\vartheta, |k-2m|) + \frac{1}{\pi} \varepsilon_{-1}(f, \vartheta|k-2m|/r). \tag{3.14}$$

If $|k-2m| \leq |k|$ we put $\sigma_0 = \infty$. From (VII.3.21, 23) we see that for $|x| \leq 1$

$$\int_{-\infty}^{+\infty} J_k(\sigma|x|) J_{k-2m}(\sigma r) \, d\sigma = 2|x|^{-1} I_{|k|,|k-2m|}(r/|x|)$$

$$\leq 2|x|^{-1} C(r/|x|) (|k|+1) (r/|x|)^{-|k|-1}$$

$$\leq 2 C(r) (|k|+1) r^{-|k|-1}$$

where we have used that $C(r)$ is decreasing, hence

$$|\hat{g}_{km}| \leq \frac{1}{\pi} C(r)(|k|+1) r^{-|k|-1} \tag{3.15}$$

for $|k-2m| \leq |k|$.

Now consider the sum

$$\sum_{(k,2m) \notin K} |\hat{g}_{km}| = \Sigma_1 + \Sigma_2 + \Sigma_3 + \Sigma_4 \tag{3.16}$$

the ranges of summation being

Σ_1: $|k| < b/\vartheta$, $\qquad |k-2m| \geq rb/\vartheta$,

Σ_2: $|k| \geq b/\vartheta$, $\qquad |k-2m| < r|k|$,

Σ_3: $|k| \geq b/\vartheta$, $\qquad |k-2m| \geq r|k|$,

Σ_4: $(1/\vartheta-1)rb \leq |k| < b/\vartheta$, $\quad |k-2m| \leq |k|$, see Fig. III.6. In Σ_1 we have $|k - 2m| > r|k|$. Hence we get from (3.14) for fixed k

$$\sum_{|k-2m|\geq rb/\vartheta} |\hat{g}_{km}| \leq \sum_{|k-2m|\geq rb/\vartheta} \left\{\frac{1}{2\pi r}\eta_1(\vartheta, |k-2m|) + \frac{1}{\pi}\varepsilon_{-1}(f, \vartheta|k-2m|/r)\right\}$$

$$\leq 2 \sum_{l \geq rb/\vartheta} \left\{\frac{1}{2\pi r}\eta_1(\vartheta, l) + \frac{1}{\pi}\varepsilon_{-1}(f, \vartheta l/r)\right\}$$

$$\leq \frac{1}{\pi r}\eta_2(\vartheta, rb/\vartheta) + \frac{2r}{\pi\vartheta}\varepsilon_0(f, b)$$

where we have used (2.7) and (2.9), the latter one with ϑ replaced by ϑ/r. Since at most $2b/\vartheta$ values of k appear in Σ_1 we get for fixed k

$$\Sigma_1 \leq \frac{2b}{\vartheta}\left\{\frac{1}{\pi r}\eta_2(\vartheta, rb/\vartheta) + \frac{2r}{\pi\vartheta}\varepsilon_0(f, b)\right\}$$

$$\leq \frac{2}{\vartheta\pi r}b\,\eta_2(\vartheta, rb/\vartheta) + \frac{4r}{\pi\vartheta^2}\varepsilon_1(f, b).$$

In Σ_2 we have $|k - 2m| < r|k|$, and the m sum contains at most $r|k|$ terms. Hence, from (3.13), (2.7)

$$\Sigma_2 \leq \sum_{|k|\geq b/\vartheta} r|k|\left\{\frac{1}{2\pi}\eta_1(\vartheta, |k|) + \frac{1}{\pi}\varepsilon_{-1}(f, \vartheta|k|)\right\}$$

$$\leq \frac{r}{\pi}\sum_{l > b/\vartheta} l\eta_1(\vartheta, l) + 2\frac{r}{\pi}\sum_{l \geq b/\vartheta}\varepsilon_0(f, \vartheta l)$$

$$\leq \frac{r}{\pi}\eta_{4,1}(\vartheta, b/\vartheta) + \frac{2r}{\pi\vartheta}\varepsilon_1(f, b).$$

In Σ_3 we have $|k - 2m| \geq r|k|$ as in Σ_1. Proceeding exactly as in Σ_1 we get for the m sum in Σ_3

$$\sum_{\substack{m \\ |k-2m|\geq r|k|}} |\hat{g}_{km}| \leq \frac{1}{\pi r}\eta_2(\vartheta, r|k|) + \frac{2}{\pi}\frac{r}{\vartheta}\varepsilon_0(f, \vartheta|k|)$$

hence

$$\Sigma_3 \leq \sum_{|k|\geq b/\vartheta}\left\{\frac{1}{\pi r}\eta_2(\vartheta, r|k|) + \frac{2r}{\pi\vartheta}\varepsilon_0(f, \vartheta|k|)\right\}$$

$$= 2\sum_{l \geq b/\vartheta}\left\{\frac{1}{\pi r}\eta_2(\vartheta, rl) + \frac{2r}{\pi\vartheta}\varepsilon_0(f, \vartheta l)\right\}$$

$$\leq \frac{2}{\pi r}\eta_3(\vartheta, rb/\vartheta) + \frac{4r}{\pi\vartheta^2}\varepsilon_1(f, b),$$

see (2.7), (2.9). Finally, in Σ_4, we have at most $|k| + 1$ terms in the m sum, and all of these terms can be estimated by (3.15). Hence, with $a = (1/\vartheta - 1)rb$

$$\Sigma_4 \leq \frac{1}{\pi} C(r) \sum_{(1/\vartheta - 1)rb \leq |k| \leq b/\vartheta} (|k| + 1)^2 r^{-|k|-1}$$

$$\leq \frac{2}{\pi} C(r) \sum_{l > a} l^2 e^{-l \ln r}$$

$$\leq \frac{2}{\pi} C(r) \frac{1}{\ln r - 2/a} a^2 e^{-a \ln r}$$

by (2.6). It follows that

$$\Sigma_4 \leq \eta(\vartheta, b \ln r)$$

where η satisfies (2.4).

Combining the estimates for $\Sigma_1, \ldots, \Sigma_4$ we get from (3.16)

$$\sum_{(k, 2m) \notin K} |\hat{g}_{km}| \leq \eta(\vartheta, b') + \frac{10r}{\pi \vartheta^2} \varepsilon_1(f, b).$$

Now we can apply Theorem 1.5 in the form of (1.12) to g, K and W, obtaining

$$\|g\|_{L_\infty(\mathbb{R}^2)} \leq \eta(\vartheta, b') + \frac{20r}{\pi \vartheta^2} \varepsilon_1(f, b)$$

and this is (3.10). □

Theorem 3.2 admits an interpretation analogous to Theorem 3.1. For the fan-beam geometry we have

$$W = \pi \begin{pmatrix} 2/p & 0 \\ 0 & 1/(2q) \end{pmatrix}, \quad 2\pi(W^{-1})^\mathrm{T} = \begin{pmatrix} p & 0 \\ 0 & 4q \end{pmatrix}.$$

From Fig. III.6 we see that the sets $K + 2(W^{-1})^\mathrm{T} l$, $l \in \mathbb{Z}^2$ are mutually disjoint if

$$p \geq 2b/\vartheta, \quad q \geq \frac{r}{2} b/\vartheta. \tag{3.17}$$

These are the sampling conditions for the fan-beam geometry. For the minimal values of p, q we have $p = (4/r)q$.

For r close to 1, a denser non-overlapping covering of the plane is possible. We enlarge K by including the four tips which have been cut off by the horizontal lines $k = \pm b/\vartheta$. The resulting set K' is shown in Fig. III.7. The translates of K' by the grid generated by

$$2\pi(W^{-1})^\mathrm{T} = r \frac{b}{\vartheta'} \begin{pmatrix} 1 & 0 \\ 0 & 2 \end{pmatrix}, \quad \vartheta' \leq \frac{\vartheta}{2 - \vartheta}$$

are mutually disjoint. The matrix

$$W = \frac{\pi \vartheta'}{rb} \begin{pmatrix} 2 & 0 \\ 0 & 1 \end{pmatrix}$$

defines a grid in the α–β plane which is identical to the PET geometry if $p = rb/\vartheta'$.

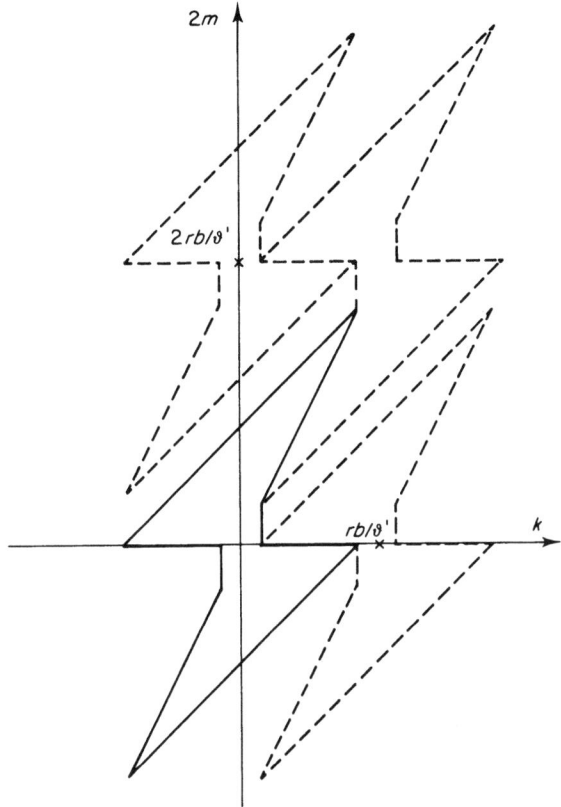

FIG. III.7 The set K' (enclosing K of (3.9)) for the PET geometry. The crosses indicate the columns of $2\pi (W^{-1})^T$. Some of the translates of K' are also drawn (dashed). r and ϑ are chosen as in Fig. III.6.

Therefore the sampling condition for the PET geometry is

$$p \geq rb/\vartheta' \tag{3.18}$$

with some $\vartheta' < 1$.

We conclude this section by a survey on the scanning geometries discussed. Table III.1 contains the sampling conditions, an optimality relation which holds if angular and lateral sampling rates are both minimal for a certain bandwidth, and the number of sampled line integrals for the optimal choice p, q. For simplicity we have replaced the numbers ϑ, ϑ' by 1.

We see that the interlaced parallel geometry needs less data than the others. Therefore its relative inefficiency is normalized to 1. Second best is the PET geometry (provided r is close to 1). We find it very satisfactory that a natural sampling scheme such as PET is also an efficient one and even the most efficient one among the fan-beam schemes. Third best is the standard parallel geometry,

TABLE III.1 Scanning geometries. The sampling conditions refer to the reconstruction of an essentially b-band-limited function with support in Ω^2.

Scanning geometry	Sampling condition	Optimal relation	Number of data	Relative inefficiency	Formula
Standard parallel	$p > b, q > b/\pi$	$p = \pi q$	$\dfrac{2}{\pi}b^2$	2	(3.5)
Interlaced parallel	$p > b, q > b/\pi$	$p = \pi q$	$\dfrac{1}{\pi}b^2$	1	(3.6)
Fan-beam	$p > 2b,$ $q > br/2$	$p = 4q/r$	$\dfrac{4r\bar{\alpha}(r)}{\pi}b^2$	$4r\bar{\alpha}(r),$ $\bar{\alpha}(r) = \arcsin(1/r)$	(3.17)
PET (r close to 1)	$p > b$	—	$\dfrac{1}{2}b^2$	$\dfrac{\pi}{2}$	(3.18)

while the fan-beam geometry has relative inefficiency between $4(r$ large) and $2\pi(r$ close to 1).

III.4 Bibliographical Notes

The material in Section III.2 is based on Louis (1981a, 1982, 1984a, 1984b). Theorem 2.1 is taken from Louis (1984b), while the proof of Theorem 2.3 is patterned after Louis (1984a). The 3-dimensional examples are taken from Louis (1982). For $n = 2$ a much more elaborate version of Theorem 2.3, with an analysis of the transition region $|\xi| \sim m$, has been obtained by Logan (1975).

The basic approach of Section III.3 goes back to Lindgren and Rattey (1981). They found that what we call the interlaced parallel geometry has the same resolution as the standard parallel geometry, with only one-half of the data. The interlaced parallel geometry has originally been suggested by Cormack (1978) based on a very nice geometrical argument. In the same way Cormack (1980) found that the PET geometry is optimal among the fan-beam geometries. The conditions (3.5) have been given by Bracewell and Riddle (1967) and by many others who have not been aware of that work. A heuristic derivation of the relation $p = \pi q$ has been given by Crowther et al. (1970), see V.2. The sampling conditions (3.17) for fan-beam scanning appear to be new. Joseph and Schulz (1980) gave the non-optimal condition $p > 2b/(1 - \sin \bar{\alpha}(r))$, while Rattey and Lindgren (1981), based on an approximation of the fan-beam geometry by a parallel one, obtained the approximate condition $p > b$ for $1 < r < 3$ and $p > 2b/(1 + 3/r)$ for $r > 3$. A treatment of the PET geometry as an interlaced parallel scheme reveals that it is the fan-beam analog of the interlaced parallel scheme. This may serve as an explanation for its favourable efficiency.

Of course, one can derive from Theorem 3.2 other fan-beam geometries simply by finding grids which lead to non-overlapping coverings of the plane by the translates of K. We have not found scanning geometries in this way which promise to be superior to the existing ones.

IV
Ill-posedness and Accuracy

All problems in CT are ill-posed, even if to a very different degree. Therefore, any serious mathematical treatment of CT requires some fundamental notions from the theory of ill-posed problems. We give in Section IV.1 a short introduction into this field. In Section IV.2 we study the accuracy we can expect for CT problems, given the accuracy of the data and the number of projections. In Section IV.3 we derive the singular value decomposition of the Radon transform. The subject of ill-posedness is taken up again in Chapter VI on incomplete data problems.

IV.1 Ill-Posed Problems

We discuss ill-posed problems only in the framework of linear problems in Hilbert spaces. Let H, K be Hilbert spaces and let A be a linear bounded operator from H into K. The problem

$$\text{given } g \in K, \text{ find } f \in H \text{ such that } Af = g \tag{1.1}$$

is called well-posed by Hadamard (1932) if it is uniquely solvable for each $g \in K$ and if the solution depends continuously on g. Otherwise, (1.1) is called ill-posed. This means that for an ill-posed problem the operator A^{-1} either does not exist, or is not defined on all of K, or is not continuous. The practical difficulty with an ill-posed problem is that even if it is solvable, the solution of $Af = g$ need not be close to the solution of $Af = g^\varepsilon$ if g^ε is close to g.

In the sequel we shall remove step by step the deficiencies of an ill-posed problem. First we define a substitute for the solution if there is none. We simply take a minimizer of $\|Af - g\|$ as such a substitute. This makes sense if $g \in \text{range}(A) + (\text{range}(A))^\perp$. Then we dispose of a possible non-uniqueness by choosing among all those minimizers that one which has minimal norm. This well defined element of K is called the (Moore–Penrose) generalized solution of (1.1) and is denoted by $A^+ g$. The linear operator $A^+ : K \to H$ with domain $\text{range}(A) + (\text{range}(A))^\perp$ is called the (Moore–Penrose) generalized inverse.

THEOREM 1.1 $f = A^+ g$ is the unique solution of

$$A^* A f = A^* g$$

in $\overline{\text{range}(A^*)}$.

Proof f minimizes $\|Af - g\|$ if and only if
$$(Af - g, Au) = 0$$
for all $u \in H$, i.e. if and only if $A^* A f = A^* g$. Among all solutions of this equation the unique element with least norm is the one in $(\ker(A))^\perp = \overline{\text{range}(A^*)}$. □

We remark that the system $A^* A f = A^* g$ is usually called the system of normal equations.

In general, A^+ is not a continuous operator. To restore continuity we introduce the notion of a regularization of A^+. This is a family $(T_\gamma)_{\gamma > 0}$ of linear continuous operators $T_\gamma \colon K \to H$ which are defined on all of K and for which
$$\lim_{\gamma \to 0} T_\gamma g = A^+ g$$
on the domain of A^+. Obviously, $\|T_\gamma\| \to \infty$ as $\gamma \to 0$ if A^+ is not bounded. With the help of a regularization we can solve (1.1) approximately in the following sense. Let $g^\varepsilon \in K$ be an approximation to g such that $\|g^\varepsilon - g\| \leq \varepsilon$. Let $\gamma(\varepsilon)$ be such that, as $\varepsilon \to 0$,

  (i) $\gamma(\varepsilon) \to 0$ (ii) $\|T_{\gamma(\varepsilon)}\| \varepsilon \to 0$.

Then, as $\varepsilon \to 0$
$$\|T_{\gamma(\varepsilon)} g^\varepsilon - A^+ g\| \leq \|T_{\gamma(\varepsilon)}(g^\varepsilon - g)\| + \|T_{\gamma(\varepsilon)} g - A^+ g\|$$
$$\leq \|T_{\gamma(\varepsilon)}\| \varepsilon + \|T_{\gamma(\varepsilon)} g - A^+ g\|$$
$$\to 0.$$

Hence, $T_{\gamma(\varepsilon)} g^\varepsilon$ is close to $A^+ g$ if g^ε is close to g.

The number γ is called a regularization parameter. Determining a good regularization parameter is one of the crucial points in the application of regularization methods. We do not discuss this matter. We rather assume that we can find a good regularization parameter by trial and error.

There are several methods for constructing a regularization.

(1) *The Truncated Singular Value Decomposition* By a singular value decomposition we mean a representation of A in the form
$$Af = \sum_{k=1}^\infty \sigma_k (f, f_k) g_k \qquad (1.2)$$
where (f_k), (g_k) are normalized orthogonal systems in H, K respectively and σ_k are positive numbers, the singular values of A. We always assume the sequence $\{\sigma_k\}$ to be bounded. Then, A is a linear continuous operator from H into K with adjoint
$$A^* g = \sum_{k=1}^\infty \sigma_k (g, g_k) f_k,$$

and the operators

$$A^* A f = \sum_{k=1}^{\infty} \sigma_k^2 (f, f_k) f_k,$$

$$A A^* g = \sum_{k=1}^{\infty} \sigma_k^2 (g, g_k) g_k$$

are self-adjoint operators in H, K respectively. The spectrum of $A^* A$ consists of the eigenvalues σ_k^2 with eigenelements f_k and possibly of the eigenvalue 0 whose multiplicity may be infinite. The same is true for AA^* with eigenelements g_k. The two eigensystems are related by

$$A^* g_k = \sigma_k f_k, \quad A f_k = \sigma_k g_k. \qquad (1.3)$$

Vice versa, if (f_k), (g_k) are normalized eigensystems of $A^* A$, $A A^*$ respectively such that (1.3) holds, then A has the singular value decomposition (1.2). In particular, compact operators always admit a singular value decomposition.

THEOREM 1.2 If A has the singular value decomposition (1.2), then

$$A^+ g = \sum_{k=1}^{\infty} \sigma_k^{-1} (g, g_k) f_k.$$

Proof First we show that the series converges if g is in the domain of A^+, i.e. if $g \in \text{range}(A) + (\text{range}(A))^\perp$. For $g = Av + u$ with $u \in (\text{range}(A))^\perp$ we have

$$(g, g_k) = (Av + u, g_k) = (Av, g_k) + (u, g_k)$$
$$= (v, A^* g_k) + (u, g_k).$$

By (1.3), $g_k \in \text{range}(A)$ and $A^* g_k = \sigma_k f_k$. Hence

$$(g, g_k) = \sigma_k (v, f_k)$$

and it follows that

$$f^+ = \sum_{k=1}^{\infty} \sigma_k^{-1} (g, g_k) f_k = \sum_{k=1}^{\infty} (v, f_k) f_k$$

converges. Applying $A^* A$ term by term we obtain

$$A^* A f^+ = \sum_{k=1}^{\infty} \sigma_k^{-1} (g, g_k) A^* A f_k$$

$$= \sum_{k=1}^{\infty} \sigma_k (g, g_k) f_k$$

$$= A^* g.$$

Since, by (1.3), $f^+ \in \overline{\text{range}(A^*)}$ it follows from Theorem 1.1 that in fact $f^+ = A^+ g$. □

We see from Theorem 1.2 that A^+ is unbounded if and only if $\sigma_k \to 0$ as $k \to \infty$.

In that case we can construct a regularization of A^+ by the truncated singular value decomposition

$$T_\gamma g = \sum_{k \leq 1/\gamma} \sigma_k^{-1} (g, g_k) f_k. \tag{1.4}$$

It follows from Theorem 1.2 that $T_\gamma g \to A^+ g$ as $\gamma \to 0$, and T_γ is bounded with

$$\|T_\gamma\| \leq \sup_{k \leq 1/\gamma} \sigma_k^{-1}.$$

More generally we can put

$$T_\gamma g = \sum_{k=1}^\infty F_\gamma(\sigma_k) (g, g_k) f_k \tag{1.5}$$

where $F_\gamma(\sigma)$ approximates σ^{-1} for σ large and tends to zero as $\sigma \to 0$. F_γ is called a filter and regularization methods based on (1.5) are referred to as digital filtering.

The singular value decomposition gives much insight into the character of the ill-posedness. Let g^ε be an approximation to g such that $\|g - g^\varepsilon\| \leq \varepsilon$. Knowing only g^ε, all we can say about the expansion coefficients for $A^+ g$ in Theorem 1.2 is

$$|\sigma_k^{-1} (g, g_k) - \sigma_k^{-1} (g^\varepsilon, g_k)| \leq \varepsilon/\sigma_k.$$

We see that for σ_k small, the contribution of g_k to $A^+ g$ cannot be computed reliably. Thus looking at the singular values and the corresponding elements g_k shows which features of the solution f of (1.1) can be determined from an approximation g^ε to g and which ones can not.

(2) *The Method of Tikhonov–Phillips* Here we put

$$T_\gamma = (A^* A + \gamma I)^{-1} A^* = A^* (AA^* + \gamma I)^{-1} \tag{1.6}$$

Equivalently, $f_\gamma = T_\gamma g$ can be defined to be the minimizer of

$$\|Af - g\|^2 + \gamma \|f\|^2.$$

We show that $f_\gamma = T_\gamma g \to f^+ = A^+ g$ as $\gamma \to 0$. From Theorem 1.1 we have

$$A^* A f^+ = A^* g, \quad f^+ \perp \ker(A).$$

It follows that

$$(A^* A + \gamma I)(f^+ - f_\gamma) = \gamma f^+. \tag{1.7}$$

Let (E_λ) be the resolution of the identity associated with the self-adjoint operator $A^* A$, see Yosida (1968), ch. XI. 5:

$$A^* A = \int \lambda \, dE_\lambda$$

$$(A^* A + \gamma I)^{-1} = \int (\lambda + \gamma)^{-1} \, dE_\lambda.$$

Note that $E_\lambda = 0$ for $\lambda < 0$. Using this integral representation in (1.7) we obtain

$$f^+ - f_\gamma = \int \frac{\gamma}{\lambda + \gamma} \, dE_\lambda f^+.$$

Hence,

$$\|f^+ - f_\gamma\|^2 = \int \left(\frac{\gamma}{\lambda+\gamma}\right)^2 d\|E_\lambda f^+\|^2$$

$$= \int_{-\infty}^{\sqrt{\gamma}} \left(\frac{\gamma}{\lambda+\gamma}\right)^2 d\|E_\lambda f^+\|^2 + \int_{\sqrt{\gamma}}^{\infty} \left(\frac{\gamma}{\lambda+\gamma}\right)^2 d\|E_\lambda f^+\|^2$$

$$\leq \int_{-\infty}^{\sqrt{\gamma}} d\|E_\lambda f^+\|^2 + \gamma \int_{\sqrt{\gamma}}^{\infty} d\|E_\lambda f^+\|^2$$

$$= \|E_{\sqrt{\gamma}} f^+\|^2 + \gamma (\|f^+\|^2 - \|E_{\sqrt{\gamma}} f^+\|^2). \tag{1.8}$$

With P the orthogonal projection on $\ker(A^*A) = \ker(A)$ we have

$$\lim_{\gamma \to 0} \|E_{\sqrt{\gamma}} f^+\|^2 = \|Pf^+\|^2$$
$$= 0$$

since $f^+ \perp \ker(A)$. Now it follows from (1.8) that in fact $f_\gamma \to f^+$ as $\gamma \to 0$.

If A has the singular value decomposition (1.2) it is readily seen that f_γ has the form (1.5) with

$$F_\gamma(\sigma) = \frac{1}{1+\gamma/\sigma^2} \frac{1}{\sigma}.$$

Thus the method of Tikhonov–Phillips is a special case of digital filtering.

(3) *Iterative Methods* Suppose we have an iterative method for the solution of $Af = g$ which has the form

$$f^{k+1} = B_k f^k + C_k g, \quad k = 0, 1, \ldots \tag{1.9}$$

with linear continuous operators B_k, C_k. Assume that f^k converges to $A^+ g$. For each $\gamma > 0$ let $k(\gamma)$ be an index such that $k(\gamma) \to \infty$ as $\gamma \to 0$. Then,

$$T_\gamma f = f^{k(\gamma)}$$

is obviously a regularization of A^+. Here, the determination of a good regularization parameter γ amounts to stopping the iteration after a suitable number of steps. In general, an iteration method (1.9) which converges for g in the domain of A^+ does not converge for all g. It rather exhibits a semi-convergence phenomenon: even if it provides a satisfactory solution after a certain number of steps, it deteriorates if the iteration goes on.

By means of regularization methods we can solve an ill-posed problem approximately. In order to find out what accuracy we can get we have to make specific assumptions on A as well as on the exact solution f. In the context of CT, the following setting will be useful: we take $H = L_2(\Omega^n)$, Ω^n the unit sphere in $\mathbb{R}^n$, and we make two assumptions:

(i) There is a number $\alpha > 0$ such that, with positive constants m, M,

$$m\|f\|_{H_0^{-\alpha}(\Omega^n)} \leq \|Af\|_K \leq M\|f\|_{H_0^{-\alpha}(\Omega^n)}. \tag{1.10}$$

(ii) The exact solution f is in $H_0^\beta(\Omega^n)$ for some $\beta > 0$, and

$$\|f\|_{H_0^\beta(\Omega^n)} \leq \rho. \tag{1.11}$$

From (1.10) it follows that A^{-1} exists but is unbounded as an operator from K into $L_2(\Omega^n)$. This means that the equation $Af = g$ is ill-posed in the $L_2(\Omega^n) - K$ setting, the degree of the ill-posedness being measured by the number α. Equation (1.11) is a smoothness requirement on the exact solution and represents a typical example of *a priori* information in the theory of ill-posed problems. In Theorem 2.2 we shall use (1.11) to restrict the variation of f so as to avoid the indeterminacy result of Theorem II.3.7.

Now assume that instead of g only an approximation g^ε with $\|g - g^\varepsilon\| \leq \varepsilon$ is available. Then, our information on the exact solution can be summarized in the inequalities

$$\|Af - g^\varepsilon\|_K \leq \varepsilon, \qquad \|f\|_{H_0^\beta(\Omega^n)} \leq \rho. \tag{1.12}$$

If f_1, f_2 are elements satisfying (1.12) it follows that

$$\|A(f_1 - f_2)\|_K \leq 2\varepsilon, \qquad \|f_1 - f_2\|_{H_0^\beta(\Omega^n)} \leq 2\rho.$$

With

$$d(\varepsilon, \rho) = \sup\{\|f\|_{L_2(\Omega^n)}: \|Af\|_K \leq \varepsilon, \|f\|_{H_0^\beta(\Omega^n)} \leq \rho\} \tag{1.13}$$

we obtain

$$\|f_1 - f_2\|_{L_2(\Omega^n)} \leq d(2\varepsilon, 2\rho). \tag{1.14}$$

Therefore $d(2\varepsilon, 2\rho)$ can be considered as the worst case error in the reconstruction of f from the erroneous data g^ε, given that (1.10), (1.11) holds. The asymptotic behaviour of $d(\varepsilon, \rho)$ as $\varepsilon \to 0$ is clarified in the following theorem.

THEOREM 1.3 *If (1.10) holds, then there is a constant $c(m, \alpha, \beta)$ such that*

$$d(\varepsilon, \rho) \leq c(m, \alpha, \beta) \varepsilon^{\beta/(\alpha+\beta)} \rho^{\alpha/(\alpha+\beta)}.$$

Proof From (VII.4.9) with $\gamma = 0$ and α replaced by $-\alpha$ we get

$$\|f\|_{L_2(\Omega^n)} \leq \|f\|_{H_0^{-\alpha}(\Omega^n)}^{\beta/(\beta+\alpha)} \|f\|_{H_0^\beta(\Omega^n)}^{\alpha/(\beta+\alpha)}.$$

If $\|Af\| \leq \varepsilon$, then

$$\|f\|_{H_0^{-\alpha}(\Omega^n)} \leq \varepsilon/m$$

from (1.10). Hence, if $\|Af\| \leq \varepsilon$ and $\|f\|_{H_0^\beta(\Omega^n)} \leq \rho$, then

$$\|f\|_{L_2(\Omega)} \leq (\varepsilon/m)^{\beta/(\alpha+\beta)} \rho^{\alpha/(\alpha+\beta)}$$

and the theorem follows. □

We observe that the right-hand side of (1.10) is irrelevant for Theorem 1.3 to hold. However, it makes sure that the estimate of Theorem 1.3 is best possible as far the exponents of ε, ρ are concerned.

We interpret Theorem 1.3 as follows. If the data error of an ill-posed problem satisfying (1.10), (1.11) is ε, then the true solution can be recovered with an accuracy $0(\varepsilon^{\beta/(\alpha+\beta)})$. Since $\beta/(\alpha+\beta) < 1$ we always have a loss in accuracy. We call the problem

Severely ill-posed   if $\beta/(\alpha+\beta)$ is closed to 0.
       In that case the loss of accuracy is catastrophic. Typically, $\alpha = \infty$, i.e. the estimate (1.10) does not hold for any finite α,

Mildly ill-posed   if $\beta/(\alpha+\beta)$ is close to 1. In that case we have only little loss in accuracy,

Modestly ill-posed   if $\beta/(\alpha+\beta)$ is neither close to zero nor close to 1.

We shall see that this classification of ill-posed problems provides a simple means for judging problems in CT. Note that the degree of ill-posedness not only depends on the properties of the operator A as expressed by (1.10) but also on the smoothness of the true solution.

A completely different approach to ill-posed problems comes from statistics. Here we think of f, g as families of random variables which are jointly normally distributed with mean values $\bar{f}, \bar{g}$ and covariances F, G, respectively, i.e.

$$F(x, x') = E(f(x) - \bar{f}(x))(f(x') - \bar{f}(x'))$$

with E the mathematical expectation, and correspondingly for G. Assume that there is linear relation

$$g = Af + n \qquad (1.15)$$

between f and g where A is a linear operator and n is a family of random variables which is normally distributed with mean value 0 and covariance Σ. We assume f and n to be independent. n represents measurement errors. Then, (f, g) has the mean value $(\bar{f}, \bar{g})$ and the covariance

$$\begin{pmatrix} F & FA^* \\ AF & AFA^* + \Sigma \end{pmatrix}.$$

As solution f_B of (1.10) we take the conditional expectation of f having observed g. In analogy to the case of finitely many variables, see Anderson (1958), we have

$$f_B = E(f|g) = \bar{f} + FA^*(AFA^* + \Sigma)^{-1}(g - A\bar{f}). \qquad (1.16)$$

f_B is known as the best linear mean square estimate for f, see Papoulis (1965), Ch. 11. Note that for $\bar{f} = 0$, $F = I$ and $\Sigma = \gamma I$, (1.16) is formally the same as the method of Tikhonov–Phillips (1.6). The choice of $\Sigma = \gamma I$ corresponds to 'white noise' and is an appropriate assumption for measurement errors. The choice of F reflects the properties of f. For f an image density a model frequently used in digital image processing is the isotropic exponential model

$$F(x,x') = \sigma e^{-\lambda|x-x'|} \qquad (1.17)$$

with constants σ, $\lambda > 0$, see Pratt (1978). This model assumes that the interrelation between the grey levels of the picture at the points x, x', as measured by the covariance between the density distributions $f(x), f(x')$, depends only on the distance between x, x' and decays exponentially as this distance increases. In the next section we shall see that (1.17) translates into a smoothness assumption for a deterministic description of pictures.

IV.2   Error Estimates

The purpose of this section is to apply Theorem 1.3 to **R** and to **P**. In view of Theorem II.5.1 these transforms satisfy (1.10) with $\alpha = (n-1)/2$, $\alpha = 1/2$, respectively. It only remains to find out what Sobolev spaces we have to take for the picture densities f we want to reconstruct.

In view of the applications we want to reconstruct at least pictures which are smooth except for jumps across smooth $(n-1)$-dimensional manifolds. A typical picture of this kind is given by the characteristic function f of Ω^n. As in (VII.1.3) we obtain

$$\hat{f}(\xi) = |\xi|^{-n/2} J_{n/2}(|\xi|)$$

with $J_{n/2}$ the Bessel function, see VII.3. Hence

$$\|f\|_{H^\beta}^2 = \int_{\mathbf{R}^n} (1+|\xi|^2)^\beta |\xi|^{-n} J_{n/2}^2(|\xi|) \, d\xi$$

$$= |S^{n-1}| \int_0^\infty (1+\sigma^2)^\beta \sigma^{-1} J_{n/2}^2(\sigma) \, d\sigma.$$

Because of (VII.3.24) this is finite if and only if $\beta < 1/2$. Hence $f \in H^\beta$ if and only if $\beta < 1/2$. We conclude that for the densities of simple pictures such as described above Sobolev spaces of order less than $1/2$ are appropriate.

On a more scientific level we come to the same conclusion. Adopting the isotropic exponential model (1.17) we think of a picture as a family $(f(x))_{x \in \mathbf{R}^2}$ of random variables such that, with $\bar{f} = Ef$,

$$E(f(x) - \bar{f}(x))(f(x') - \bar{f}(x')) = \sigma(x)\sigma(x') e^{-\lambda|x-x'|} \qquad (2.1)$$

where we have added the C_0^∞ function σ to express that the picture is of finite extent. We want to compute $E|(f-\bar{f})^{\wedge}|^2$ for a real function f. We have

$$|(f-\bar{f})^{\wedge}(\xi)|^2 = (2\pi)^{-n} \int_{\mathbf{R}^n} \int_{\mathbf{R}^n} e^{-i(x-x')\cdot\xi} (f-\bar{f})(x)(f-\bar{f})(x') \, dx \, dx'.$$

Applying E we get from (2.1)

$$E|(f-\bar{f})\hat{\,}(\xi)|^2 = (2\pi)^{-n} \int_{R^n} \int_{R^n} e^{-i(x-x')\cdot\xi} \sigma(x)\sigma(x') e^{-\lambda|x-x'|} dx\, dx'$$

With $k(x) = e^{-\lambda|x|}$ we obtain with rules R2 and R4 of VII.1 after some algebra

$$E|(f-\bar{f})\hat{\,}|^2 = (2\pi)^{-n/2} \hat{k} * |\hat{\sigma}|^2. \qquad (2.2)$$

For $\hat{k}$ we obtain

$$\hat{k}(\xi) = (2\pi)^{-n/2} \int_{R^n} e^{-ix\cdot\xi - \lambda|x|} dx$$

$$= (2\pi)^{-n/2} \int_0^\infty r^{n-1} e^{-\lambda r} \int_{S^{n-1}} e^{-ir\rho\theta\cdot\omega} d\theta\, dr$$

where we have put $x = r\theta$, $\xi = \rho\cdot\omega$. The integral over S^{n-1} is the case $l = 0$ of (VII.3.19):

$$\int_{S^{n-1}} e^{-ir\rho\theta\cdot\omega} d\omega = (2\pi)^{n/2} (r\rho)^{(2-n)/2} J_{(n-2)/2}(r\rho).$$

This leads to

$$\hat{k}(\rho\omega) = \rho^{(2-n)/2} \int_0^\infty r^{n/2} e^{-\lambda r} J_{n/2-1}(r\rho)\, dr.$$

The latter integral is the case $v = n/2 - 1$ of (VII.3.26). We finally obtain

$$\hat{k}(\rho\omega) = c_1(n)\lambda(\lambda^2 + \rho^2)^{-(n+1)/2} \qquad (2.3)$$

with some constant $c_1(n)$. From (2.2) we obtain

$$E\|f-\bar{f}\|_{H^\beta}^2 = E\int_{R^n} (1+|\xi|^2)^\beta |(f-\bar{f})\hat{\,}(\xi)|^2\, d\xi$$

$$= \int_{R^n} (1+|\xi|^2)^\beta E|(f-\bar{f})\hat{\,}(\xi)|^2\, d\xi$$

$$= (2\pi)^{-n/2} \int_{R^n} (1+|\xi|^2)^\beta (\hat{k} * |\hat{\sigma}|^2)(\xi)\, d\xi$$

$$= (2\pi)^{-n/2} \int_{R^n} |\hat{\sigma}(\eta)|^2 \int_{R^n} (1+|\xi|^2)^\beta \hat{k}(\xi-\eta)\, d\xi\, d\eta.$$

In view of (2.3) this is finite if and only if $\beta < 1/2$.

These observations suggest one thinks of picture densities as functions in the Sobolev space $H_0^\beta(\Omega^n)$ with β close to $1/2$. Since we are working with C^∞ functions only we assume a picture density to be a function $f \in C_0^\infty(\Omega^n)$ such that

$$\|f\|_{H_0^\beta(\Omega^n)} \le \rho \tag{2.4}$$

with β close to $1/2$ and ρ not too large.

Now let

$$d^R(\varepsilon, \rho) = \sup\left\{\|f\|_{L_2(\Omega^n)} : \|\mathbf{R}f\|_{L_2(Z)} \le \varepsilon, \|f\|_{H_0^\beta(\Omega^n)} \le \rho\right\}$$

$$d^P(\varepsilon, \rho) = \sup\left\{\|f\|_{L_2(\Omega^n)} : \|\mathbf{P}f\|_{L_2(T)} \le \varepsilon, \|f\|_{H_0^\beta(\Omega^n)} \le \rho\right\}.$$

Remember that $d^R(2\varepsilon, 2\rho)$, $d^P(2\varepsilon, 2\rho)$ can be considered as worst case errors for our reconstruction problems with data error ε and *a priori* information (2.4).

THEOREM 2.1 There is a constant $c(\beta, n)$ such that

$$d^R(\varepsilon, \rho) \le c(\beta, n) \varepsilon^{2\beta/(n-1+2\beta)} \rho^{(n-1)/(n-1+2\beta)},$$

$$d^P(\varepsilon, \rho) \le c(\beta, n) \varepsilon^{2\beta/(1+2\beta)} \rho^{1/(1+2\beta)}.$$

Proof Since **R**, **P** satisfy (1.10) with $\alpha = (n-1)/2$, $\alpha = 1/2$, respectively it suffices to apply Theorem 1.3 for these values of α. □

Of course the estimates for **R**, **P** are the same for $n = 2$. We are interested in values for β close to $1/2$. Putting $\beta = 1/2$ for simplicity we obtain

$$d^R(\varepsilon, \rho) \le c(n) \varepsilon^{1/n} \rho^{1-1/n}, \tag{2.5}$$

$$d^P(\varepsilon, \rho) \le c(n) \varepsilon^{1/2} \rho^{1/2}. \tag{2.6}$$

In the terminology of Section IV.1, both reconstruction problems are modestly ill-posed (for dimensions 2, 3). Note that the degree of ill-posedness is dimension dependent for **R** but not for **P**. While a data error of size ε leads to an error in the reconstruction from line integrals of order $\varepsilon^{1/2}$, the error in the reconstruction from plane integrals is of order $\varepsilon^{1/3}$.

Besides inaccurate measurements a further source of errors is discrete sampling. Let us assume that $\mathbf{R}f$ is known only for a finite number of directions $\theta_1, \ldots, \theta_p$ and real numbers $s_1, \ldots, s_q$. We assume that the (θ_j, s_l) cover $S^{n-1} \times [-1, +1]$ uniformly in the sense that

$$\sup_{-1 \le s \le 1} \inf_{l=1}^{q} |s_l - s| \le h$$

$$\sup_{\theta \in S^{n-1}} \inf_{j=1}^{p} |\theta_j - \theta| \le h/\pi \tag{2.7}$$

where the factor of π has been introduced in order to be in agreement with

(V.2.14). In analogy with the definition of $d^R(\varepsilon, \rho)$ we put

$$d^R(h, \rho) = \sup\left\{\|f\|_{L_2(\Omega^r)}: Rf(\theta_j, s_l) = 0,\right.$$
$$\left. j = 1, \ldots, p, l = 1, \ldots, q, \|f\|_{H_0^\beta(\Omega^r)} \leq \rho\right\}.$$

Then, $d^R(h, 2\rho)$ can be considered as worst case error for the reconstruction of f from Rf given at the points θ_j, s_l satisfying (2.7) under the *a priori* information (2.4).

THEOREM 2.2 Let $\beta > 1/2$. Then there is a constant $c(\beta, n)$ such that

$$d^R(h, \rho) \leq c(\beta, n) h^\beta \rho.$$

Proof Let $\|f\|_{H^\beta(\Omega^r)} \leq \rho$ and let $g = Rf$ vanish on (θ_j, s_l), $j = 1, \ldots, p$, $l = 1, \ldots, q$. According to Theorem II.5.3 we have

$$\|g\|_{\bar{H}^{\beta + (n-1)/2}(Z)} \leq c_1(\beta, n) \rho$$

with some constant $c_1(\beta, n)$. We now apply Lemma VII.4.8 to $\Omega = S^{n-1} \times (-1, +1)$ and $\Omega_h = \{(\theta_j, s_l): j = 1, \ldots, p, l = 1, \ldots, q\}$. This is possible by means of local coordinates, identifying the Sobolev spaces $\bar{H}^{\beta + (n-1)/2}(Z)$ and $H^{\beta + (n-1)/2}(\Omega)$. Since $\beta + (n-1)/2 > n/2$ we obtain

$$\|g\|_{L_2(Z)} \leq c_2(\beta, n) h^{\beta + (n-1)/2} \rho$$

with some constant $c_2(\beta, n)$. Now we have

$$\|Rf\|_{L_2(Z)} \leq \varepsilon = c_2(\beta, n) h^{\beta + (n-1)/2} \rho, \qquad \|f\|_{H_0^\beta(\Omega^r)} \leq \rho.$$

Applying Theorem 2.1 we obtain

$$\|f\|_{L_2(\Omega^r)} \leq c(\beta, n) \varepsilon^{2\beta/(n-1+2\beta)} \rho^{(n-1)/(n-1+2\beta)}$$
$$\leq c_3(\beta, n) h^\beta \rho,$$

hence the theorem. □

It is interesting to compare Theorem 2.2 with Theorem II.3.7. While the latter theorem tells us that a function is essentially undetermined by finitely many projections—even if it is C^∞—, Theorem 2.2 states that this indeterminacy disappears as soon as the variation of the function—as measured by its norm in $H_0^\beta(\Omega)$—is restricted.

We remark that the estimates of the last two theorems are sharp as far as the exponents are concerned. This is easily shown in the case of Theorem 2.1. It follows from Natterer (1980a), Louis (1981a, 1984a) for Theorem 2.2.

IV.3 The Singular Value Decomposition of the Radon Transform

In Section IV.1 we have seen that the singular value decomposition is a valuable tool in the study of ill-posed problems. After some preparations we shall derive the singular value decomposition of the Radon transform as an operator from $L_2(\Omega^n)$ into $L_2(Z, w^{1-n})$, where $w(s) = (1-s^2)^{1/2}$, see Theorem II.1.6.

To begin with we show that for $\theta_1, \theta_2 \in S^{n-1}$

$$R_{\theta_1} R_{\theta_2}^{\#} g(s) = |\Omega^{n-2}| \int_{|t| \leq \sqrt{(1-s^2)}} g(t \sin \varphi + s \cos \varphi) w^{n-2}(\sqrt{(s^2+t^2)}) dt \quad (3.1)$$

where $\varphi \in [0, \pi]$ is the angle between θ_1, θ_2, i.e. $\cos \varphi = \theta_1 \cdot \theta_2$. For the proof we may assume that $\theta_1 = (0, \ldots, 0, 1)^T$ and $\theta_2 = (\theta', \cos \varphi)^T$ with $|\theta'| = \sin \varphi$. Then, with $x = (x', x_n)^T$,

$$R_{\theta_2}^{\#} g(x) = g(x \cdot \theta_2) = g(x' \cdot \theta' + x_n \cos \varphi)$$

and

$$R_{\theta_1} R_{\theta_2}^{\#} g(s) = \int_{|x'| \leq \sqrt{(1-s^2)}} R_{\theta_2} g(x', s) dx'$$

$$= \int_{|x'| \leq \sqrt{(1-s^2)}} g(x' \cdot \theta' + s \cos \varphi) dx'.$$

Since the measure of $\{x' \in \mathbb{R}^{n-1} : |x'| \leq \sqrt{(1-s^2)}, x' \cdot \theta' = t|\theta'|\}$ for $n > 2$ is

$$|\Omega^{n-2}|(1-s^2-t^2)^{(n-2)/2}$$

for $|t| \leq \sqrt{(1-s^2)}$ we obtain from Fubini's theorem

$$R_{\theta_1} R_{\theta_2}^{\#} g(s) = \int_{|t| \leq \sqrt{(1-s^2)}} g(t|\theta'| + s \cos \varphi) |\Omega^{n-2}|(1-s^2-t^2)^{(n-2)/2} dt.$$

This holds also for $n = 2$ since $|\Omega^0| = 1$. Since $|\theta'| = \sin \varphi$, (3.1) is proved.

Next we apply (3.1) to the Gegenbauer polynomials $C_m^{n/2}$, i.e. the orthogonal polynomials in $[-1, +1]$ with weight w^{n-1} which we have normalized such that $C_m^{n/2}(1) = 1$. $C_m^{n/2}(t \sin \varphi + s \cos \varphi)$ is a linear combination of terms of the form

$$t^j s^{k-j}, \quad 0 \leq j \leq k \leq m.$$

Substituting $(1-s^2)^{1/2} u$ for t we obtain for each of these terms

$$\int_{|t| \leq \sqrt{(1-s^2)}} t^j s^{k-j} (1-s^2-t^2)^{(n-2)/2} dt = s^{k-j} (1-s^2)^{j/2 + (n-2)/2 + 1/2}$$

$$\times \int_{-1}^{+1} u^j (1-u^2)^{(n-2)/2} du.$$

For j odd, this is zero. For j even, this is of the form

$$w^{n-1}(s) P_k(s)$$

with some polynomial P_k of degree k. Hence,

$$\mathbf{R}_{\theta_1}\mathbf{R}^{\#}_{\theta_2}C_m^{n/2} = w^{n-1} P_m \tag{3.2}$$

with P_m a polynomial of degree m. From the orthogonality properties of the Gegenbauer polynomials it follows that

$$(\mathbf{R}_{\theta_1}\mathbf{R}^{\#}_{\theta_2}C_m^{n/2}, C_l^{n/2})_{L_2(-1,+1)} = \int_{-1}^{+1} w^{n-1} P_m C_l^{n/2}\, ds = 0 \tag{3.3}$$

for $l > m$. From (3.1) we see that $R_{\theta_1}R^{\#}_{\theta_2}$ is a symmetric operator, hence (3.3) holds also for $l < m$. Thus P_m is orthogonal, in the sense of $L_2([-1, +1], w^{n-1})$, to $C_l^{n/2}$ for $l \neq m$, i.e. P_m coincides, up to a constant factor, with $C_m^{n/2}$. Now (3.2) assumes the form

$$\mathbf{R}_{\theta_1}\mathbf{R}^{\#}_{\theta_2}C_m^{n/2} = \alpha_m(\theta_1\cdot\theta_2)w^{n-1}C_m^{n/2} \tag{3.4}$$

with some constant $\alpha_m(\theta_1\cdot\theta_2)$ which we now determine by letting $s \to 1$. We obtain from (3.1)

$$\alpha_m(t) = c(n)\,C_m^{n/2}(t),$$

$$c(n) = |\Omega^{n-2}| \int_{-1}^{+1} (1-u^2)^{(n-2)/2}\,du = \frac{\pi^{(n-1)/2}}{\Gamma\left(\dfrac{n+1}{2}\right)}. \tag{3.5}$$

For later use we record the following consequence of (3.3): putting

$$C_{m,\theta}^{n/2}(x) = C_m^{n/2}(x\cdot\theta) \tag{3.6}$$

in Ω^n we have

$$\left(C_{m,\theta_1}^{n/2}, C_{l,\theta_2}^{n/2}\right)_{L_2(\Omega^n)} = \begin{cases} 0, & m \neq l \\ c(m,n)C_m^{n/2}(\theta_1\cdot\theta_2), & m = l \end{cases} \tag{3.7}$$

$$c(m,n) = |\Omega^{n-2}| \int_{-1}^{+1} (1-u^2)^{(n-2)/2}\,du$$

$$\times \int_{-1}^{+1} w^{n-1}(s)\,(C_m^{n/2}(s))^2\,ds$$

$$= \frac{\pi^{(n-1)/2}\, 2^{n-1}\,\Gamma\left(\dfrac{n+1}{2}\right)}{\left(m+\dfrac{n}{2}\right)(m+1)\ldots(m+n-1)}.$$

In the evaluation of the constant we have made use of (VII.3.1) and of well-known formulas for the Γ-function.

After these preparations we derive the singular value decomposition of **R** by considering the operator **RR*** where the adjoint is formed with respect to the inner product in the space $L_2(Z, w^{1-n})$. We obtain as in II.1

$$\mathbf{R}_\theta^* h = \mathbf{R}_\theta^\# (w^{1-n} h),$$

$$\mathbf{R}^* g = \int_{S^{n-1}} \mathbf{R}_\theta^* g \, d\theta,$$

hence

$$\mathbf{R}\mathbf{R}^* g(\omega, s) = \int_{S^{n-1}} \mathbf{R}_\omega \mathbf{R}_\theta^* g(s) \, d\theta.$$

Putting

$$u_m = w^{n-1} C_m^{n/2},$$

(3.4) assumes the form

$$\mathbf{R}_{\theta_1} \mathbf{R}_{\theta_2}^* u_m = \alpha_m(\theta_1 \cdot \theta_2) u_m,$$

i.e. u_m is an eigenfunction of the self-adjoint operator $\mathbf{R}_{\theta_1} \mathbf{R}_{\theta_2}^*$ with eigenvalue $\alpha_m(\theta_1 \cdot \theta_2)$. For h a function on S^{n-1} we therefore obtain

$$\mathbf{R}\mathbf{R}^*(h \, u_m)(\omega, s) = \int_{S^{n-1}} (\mathbf{R}_\omega \mathbf{R}_\theta^* u_m)(s) h(\theta) \, d\theta$$

$$= \int_{S^{n-1}} \alpha_m(\omega \cdot \theta) h(\theta) \, d\theta \, u_m(s)$$

$$= A_m h(\omega) u_m(s)$$

where A_m is the integral operator

$$A_m h(\omega) = \int_{S^{n-1}} \alpha_m(\omega \cdot \theta) h(\theta) \, d\theta.$$

For $h = Y_l$ a spherical harmonic of degree l we obtain with the Funk–Hecke theorem (VII.3.12)

$$A_m Y_l(\omega) = \int_{S^{n-1}} \alpha_m(\omega \cdot \theta) Y_l(\theta) \, d\theta = \sigma_{ml}^2 Y_l(\theta)$$

$$\sigma_{ml}^2 = |S^{n-2}| \int_{-1}^{+1} \alpha_m(t) C_l^{(n-2)/2}(t)(1-t^2)^{(n-3)/2} \, dt. \tag{3.8}$$

This means that the spherical harmonics of degree l are in the eigenspace of A_m with eigenvalue σ_{ml}^2. Thus the operator RR^* which is self-adjoint on $L_2(Z, w^{1-n})$

has eigenfunctions $Y_l u_m$ with eigenvalues σ_{ml}^2, and since the functions $Y_l u_m$ constitute a basis of $L_2(Z, w^{1-n})$ we have found all eigenfunctions and eigenvalues of RR^*.

Since α_m is a polynomial of degree m, we have, in view of the orthogonality properties of the Gegenbauer polynomials, $\sigma_{ml} = 0$ for $l > m$. Also, $\alpha_{ml} = 0$ if $l + m$ odd since $C_l^{(n-2)/2}$ is even for l even and odd for l odd. Inserting α_m from (3.5) into (3.8) we find for the positive eigenvalues

$$\sigma_{ml}^2 = |S^{n-2}| \frac{\pi^{(n-1)/2}}{\Gamma\left(\frac{n+1}{2}\right)} \int_{-1}^{+1} C_m^{n/2}(t) C_l^{(n-2)/2}(t)(1-t^2)^{(n-3)/2}\, dt, \qquad (3.9)$$

$$m = 0, 1, 2, \ldots, \quad l = m, m-2, \ldots.$$

Now let

$$g_{ml} = c(m) Y_l u_m, \qquad (3.10)$$

$$c(m) = \left(\int_{-1}^{+1} w^{1-n} u_m^2\, ds\right)^{-1/2}, \quad \int_{S^{n-1}} Y_l^2(\theta)\, d\theta = 1$$

be a normalized eigenfunction of RR^*. In agreement with the general procedure of Section IV.1 we compute the functions

$$f_{ml}(x) = \frac{1}{\sigma_{ml}} R^* g_{ml}(x)$$

$$= \frac{c(m)}{\sigma_{ml}} \int_{S^{n-1}} Y_l(\theta) C_m^{n/2}(x \cdot \theta)\, d\theta.$$

Again we use the Funk–Hecke theorem (VII.3.12) to obtain

$$f_{ml}(x) = Q_{ml}(|x|) Y_l(x/|x|),$$

$$Q_{ml}(r) = \frac{c(m)}{\sigma_{ml}} |S^{n-2}| \int_{-1}^{+1} C_m^{n/2}(rt) C_l^{(n-2)/2}(t)(1-t^2)^{(n-3)/2}\, dt.$$

Let

$$C_m^{n/2}(t) = a_m t^m + a_{m-2} t^{m-2} + \ldots + a_l t^l + \ldots.$$

Then, because of the orthogonality properties of the Gegenbauer polynomials,

$$Q_{ml}(r) = \frac{c(m)}{\sigma_{ml}} |S^{n-2}| \int_{-1}^{+1} (a_m r^m t^m + a_{m-2} r^{m-2} t^{m-2} + \ldots + a_l r^l t^l)$$

$$\times C_l^{(n-2)/2}(t)(1-t^2)^{(n-3)/2}\, dt$$

$$= r^l q_{ml}(r^2)$$

where q_{ml} is a polynomial of degree $(m-l)/2$. Since the functions g_{ml} are orthogonal in $L_2(Z, w^{1-n})$, the functions f_{ml} are orthogonal in $L_2(\Omega^n)$. From

$$(f_{ml}, f_{kl})_{L_2(\Omega^n)} = \int_0^1 r^{n-1} \int_{S^{n-1}} f_{ml}(r\theta) f_{kl}(r\theta) \, d\theta \, dr$$

$$= \int_0^1 r^{2l+n-1} q_{ml}(r^2) q_{kl}(r^2) \int_{S^{n-1}} |Y(\theta)|^2 \, d\theta \, dr$$

$$= \frac{1}{2} \int_0^1 t^{l+(n-2)/2} q_{ml}(t) q_{kl}(t) \, dt = \begin{cases} 1, & m = k, \\ 0, & \text{otherwise} \end{cases}$$

we see that

$$q_{ml} = 2^{1/2} P_{(m-l)/2, l+(n-2)/2}$$

where $P_{k,l}$, $k = 0, 1, \ldots$ are the polynomials of degree k with

$$\int_0^1 t^l P_{k,l}(t) P_{m,l}(t) \, dt = \begin{cases} 1, & k = m, \\ 0, & \text{otherwise.} \end{cases} \qquad (3.11)$$

Up to normalization $P_{k,l}(t)$ coincides with the Jacobi polynomial $G_k(l+(n-2)/2, l+(n-2)/2, t)$, see formula 22.2.2 of Abramowitz and Stegun (1970). For f_{ml} we finally obtain

$$f_{ml}(x) = 2^{1/2} P_{(m-l)/2, l+(n-2)/2}(|x|^2) |x|^l Y_l(x/|x|). \qquad (3.12)$$

Combining (3.10), (3.12), (3.8) yields the singular value decomposition of **R**. Note that each singular value has multiplicity $N(m, l)$, see (VII.3.11). With Y_{lk}, $k = 1, \ldots, N(m, l)$ a normalized orthogonal basis for the spherical harmonics of degree l, with

$$f_{mlk}(x) = 2^{1/2} P_{(m-l)/2, l+(n-2)/2}(|x|^2) |x|^l Y_{lk}(x/|x|),$$
$$g_{mlk}(\theta, s) = c(m) Y_{lk}(\theta) u_m(s),$$

compare (3.10), the singular value decomposition of the Radon transform reads

$$Rf = \sum_{m=0}^{\infty} \sideset{}{'}\sum_{l \le m} \sigma_{ml} \sum_{k=1}^{N(m,l)} (f, f_{mlk})_{L_2(\Omega^n)} g_{mlk}. \qquad (3.13)$$

The dash indicates that the l-sum extends only over those l with $l+m$ even.

Incidentally, Theorem 1.2 leads to the following inversion formula: if $g = Rf$, then

$$f = \sum_{m=0}^{\infty} \sideset{}{'}\sum_{l \le m} \sigma_{ml}^{-1} \sum_{k=1}^{N(m,l)} (g, g_{mlk})_{L_2(Z, w^{1-n})} f_{mlk}. \qquad (3.14)$$

Note that f_{mlk} is a polynomial of order m. Hence truncated versions of (3.14) provide us with polynomial approximations to f.

We conclude this section by computing explicitly the singular values for $n = 2$. From (3.9), (VII.3.2–3),

$$\sigma_{ml}^2 = 2 \frac{\pi^{1/2}}{\Gamma(3/2)} \frac{1}{m+1} \int_{-1}^{+1} U_m(t) T_l(t) (1-t^2)^{-1/2} \, dt.$$

With $\Gamma(3/2) = \pi^{1/2}/2$ and $t = \cos\varphi$ we get

$$\sigma_{ml}^2 = \frac{4}{m+1} \int_0^\pi \frac{\sin(m+1)\varphi}{\sin\varphi} \cos l\varphi \, d\varphi.$$

Using

$$\frac{\sin(m+1)\varphi}{\sin\varphi} = \begin{cases} 2(\cos m\varphi + \cos(m-2)\varphi + \ldots + \cos\varphi), & m \text{ odd}, \\ 2(\cos m\varphi + \cos(m-2)\varphi + \ldots + \cos 2\varphi) + 1, & m \text{ even} \end{cases}$$

we finally obtain for $0 < l \le m$, $m+l$ even

$$\begin{aligned}\sigma_{ml}^2 &= \frac{8}{m+1} \int_0^\pi \cos^2 l\varphi \, d\varphi \\ &= \frac{4\pi}{m+1},\end{aligned} \quad (3.15)$$

and the same result holds for $l = 0$.

We see that $\sigma_{ml} \to 0$ as $m \to \infty$, but the decay is rather gentle, indicating that the ill-posedness of Radon's integral equation is not pronounced very much. This agrees with our findings in Section IV.2.

IV.4 Bibliographical Notes

For a thorough treatment of ill-posed problems see Tikhonov and Arsenin (1977), Groetsch (1984). For an error analysis for the Tikhonov–Phillips method in a Hilbert scale framework see Natterer (1984b).

The results of Section IV.2 have been obtained in Natterer (1980a) for $n = 2$, see also Bertero et al. (1980). A result related to Theorem 2.2—with a different measure for the variation of f—can be found in Madych (1980).

For the singular value decomposition of the Radon transform see Davison (1981) and Louis (1985). These papers consider also more general weight functions. The singular value decomposition for the exterior problem (compare VI.3) has been given by Quinto (1985). Louis (1985) gives a singular value analysis of the Tikhonov–Phillips method with a Sobolev norm for the Radon transform.

V
Reconstruction Algorithms

In this chapter we give a detailed description of some well-known reconstruction algorithms. We start with the widely used filtered backprojection algorithm and study the possible resolution. In Section V.2 we give an error analysis of the Fourier algorithm which leads to an improved algorithm comparable in accuracy with filtered backprojection. In Section V.3 we analyse the convergence properties of the Kaczmarz method for the iterative solution of under- and overdetermined linear systems. The Kaczmarz method is used in Section V.4 to derive several versions of the algebraic reconstruction technique (ART). The direct algebraic method in Section V.5 exploits invariance properties of the sampling scheme by using FFT techniques for the solution of the large linear systems arising from natural discretizations of the integral transforms. In Section V.6 we survey some further algorithms which are either interesting from a theoretical point of view or which are of possible interest in specific applications.

V.1 Filtered Backprojection

The filtered backprojection reconstruction algorithm is presently the most important algorithm, at least in the medical field. It can be viewed as a computer implementation of the inversion formula

$$f = \frac{1}{2}(2\pi)^{1-n} \mathbf{R}^{\#} \mathbf{H}^{n-1} (\mathbf{R}f)^{(n-1)}, \tag{1.1}$$

see (II.2.4). However, a different approach based on the formula

$$W_b * f = \mathbf{R}^{\#}(w_b * \mathbf{R}f), \qquad W_b = \mathbf{R}^{\#} w_b \tag{1.2}$$

of Theorem II.1.3 gives much more insight. The basic idea is to choose w_b such that W_b approximates the δ-distribution. More precisely we assume W_b to be a low-pass filter with cut-off frequency b which we write as

$$\hat{W}_b(\xi) = (2\pi)^{-n/2} \hat{\Phi}(|\xi|/b) \tag{1.3}$$

where $0 \le \hat{\Phi} \le 1$ and $\hat{\Phi}(\sigma) = 0$ for $\sigma \ge 1$. An example is the ideal low-pass filter $\hat{\Phi}(\sigma) = 1$ for $\sigma \le 1$, for which

$$W_b(x) = (2\pi)^{-n/2} b^n \frac{J_{n/2}(b|x|)}{(b|x|)^{n/2}}, \tag{1.4}$$

see (VII.1.3) and $W_b \to \delta$ for $b \to \infty$.

Theorem II.1.4 gives the relation between W_b and w_b in terms of Fourier transforms:

$$\hat{W}_b(\xi) = (2\pi)^{(n-1)/2} |\xi|^{1-n} \left(\hat{w}_b\left(\frac{\xi}{|\xi|}, |\xi|\right) + \hat{w}_b\left(-\frac{\xi}{|\xi|}, -|\xi|\right) \right).$$

Since $\hat{W}_b$ is a radial function we drop the first argument in $\hat{w}_b$. For $\hat{w}_b$ even we obtain

$$\hat{w}_b(\sigma) = \frac{1}{2} (2\pi)^{1/2-n} |\sigma|^{n-1} \hat{\Phi}(|\sigma|/b). \tag{1.5}$$

From our assumptions on $\hat{\Phi}$ it follows that

$$0 \leq \hat{w}_b(\sigma) \leq \frac{1}{2} (2\pi)^{1/2-n} |\sigma|^{n-1}. \tag{1.6}$$

The evaluation of (1.2) calls for performing the one-dimensional convolution or filtering operation $w_b * \mathbf{R}f$ for each direction in S^{n-1}, followed by the application of the backprojection operator $\mathbf{R}^\#$. This explains the name of the algorithm.

The filtered backprojection algorithm is a discrete version of (1.2). Let $f \in C_0^\infty(\Omega^n)$, and let $g = \mathbf{R}f$ be sampled at (θ_j, s_l), $j = 1, \ldots, p$, $l = -q, \ldots, q$, where $\theta_j \in S^{n-1}$ and $s_l = hl$, $h = 1/q$. Then, the convolution $w_b * g$ can be replaced by the discrete convolution

$$w_b \overset{h}{*} g(\theta_j, s) = h \sum_{l=-q}^{q} w_b(s - s_l) g(\theta_j, s_l). \tag{1.7}$$

For computing the backprojection in (1.2) we need a quadrature rule on S^{n-1} based on the nodes $\theta_1, \ldots, \theta_p$ and having positive weights α_{pj}. We shall assume that this rule is exact in H'_{2m}, the even spherical harmonics of degree $2m$ (see III.2) for some m, i.e.

$$\int_{S^{n-1}} v(\theta) \, d\theta = \sum_{j=1}^{p} \alpha_{pj} v(\theta_j) \tag{1.8}$$

for $v \in H'_{2m}$. The backprojection in (1.2) can now be replaced by the discrete backprojection

$$\mathbf{R}_p^\# v(x) = \sum_{j=1}^{p} \alpha_{pj} v(\theta_j, x \cdot \theta_j). \tag{1.9}$$

The complete filtered backprojection algorithm now reads

$$f_{FB} = \mathbf{R}_p^\# w_b \overset{h}{*} g. \tag{1.10}$$

Before giving more explicit versions of (1.10) we study the effect of the various discretizations.

THEOREM 1.1 Let $f \in C_0^\infty(\Omega^n)$. Assume that (1.8) holds on H'_{2m} and that, for some ϑ with $0 < \vartheta < 1$,

$$b \leq \vartheta m, \quad b \leq \pi/h. \tag{1.11}$$

Then, with η defined as in (III.2.4), we have

$$f_{FB} = W_b * f + e_1 + e_2,$$

$$|e_1| \leq \frac{1}{2}(2\pi)^{-n/2} \varepsilon_0^*(f, b), \quad \varepsilon_0^*(f, b) = |S^{n-1}| \sup_{\theta \in S^{n-1}} \int_{|\sigma| \geq b} |\sigma|^{n-1} |\hat{f}(\sigma\theta)| \, d\sigma,$$

$$|e_2| \leq \|f\|_{L_\infty(\Omega^n)} \eta(\vartheta, m).$$

Proof We have

$$f_{FB} = \mathbf{R}^\# w_b * g + e_1 + e_2 = W_b * f + e_1 + e_2,$$

$$e_1 = \mathbf{R}_p^\# (w_b \overset{h}{*} g - w_b * g),$$

$$e_2 = (\mathbf{R}_p^\# - \mathbf{R}^\#)(w_b * g).$$

From (III.1.7) we obtain

$$(w_b \overset{h}{*} g - w_b * g)\hat{\,}(\theta, \sigma) = (2\pi)^{1/2} \hat{w}_b(\sigma) \sum_{l \neq 0} \hat{g}\left(\theta, \sigma - \frac{2\pi}{h} l\right),$$

hence, by taking the inverse Fourier transform,

$$|w_b \overset{h}{*} g - w_b * g|(\theta, s) \leq \int_{-b}^{b} |\hat{w}_b(\sigma)| \sum_{l \neq 0} \left|\hat{g}\left(\theta, \sigma - \frac{2\pi}{h} l\right)\right| d\sigma.$$

Since $b \leq \pi/h$ we obtain from (1.6)

$$|w_b \overset{h}{*} g - w_b * g|(\theta, s) \leq \frac{1}{2}(2\pi)^{1/2-n} \int_{|\sigma| \geq b} |\sigma|^{n-1} |\hat{g}(\theta, \sigma)| \, d\sigma$$

$$= \frac{1}{2}(2\pi)^{-n/2} \int_{|\sigma| \geq b} |\sigma|^{n-1} |\hat{f}(\sigma\theta)| \, d\sigma$$

where we have used Theorem II.1.1. Applying $\mathbf{R}_p^\#$ and observing that, because of $\alpha_{pj} > 0$ and (1.8) with $v = 1$, i.e.

$$\sum_{j=1}^{p} \alpha_{pj} = |S^{n-1}|, \tag{1.12}$$

we obtain the estimate on e_1.

Next we consider the error e_2 which comes from discretizing the backprojection. We expand $w_b * g$ in terms of spherical harmonics, see VII.3:

$$(w_b * g)(\theta, x \cdot \theta) = \sum_{l=0}^{\infty} \frac{1}{c(n,l)} \sum_k Y_{2l,k}(\theta) v_{l,k}(x),$$

$$v_{l,k}(x) = \int_{S^{n-1}} Y_{2l,k}(\theta) (w_b * g)(\theta, x \cdot \theta) d\theta.$$

Here, the k-sum runs over all $N(n, l)$ spherical harmonics, and the $Y_{2l,k}$ are normalized such that

$$\int_{S^{n-1}} |Y_{2l,k}(\theta)|^2 d\theta = c(n,l)$$

with $c(n, l)$ from (VII.3.13).

We then have from (VII.3.13) that $|Y_{2l,k}| \leq 1$.

Note that the spherical harmonics of odd degree dropped out since $w_b * g(\theta, x \cdot \theta)$ is an even function of θ.

Using the Fourier integral for $w_b * g$, the rule R4 of VII.1, Theorem II.1.1 and the Fourier integral for $\hat{f}$ we obtain

$$v_{l,k}(x) = \int_{S^{n-1}} Y_{2l,k}(\theta) (2\pi)^{-1/2} \int_{R^1} e^{i\sigma x \cdot \theta} \widehat{(w_b * g)}(\theta, \sigma) d\sigma d\theta$$

$$= \int_{S^{n-1}} Y_{2l,k}(\theta) \int_{-b}^{b} e^{i\sigma x \cdot \theta} \hat{w}_b(\sigma) \hat{g}(\theta, \sigma) d\sigma d\theta$$

$$= (2\pi)^{(n-1)/2} \int_{S^{n-1}} Y_{2l,k}(\theta) \int_{-b}^{b} e^{i\sigma x \cdot \theta} \hat{w}_b(\sigma) \hat{f}(\sigma\theta) d\sigma d\theta$$

$$= (2\pi)^{-1/2} \int_{\Omega^*} f(y) \int_{-b}^{b} \hat{w}_b(\sigma) \int_{S^{n-1}} Y_{2l,k}(\theta) e^{i\sigma(x-y) \cdot \theta} d\theta d\sigma dy.$$

The inner integral can be evaluated by (VII.3.19) to yield

$$(2\pi)^{n/2} i^{2l} (\sigma|x-y|)^{(2-n)/2} J_{2l+(n-2)/2}(\sigma|x-y|) Y_{2l,k}\left(\frac{x-y}{|y-x|}\right).$$

Combining this with (1.6) and remembering that $|Y_{2l,k}| \leq 1$ we obtain

$$|v_{l,k}(x)| \leq \frac{1}{2}(2\pi)^{-n/2} \int_{\Omega^*} |f(y)| |x-y|^{(2-n)/2} \int_{-b}^{b} \sigma^{n/2} J_{2l+(n-2)/2}(\sigma|x-y|) d\sigma dy.$$

Now let $l > m$. Then, because of $b \leq \vartheta m < \vartheta l$ and $|x - y| \leq 2$, we obtain for the inner integral the upper bound

$$\frac{1}{2} l^{n/2} \eta_1(\vartheta, 2l)$$

see (III.2.5). It follows that for $l > m$ with some constant $c(n)$

$$|v_{l,k}(x)| \leq c(n) \|f\|_{L_\infty(\Omega^r)} l^{n/2} \eta_1(\vartheta, 2l).$$

Hence, with $(w_b * g)_m$ the series for $w_b * g$ truncated after the mth term, we have

$$\|w_b * g - (w_b * g)_m\|_{L_\infty(Z)} \leq \sum_{l>m} \frac{1}{c(n,l)} \sum_k \|v_{l,k}\|_{L_\infty(\Omega^r)}$$

$$\leq c(n) \|f\|_{L_\infty(\Omega^r)} \sum_{l>m} \frac{N(n,l)}{c(n,l)} l^{n/2} \eta_1(\vartheta, 2l)$$

$$\leq \|f\|_{L_\infty(\Omega^r)} \eta(\vartheta, m)$$

where we have used (VII.3.11), (VII.3.13) and (III.2.7).

Since (1.8) is exact on H'_{2m} we obtain for e_2 from (1.12)

$$|e_2| = |(R_p^\# - R^\#)(w_b * g - (w_b * g)_m)|$$

$$\leq 2|S^{n-1}| \|w_b * g - (w_b * g)_m\|_{L_\infty(Z)}$$

$$\leq 2|S^{n-1}| \|f\|_{L_\infty(\Omega^r)} \eta(\vartheta, m)$$

and this is the estimate of the theorem. □

A few remarks are in order.

(1) The crucial parameter in the filtered backprojection algorithm is b. It obviously controls the resolution. If f is essentially b — band-limited in the sense that $\varepsilon_0^*(f, b)$ is negligible, then f_{FB} is a reliable reconstruction of f provided b satisfies (1.11) and is sufficiently large.

(2) The cut-off frequency b is subject to two restrictions: $b \leq \pi/h$ guarantees that the convolutions are properly discretized, while $b \leq \vartheta m$ excludes those high frequencies in $w_b * g$ which cannot be integrated accurately by the quadrature rule (1.8).

(3) There is obviously a connection between the existence of quadrature rules exact on H'_{2m} and resolution.

Since

$$\dim H'_{2m} = \binom{2m+n-1}{n-1}$$

and since the quadrature rule (1.8) contains np free parameters $\alpha_1, \ldots, \alpha_p, \theta_1, \ldots, \theta_p$ one might guess that one can find a quadrature rule exact on H'_{2m} if

$$np \geq \binom{2m+n-1}{n-1}.$$

Below we shall see that this is in fact the case for $n = 2$, but for $n = 3$ we shall need $p = (m+1)^2$ nodes what is roughly $\frac{3}{2}$ times the optimal number $p = \frac{1}{3}$

$(m+1)(2m+1)$. What is known about optimal quadrature on S^{n-1} can be seen from Neutsch (1983) and McLaren (1963), for a discussion of the subject in the present context see Grünbaum (1981).

(4) The evaluation of $f_{FB}(x)$ requires the computation of $w \overset{h}{*} g(\theta_j, x \cdot \theta_j)$ for $j = 1, \ldots, p$. Thus we need $0(pq)$ operations for each x at which we want to reconstruct. In order to reduce this number to $0(p)$ we evaluate (1.7) for $s = s_l$, $l = -q, \ldots, q$ only and insert an interpolation step I_h in (1.10), i.e. we compute

$$f_{FBI} = \mathbf{R}_p^\# I_h(w \overset{h}{*} g) \tag{1.13}$$

rather than (1.10). For I_h we take the B-spline approximation

$$I_h g(s) = \sum_l g(s_l) B_{1/h}(s - s_l)$$

of order k (see III.1.9).

In Theorem 1.2 below we study the effect of interpolation independently of the other discretization errors, i.e. we investigate the expression $\mathbf{R}^\# I_h(w * g)$.

THEOREM 1.2 We have for $b \leq \pi/h$

$$\mathbf{R}^\# I_h(w_b * g) = G_h * W_b * f + e_3$$

where the filter G_h is given by

$$\hat{G}_h(\xi) = (2\pi)^{-n/2} \begin{cases} (\text{sinc}((h/2)|\xi|))^k, & |\xi| \leq \pi/h, \\ 0, & \text{otherwise} \end{cases}$$

and the error e_3 satisfies $\hat{e}_3(\xi) = 0$ for $|\xi| \leq \pi/h$ and

$$\|e_3\|_{L_2(\Omega^r)} \leq \left(\frac{2}{\pi}\right)^{k-1} h^\alpha \|f\|_{H_0^\alpha(\Omega^r)}.$$

Proof From Theorem III.1.4 we get for $b \leq \pi/h$ and $\alpha \geq 0$

$$I_h(w_b * g) = F_h * w_b * g + a_h, \tag{1.14}$$

$$|a_h|_{H^{(1-n)/2}(\mathbf{R}^1)} \leq \left(\frac{2}{\pi}\right)^{k-1} h^{(n-1)/2-\alpha} |w_b * g|_{H^{-\alpha}(\mathbf{R}^1)} \tag{1.15}$$

$$\leq \frac{1}{2}(2\pi)^{1-n} \left(\frac{2}{\pi}\right)^{k-1} h^{(n-1)/2-\alpha} |g|_{H^{n-1-\alpha}(\mathbf{R}^1)}$$

where we have used R4 of VII.1 and (1.6). From Theorem II.1.4 we obtain for any even function a on Z

$$\|\mathbf{R}^\# a\|_{L_2(\mathbf{R}^n)}^2 = 4(2\pi)^{n-1} \int_{\mathbf{R}^n} |\xi|^{2(1-n)} \left|\hat{a}\left(\frac{\xi}{|\xi|}, |\xi|\right)\right|^2 d\xi$$

$$= 2(2\pi)^{n-1} \int_{S^{n-1}} \int_{\mathbf{R}^1} |\sigma|^{1-n} |\hat{a}(\theta, \sigma)|^2 d\sigma \, d\theta$$

$$= 2(2\pi)^{n-1} |a|_{H^{(1-n)/2}(Z)}^2.$$

Using this for $a = a_h$ and integrating over S^{n-1} we get from (1.15) and Theorem II.1.1

$$\|\mathbf{R}^\# a_h\|_{L_2(\mathbf{R}^n)} \leq (2\pi)^{(1-n)/2} \left(\frac{2}{\pi}\right)^{k-1} h^{(n-1)/2-\alpha} |g|_{H^{n-1-\alpha}(Z)}$$

$$\leq \left(\frac{2}{\pi}\right)^{k-1} h^{(n-1)/2-\alpha} \|f\|_{H_0^{(n-1)/2-\alpha}(\Omega^r)}.$$

(1.16)

Applying $\mathbf{R}^\#$ to (1.14) we get

$$\mathbf{R}^\# I_h (w_b * g) = \mathbf{R}^\# (F_h * w_b * g) + e_3, \qquad e_3 = \mathbf{R}^\# a_h.$$

Since $\hat{a}_h(\sigma) = 0$ for $|\sigma| \leq \pi/h$ it follows from Theorem II.1.4 that $\hat{e}_3(\xi) = 0$ for $|\xi| \leq \pi/h$, and the estimate on e_3 of the theorem follows from (1.16) with $(n-1)/2 - \alpha$ replaced by α. With $F_h = \mathbf{R} G_h$ we have from Theorem II.1.1.

$$\hat{G}_h(\xi) = (2\pi)^{(1-n)/2} \hat{F}_h(|\xi|)$$

and from Theorem II.1.2

$$F_h * g = \mathbf{R} G_h * \mathbf{R} f = \mathbf{R} (G_h * f).$$

Finally, from (1.2) applied to $G_h * f$, we see that

$$\mathbf{R}^\# (F_h * w_b * g) = \mathbf{R}^\# (w_b * \mathbf{R} (G_h * f))$$
$$= W_b * G_h * f$$

and the proof is finished. □

From Theorem 1.2 we see that, apart from a highly oscillating additive error e_3, interpolation has the same effect as applying the filter G_h. The error e_3 has the same order of magnitude, namely $h^\alpha \|f\|_{H^\alpha(\Omega^r)}$, as the discretization error in the data which we found in Theorem IV.2.2 as long as $\alpha \leq (n-1)/2$. This result is quite satisfactory. Note that the order k of the splines does not enter decisively. In practical tests it has been found (Rowland, 1979) that $k = 2$ (broken line interpolation) is satisfactory but $k = 1$ (nearest neighbour interpolation) is not.

Now we give a detailed description of the algorithm for special scanning geometries.

V.1.1. The Parallel Geometry in the Plane

Here, $g = \mathbf{R}f$ is available for $(\theta_j, s_l), j = 1, \ldots, p, l = -q, \ldots, q,$

$\theta_j = \begin{pmatrix} \cos \varphi_j \\ \sin \varphi_j \end{pmatrix}, \varphi_j = \pi (j-1)/p, s_l = hl, h = 1/q.$

As quadrature rule on S^1 we take the trapezoidal rule (VII.2.9) with p nodes which is exact on H'_{2p-2} and we use linear (broken line) interpolation. Then the filtered backprojection algorithm (1.13) with interpolation goes as follows.

Step 1: For $j = 1, \ldots, p$ carry out the convolutions

$$v_{j,k} = h \sum_{l=-q}^{q} w_b (s_k - s_l) g (\theta_j, s_l), \quad k = -q, \ldots, q. \tag{1.17a}$$

For the function w_b see (1.20)–(1.23) below.

Step 2: For each reconstruction point x, compute the discrete backprojection

$$f_{FBI}(x) = \frac{2\pi}{p} \sum_{j=1}^{p} ((1-u)v_{j,k} + uv_{j,k+1}) \tag{1.17b}$$

where, for each x and j, k and u are determined by

$$s = \theta_j \cdot x, \quad k \leq s/h < k+1, \quad u = s/h - k.$$

The function w_b depends on the choice of the filter Φ in (1.3) or (1.5). For the filter

$$\hat{\Phi}(\sigma) = \begin{cases} 1 - \varepsilon\sigma, & \sigma \leq 1, \\ 0, & \sigma > 1 \end{cases}$$

containing the parameter $\varepsilon \in [0, 1]$ we obtain from (1.5)

$$w_b(s) = \frac{1}{8\pi^2} \int_{-b}^{b} |\sigma| \left(1 - \varepsilon \frac{|\sigma|}{b}\right) e^{i s\sigma} \, d\sigma$$

$$= \frac{1}{4\pi^2} \int_{0}^{b} \sigma \left(1 - \varepsilon \frac{\sigma}{b}\right) \cos(s\sigma) \, d\sigma.$$

An integration by parts yields

$$w_b(s) = \frac{b^2}{4\pi^2} \{u(bs) - \varepsilon v(bs)\},$$

$$u(s) = \begin{cases} \dfrac{\cos s - 1}{s^2} + \dfrac{\sin s}{s}, & s \neq 0, \\ 1/2, & s = 0, \end{cases} \tag{1.20}$$

$$v(s) = \begin{cases} \dfrac{2 \cos s}{s^2} + \left(1 - \dfrac{2}{s^2}\right) \dfrac{\sin s}{s}, & s \neq 0, \\ 1/3, & s = 0. \end{cases}$$

See Fig. V.1 for a graph of w_b.

If b is tied to h by $b = \pi/h$, which is the maximal value of b in Theorem 1.1, and

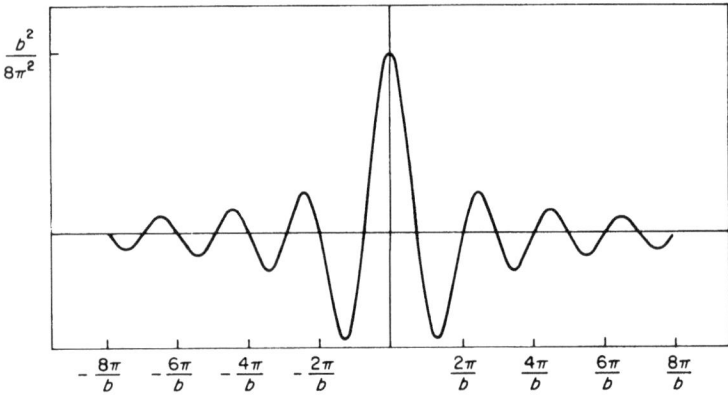

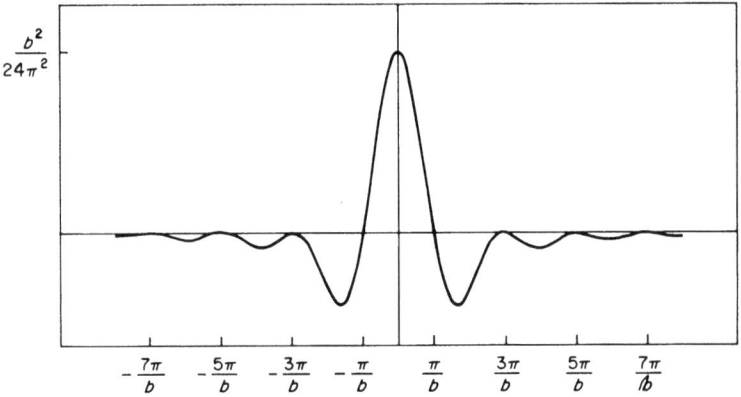

Fig. V.1 Graph of the filter w_b in the filtered backprojection algorithm for $\varepsilon = 0$ (top) and $\varepsilon = 1$ (bottom).

if w_b is evaluated for $s = s_l$ only, considerable simplification occurs:

$$w_b(s_l) = \frac{b^2}{2\pi^2} \begin{cases} 1/4 - \varepsilon/6, & l = 0, \\ -\varepsilon/(\pi^2 l^2), & l \neq 0 \text{ even}, \\ -(1-\varepsilon)/(\pi^2 l^2), & l \text{ odd}. \end{cases} \qquad (1.21)$$

For $\varepsilon = 0$, this is the function suggested by Ramachandran and Lakshminarayanan (1971). The filter W_b which belongs to this choice has been given in (1.4). Shepp and Logan (1974) suggested the filter

$$\hat{\Phi}(\sigma) = \begin{cases} \text{sinc}(\sigma\pi/2), & \sigma \leq 1, \\ 0, & \sigma > 1. \end{cases}$$

This leads to

$$w_b(s) = \frac{1}{8\pi^2} \int_{-b}^{b} |\sigma| \operatorname{sinc}\left(\frac{|\sigma|\pi}{2b}\right) e^{is\sigma} d\sigma$$

$$= \frac{b}{2\pi^3} \int_{0}^{b} \sin\left(\frac{\sigma\pi}{2b}\right) \cos(\sigma s) d\sigma$$

$$= \frac{b^2}{2\pi^3} u(bs), \tag{1.22}$$

$$u(s) = \frac{\frac{\pi}{2} - s \sin s}{\left(\frac{\pi}{2}\right)^2 - s^2}$$

with the usual modification for $s = \pm \pi/2$. Again, for $b = \pi/h$ and $s = s_l$ we simply obtain

$$w_b(s_l) = \frac{b^2}{\pi^4} \frac{1}{1 - 4l^2}. \tag{1.23}$$

From our error analysis in Theorem 1.1 and Theorem 1.2 we can expect the algorithm (1.17), with either of the choices (1.21), (1.23) for w_b, to reconstruct reliably an essentially b-band-limited function f, provided $b < p$ and $h \le \pi/b$, b sufficiently large. This coincides with what we found out about the resolution of the parallel scanning geometry in III.3.

The number of the operations of the filtered backprojection algorithm (1.17) is as follows. For the convolutions we need $0(pq^2)$ operations what can be reduced to $0(pq \log q)$ if FFT is used, see VII.5. The backprojection requires $0(p)$ operations for each x, totalling up to $0(pq^2)$ operations if f_{FBI} is computed on a $(2q+1) \times (2q+1)$-grid which corresponds to the sampling of $\mathbf{R}_{\theta_j} f$. For the optimal relation $p = \pi q$ of III.3 we thus arrive at $0(q^3)$ operations, regardless of whether we use FFT or not.

The corresponding work estimate in n dimensions is $0(pq \log q)$ for the convolutions and $0(pq^n)$ for the backprojection. If $p = c q^{n-1}$ as suggested in (III.2.15) the total work is $0(q^{2n-1})$.

V.1.2. The Fan-beam Geometry in the Plane

The simplest way to deal with fan-beam data is to compute the parallel data from the fan-beam data by suitable interpolations ('rebinning' the data, see Herman (1980)). In the following we adapt the filtered backprojection algorithm to fan-beam data. Again we start out from (1.2) which we write explicitly as

$$F_b * f(x) = \int_{S^1} \int_{-1}^{+1} w_b(x \cdot \theta - s) \mathbf{R} f(\theta, s) \, ds \, d\theta. \tag{1.24}$$

We use the same notation as in III.3, i.e. the parallel coordinates s, $\theta = \begin{pmatrix} \cos\varphi \\ \sin\varphi \end{pmatrix}$ are related to the fan-beam coordinates α, β by

$$s = r \sin\alpha, \qquad \varphi = \beta + \alpha - \pi/2,$$

and $g(\beta, \alpha) = \mathbf{R}f(\theta, s)$. The Jacobian of the transformation is

$$\frac{\partial(s, \varphi)}{\partial(\alpha, \beta)} = \begin{vmatrix} r\cos\alpha & 0 \\ 1 & 1 \end{vmatrix} = r\cos\alpha.$$

We have to express $|x \cdot \theta - s|$ in terms of α, β. This is the distance between x and the straight line $L(\alpha, \beta)$ which is the dashed line in Fig. V.2. Let y be the orthogonal projection of x onto $L(\alpha, \beta)$ and let γ be the angle between $x - a$ and $-a$, i.e.

$$\cos(\pm\gamma) = \frac{(a-x, a)}{|a-x||a|}, \quad +\text{for } a^\perp \cdot x \leq 0, \quad -\text{for } a^\perp \cdot x \geq 0.$$

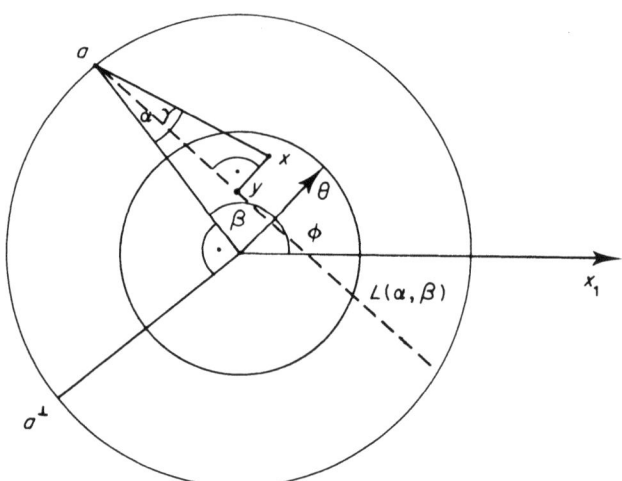

FIG. V.2 Transformation of (1.24) to fan-beam coordinates. Compare Fig. III.4.

Note that γ depends only on x and β, but not on α. Considering the triangle xya we find that

$$|x - y| = |x \cdot \theta - s| = |x - a||\sin(\gamma - \alpha)|.$$

Now we can carry out the transformation in (1.24), obtaining

$$F_b * f(x) = r \int_0^{2\pi} \int_{-\pi/2}^{\pi/2} w_b(|x - a|\sin(\gamma - \alpha)) g(\beta, \alpha) \cos\alpha \, d\alpha \, d\beta.$$

At a first glance the inner integral looks as if it could be done by convolutions. Unfortunately, due to the presence of the factor $|x - a|$, the convolution kernel varies with β and x. This means that the inner integral has to be computed for each pair β, x, making the procedure much less efficient than in the parallel case. In order to circumvent this nuisance we remark that, in view of (1.5), we have

$$w_b(\rho s) = \rho^{-n} w_{\rho b}(s)$$

as is easily verified. Using this with $n = 2$ and $\rho = |x - a|$ we obtain

$$F_b * f(x) = r \int_0^{2\pi} |x-a|^{-2} \int_{-\pi/2}^{\pi/2} w_{|x-a|b}(\sin(\gamma - \alpha)) g(\beta, \alpha) \cos \alpha \, d\alpha \, d\beta.$$

(1.25)

At this point make an approximation: the number $|x - a|b$ in (1.25) plays the role of a cut-off frequency and the inner integral depends only slightly on this cut-off frequency if it is only big enough. Therefore, we can replace $|x - a|b$ by a sufficiently large cut-off frequency c which does not depend on x, β. We obtain

$$F_b * f(x) \sim r \int_0^{2\pi} |x-a|^{-2} \int_{-\pi/2}^{\pi/2} w_c(\sin(\gamma - \alpha)) g(\beta, \alpha) \cos \alpha \, d\alpha \, d\beta \quad (1.26)$$

and we expect this to be a good approximation for essentially b-band-limited functions f if $c \geq |x - a|b$ for all x, β, e.g. for $c = (1 + r)b$.

The implementation of (1.26) is now analogous to the parallel case: assume g to be sampled for $\beta_j = 2\pi(j-1)/p$, $j = 1, \ldots, p$ and $\alpha_l = hl$, $l = -q, \ldots, q$, $h = \pi/2q$. Then, the filtered backprojection algorithm reads:

Step 1: For $j = 1, \ldots, p$ carry out the convolutions

$$v_{j,k} = h \sum_{l=-q}^{q} w_c(\sin(\alpha_k - \alpha_l)) g(\beta_j, \alpha_l) \cos \alpha_l, \quad k = -q, \ldots, q. \quad (1.27a)$$

For the function w_c see (1.20), (1.22).

Step 2: For each reconstruction point x compute the discrete backprojection

$$f_R(x) = \frac{2r\pi}{p} \sum_{j=1}^{p} |x - a_j|^{-2} ((1-u) v_{j,k} + u v_{j,k+1}) \quad (1.27b)$$

where, for each x and j, k and u are determined by

$$\gamma = \pm \arccos \frac{(a_j - x, a_j)}{|a_j - x| |a_j|}, \quad k \leq \gamma/h < k+1, \quad u = \gamma/h - k.$$

The sign is '+' if $a_j^\perp \cdot x \leq 0$ and '−' otherwise.

In accordance with our findings in III.3 we expect this algorithm to reconstruct reliably essentially b-band-limited functions f provided that $c < p/2$, $c < 2q/r$ and $c = (1 + r)b$ sufficiently large.

The algorithm as described in (1.27) needs data from sources distributed over the whole circle. Looking at Fig. V.2 we see that it should suffice to have sources on an angular range of $\pi + 2\tilde{\alpha}(r)$ since all lines hitting the reconstruction region Ω^2 can be obtained from sources on such an arc. $\tilde{\alpha}(r)$ is the maximal angle for which $L(\beta, \alpha)$ meets Ω^2, i.e. $\tilde{\alpha}(r) = \arcsin(1/r)$.

It is very easy to derive such an algorithm. We go back to (1.24), replacing it by the equivalent formula

$$F_b * f(x) = 2 \int_0^{\pi} \int_{-1}^{+1} w_b(w \cdot \theta - s) \mathbf{R} f(\theta, s) \, ds \, d\theta.$$

The image in the α–β plane of the rectangle $[-1, +1] \times [0, \pi]$ in the s–φ plane is (see Fig. V.3)

$$\frac{\pi}{2} - \tilde{\alpha}(r) \leq \beta \leq \frac{3\pi}{2} + \tilde{\alpha}(r)$$

$$\alpha_-(\beta) \leq \alpha \leq \alpha_+(\beta),$$

$$\alpha_-(\beta) = \max\left\{-\tilde{\alpha}(r), \frac{\pi}{2} - \beta\right\}, \quad \alpha_+(\beta) = \min\left\{\tilde{\alpha}(r), \frac{3\pi}{2} - \beta\right\}.$$

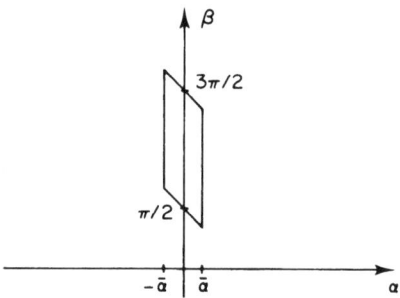

FIG. V.3 Image in the α–β plane of the rectangle $[-1, +1] \times [0, \pi]$ in the s–φ plane.

Therefore (1.25) assumes the form

$$W_b * f(x) = 2 \int_{(\pi/2) - \tilde{\alpha}(r)}^{(3\pi/2) + \tilde{\alpha}(r)} |x - a|^{-2} \int_{\alpha_-(\beta)}^{\alpha_+(\beta)} w_{|x-a|b}(\sin(\gamma - \alpha)) g(\beta, \alpha) \cos \alpha \, d\alpha \, d\beta$$

(1.28)

and this formula is implemented exactly in the same way as (1.25), leading to an algorithm with the desired property.

V.1.3. The Three-dimensional Case

Let the $(m+1)^2$ direction $\theta_{ji} \in S^2$ have spherical coordinates Ψ_j, φ_i where

$$0 \leq \psi_0 < \psi_1 < \ldots < \psi_m < \pi,$$
$$\varphi_i = i\pi/(m+1), \quad i = 0, \ldots, m, \tag{1.29}$$
$$s_l = hl, \, l = -q, \ldots, q, \, h = 1/q.$$

From (III.2.13) we know that the directions in (1.29) form a m-resolving set, allowing the reconstruction of a function f with essential bandwidth ϑm, $0 < \vartheta < 1$, if the functions $\mathbf{R}_{\theta_{ji}} f$ are given. We adapt the step-size h to this resolution by requiring that $h \leq \pi/m$.

The problem is to reconstruct f from the data $g(\theta_{ji}, s_l) = \mathbf{R}f(\theta_{ji}, s_l)$. There are two possibilities.

The two-stage algorithm

This algorithm uses the decomposition of the three-dimensional Radon transform $\mathbf{R}_3$ into the product of two-dimensional Radon transforms $\mathbf{R}_2$. Let $\theta \in S^2$ have the spherical coordinates ψ, φ and let $\omega = \begin{pmatrix} \cos \varphi \\ \sin \varphi \end{pmatrix}$, $\eta = \begin{pmatrix} \cos \psi \\ \sin \psi \end{pmatrix}$. For each $z \in \mathbb{R}^1$, define the function f_z on $\mathbb{R}^2$ by

$$f_z(x_1, x_2) = f(x_1, x_2, z).$$

Also, for each $\omega \in S^1$, define the function g_ω on $\mathbb{R}^2$ by

$$g_\omega(t, z) = \mathbf{R}_2 f_z(\omega, t) \tag{1.30}$$

where $t \in \mathbb{R}^1$. Then we have for $s \in \mathbb{R}^1$

$$\mathbf{R}_2 g_\omega(\eta, s) = \mathbf{R}_3 f(\theta, s). \tag{1.31}$$

This can be seen from Fig. V.4 which shows the plane spanned by the x_3-axes and θ. For each $(t, z) \in \mathbb{R}^2$, $g_\omega(t, z)$ is the integral of f along the line through (t, z) perpendicular to that plane. Hence, integrating g_ω along the orthogonal

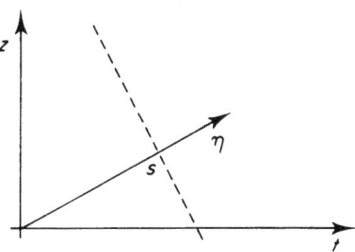

FIG. V.4 Orthogonal projection of the plane $x \cdot \theta = s$ onto the plane spanned by the x_3-axes and θ.

projection of $x \cdot \theta = s$ onto that plane, i.e. along the line $\begin{pmatrix} t \\ z \end{pmatrix} \cdot \eta = s$ (the dashed line in Fig. V.4) yields precisely the integral of f over $x \cdot \theta = s$.

The two-stage algorithm works as follows. In the first stage we solve (1.31) for each of the directions θ. In the second stage we solve (1.30) for z fixed, obtaining f in the plane $x_3 = z$.

Of course the algorithm has to be carried out in a discrete setting. This is very easy if the Ψ_j are equally spaced. Then we can run the algorithm (1.17) on (1.31) as well as on (1.30) without any changes. In view of the resolution property of (1.17), the resolution of the two-stage algorithm is precisely what we expected above.

The direct algorithm

This is an implementation of the formula (1.2) analogous to the two-dimensional case. For the evaluation of f_{FBI} in (1.13) we take the quadrature rule (VII.2.13) which is exact on H'_{2m} for m odd. Note that the $m+1$ angles Ψ_j in (VII.2.13) are arranged in an order different from the one in (1.29), requiring a slight change in the notation. Again we chose broken line interpolation ($k = 2$) for I_h. Following Marr (1974a), we take as filter

$$\hat{\Phi}(\sigma) = \begin{cases} (\text{sinc}(\sigma\pi/2))^2, & \sigma \le 1, \\ 0 & \sigma \ge 1. \end{cases}$$

Then we get from (1.5) for $n = 3$

$$w_b(s) = \frac{1}{16\pi^3} \int_{-b}^{b} \sigma^2 \left(\text{sinc} \frac{\sigma\pi}{2b} \right)^2 e^{is\sigma} d\sigma$$

$$= \frac{b^2}{2\pi^5} \int_0^b \left(\sin \frac{\sigma\pi}{2b} \right)^2 \cos s\sigma \, d\sigma$$

$$= \frac{b^3}{2\pi^6} \int_0^\pi \left(\sin \frac{\sigma}{2} \right)^2 \cos \frac{bs}{\pi} \sigma \, d\sigma$$

$$= \frac{b^3}{4\pi^6} \int_0^\pi (1 - \cos \sigma) \cos \frac{bs}{\pi} \sigma \, d\sigma.$$

For $b = \pi/h$ and $s = s_l$ we simply obtain

$$w_b(s_l) = \frac{b^3}{8\pi^5} \begin{cases} 0, & |l| > 1, \\ 2, & l = 0, \\ -1, & |l| = 1. \end{cases}$$

We see that with this choice of Φ, discrete convolution with w_b amounts to taking second order differences. This makes sense since for $n = 3$, the operator-$\mathbf{H}^2$ is the identity and (1.1) simply backprojects the second order derivative.

The complete direct algorithm now reads, with $b = \pi/h$:

$$v_{ji,l} = \frac{b^3}{8\pi^5}(2g(\theta_{ji}, s_l) - g(\theta_{ji}, s_{l-1}) - g(\theta_{ji}, s_{l+1})),$$

$$|j| = 1, \ldots, (m+1)/2, \quad i = 0, \ldots, m, \quad l = 0, \ldots, m \qquad (1.32)$$

$$f_{FBI}(x) = \frac{2\pi}{m+1} \sum_{j=-(m+1)/2}^{(m+1)/2} A_j \sum_{i=0}^{m} ((1-u)v_{ji,l} + uv_{ji,l+1})$$

where, for each x, j and i, u and l are determined by

$$s = \theta_{ji} \cdot x, \quad l \le s/h < l+1, \quad u = s/h - l.$$

As in the two-dimensional case we can expect this algorithm to reconstruct reliably essentially b-band-limited functions if $b < m$ and b sufficiently large. Our analysis depends on the angles ψ_j and the A_j being the nodes and weights of the Gauss formula (VII.2.11), but from a practical point of view we can as well take the ψ_j equally distributed and $A_j = \pi/m+1 \sin\psi_j$, compare the discussion in VII.2.

We conclude this section by doing some reconstructions in $\mathbb{R}^2$ with the filtered backprojection algorithm. The function f we want to recover is the approximate δ-function (VII.1.3), i.e.

$$f(x) = \frac{1}{2\pi} c^2 \frac{J_1(c|x|)}{c|x|}, \quad c = 64$$

This function has bandwidth c, but it is clearly not supported in Ω^2. However it decays fast enough to consider it approximately as a function which has a peak at the origin and vanishes elsewhere, see Fig. V.5(a). The Radon transform $g = \mathbf{R}f$ is easily computed from VII.1.2, Theorem I.1.1 and III.1. We obtain

$$g = c/\pi \operatorname{sinc}_c.$$

In Fig. V.5(b)–(d) we display reconstructions of f by the filtered backprojection algorithm (1.17) for a parallel scanning geometry, using the filter (1.20) with $\varepsilon = 0$. The number p of directions and the stepsize h have been chosen as follows:

(b) $p = 64$, $\quad h = \dfrac{1}{20}$

(c) $p = 32$, $\quad h = \dfrac{1}{20}$

(d) $p = 64$, $\quad h = \dfrac{1}{16}$

In all three cases, the cut-off frequency b in the algorithm has been adjusted to the stepsize h, i.e. we have put $b = \pi/h$.

In reconstruction (b), p, h satisfy the conditions $p \geq b$, $h \leq \pi/b$ of Theorem 1.1 (we have $p = m$, see the discussion following (1.23), and we have put $\theta = 1$). So we expect the reconstruction (b) in Fig. V.3(b) to be accurate, and this is in fact the case.

In reconstruction (c), p does not satisfy the condition $p \geq b$. This angular undersampling produces the artefacts at the boundary of the reconstruction region Ω^2 in Fig. V.3(c). The reason why these artefacts show up only for $p = 32$ but not for values of p between 32 and 64 lies in the fact that our object as given by f does not fill out the whole reconstruction region but only a little part around the midpoint. A quick perusal of the proof of Theorem 1.1 shows that in that case the condition $b \leq 9m$ can be relaxed to $b \leq 2 \cdot 9m$.

In reconstruction (d), h does not satisfy the condition $h \leq \pi/b$. This results in a serious distortion of the original, see Fig. V.3(d). Note that the distortions are not made up solely of high frequency artefacts but concern also the overall features. This is an example of aliasing as discussed in III.1.

The effect of violating the optimality relation $p = \pi q$ of Table III.1 is demonstrated in Fig. V.6. A simple object consisting of three circles has been reconstructed by the filtered backprojection algorithm (1.17) with w_b as in (1.21) from $p = 120$ projections consisting of $2q + 1$ line integrals each, q varying from 20 to 120. The reconstruction error as measured by the L_2-norm is plotted in Fig. V.6. The optimal value for q is $p/\pi \sim 38$. We see that in fact the L_2 error decreases as q increases from 20 to 38 and is almost constant for $q > 38$. Thus there is no point in increasing q beyond its optimal value as given by p/π.

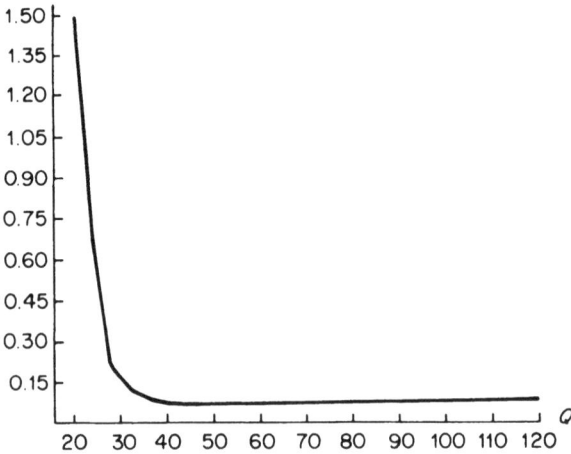

FIG. V.6 Dependence of the reconstruction error in a parallel geometry with $p = 120$ on q. The saturation if q exceeds the optimal value of 38 is apparent.

V.2 Fourier Reconstruction

By Fourier reconstruction we mean a direct numerical implementation of the projection theorem

$$\hat{f}(\sigma\theta) = (2\pi)^{(1-n)/2} (\mathbf{R}f)\hat{\;}(\theta,\sigma), \tag{2.1}$$

see Theorem II.1.1. Other methods such as those in Section V.1 and Section V.5 also use Fourier techniques but this is not what is meant by Fourier reconstruction.

Using the Fourier inversion formula

$$f(x) = (2\pi)^{-n/2} \int_{R^n} e^{ix\cdot\xi} \hat{f}(\xi)\,d\xi \tag{2.2}$$

in (2.1) we immediately obtain an inversion formula for the Radon transform in terms of Fourier transforms. The problem with this obvious procedure comes with the discretization.

Let $f \in C_0^\infty(\Omega^n)$ and let $g = \mathbf{R}f$ be sampled at (θ_j, s_l), $j = 1, \ldots, p$, $l = -q, \ldots, q$ where $\theta_j \in S^{n-1}$ and $s_l = hl$, $h = 1/q$. A straightforward discretization of (2.1), (2.2) leads to the standard Fourier reconstruction algorithm in which the polar coordinate grid

$$G_{p,q} = \{\pi r \theta_j : r = -q, \ldots, q-1,\; j = 1, \ldots, p\}$$

plays an important role.

The standard Fourier algorithm consists of three steps:

Step 1: For $j = 1, \ldots, p$, compute approximations $\hat{g}_{jr}$ to $\hat{g}(\theta_j, r\pi)$ by

$$\hat{g}_{jr} = (2\pi)^{-1/2} h \sum_{l=-q}^{q-1} e^{-i\pi l r/q} g(\theta_j, s_l), \; r = -q, \ldots, q-1.$$

From (2.1) we see that the first step provides an approximation to $\hat{f}$ on $G_{p,q}$: $\hat{f}(r\pi\theta_j) = (2\pi)^{(1-n)/2} \hat{g}_{rj}$ up to discretization errors.

An essential feature of Fourier reconstruction is the use of the fast Fourier transform (FFT), see VII.5. Without FFT, Fourier reconstruction could not compete in efficiency with other algorithms. Since we cannot do the FFT on $G_{p,q}$ we have to switch to an appropriate cartesian grid by an interpolation procedure. This is done in

Step 2: For each $k \in \mathbb{Z}^n$, $|k| < q$, find a point $\xi_k = \pi r \theta_j \in G_{p,q}$ closest to πk and put

$$\hat{f}_k = (2\pi)^{(1-n)/2} \hat{g}_{jr}.$$

$\hat{f}_k$ is an approximation to $\hat{f}(\pi k)$ obtained by nearest neighbour interpolation in the polar coordinate grid. Up to discretization errors made in step 1 it coincides with $\hat{f}(\xi_k)$.

Step 3: Compute an approximation f_m to $f(hm)$, $m \in \mathbb{Z}^n$ by

$$f_m = \left(\frac{\pi}{2}\right)^{n/2} \sum_{|k|<q} e^{i\pi m\cdot k/q} \hat{f}_k, \; |m| < q.$$

This is a discrete form of the n-dimensional inverse Fourier transform.

Incidentally, the standard Fourier algorithm provides a heuristic derivation of the optimality relation $p = \pi q$ between the number p of directions and the number $2q + 1$ of readings per direction in the standard parallel geometry in the plane: the largest cells of the polar coordinate grid G_{pq} are rectangles with sidelengths $\pi, (\pi/p) \cdot \pi q$ respectively. These rectangles become squares for $p = \pi q$.

Employing the FFT algorithm for the discrete Fourier transforms in steps 1 and 3 and neglecting step 2 we come to the following work estimate for the standard Fourier algorithm: the p discrete Fourier transforms of length $2q$ in step 1 require $0(pq \log q)$ operations, the n-dimensional discrete Fourier transform in step 3 requires $0(q^n \log q)$ operations. If p, q are tied to each other by the relation $p = cq^{n-1}$ from (III.2.15), the total work is $0(q^n \log q)$. This is much better than the $0(q^{2n-1})$ work estimate we found in Section V.1 for the filtered backprojection algorithm. This efficiency is the reason for the interest in Fourier reconstruction.

Unfortunately, Fourier reconstruction in its standard form as presented above produces severe artefacts and cannot compete with other reconstruction techniques as far as accuracy is concerned. In order to find out the source of the trouble we make a rigorous error analysis. The algorithm as it stands is designed to reconstruct functions f with essential bandwidth πq. By (III.1.6) the error in step 1 can be estimated by

$$\sum_{l \neq 0} |\hat{g}(\theta_j, \pi r - 2\pi q l)|, \qquad |r| < q$$

which is negligible if f, hence g, is essentially πq-band-limited in an appropriate sense. Likewise, the sampling of $\hat{f}$ in step 3 with step-size π is correct in the sense of the sampling Theorem III.1.1 since f has bandwidth 1, and since all frequencies up to πq are included the truncation error in step 3 is negligible for f essentially πq-band-limited in an appropriate sense. Hence step 1 and step 3 are all right, so the trouble must come from the interpolation step 2. In fact we shall see that this is the case.

Before we analyse the interpolation error what leads to a better choice of the points ξ_k in step 2 and eventually to a competitive algorithm we give a heuristic argument showing that the interpolation error is unduly large and explaining the artefacts observed in practical calculations.

From Theorem III.1.4 we know that we can describe the effect of interpolation in terms of convolutions. More specifically, if the function $\hat{f}$ on $\mathbb{R}^n$ is interpolated with B-splines of order k and step-size π the result is

$$I_\pi \hat{f} = F_\pi * \hat{f} + a_\pi$$

where $\hat{a}_\pi(x) = 0$ for $|x| \leq 1$ and

$$\hat{F}_\pi(x) = \begin{cases} (2\pi)^{-n/2} (\operatorname{sinc} \tfrac{\pi}{2} x)^k, & |x_i| \leq 1, i = 1, \ldots, n, \\ 0, \text{otherwise.} \end{cases}$$

It follows that in Ω^n
$$(I_\pi \hat{f})\check{\ }(x) = (2\pi)^{n/2} \tilde{F}_\pi(x) f(x) + \tilde{a}_\pi(x)$$
$$= (\text{sinc}\frac{\pi}{2}x)^k f(x).$$

Hence, in Ω^n, the inverse Fourier transform of the interpolated Fourier transform of f is (sinc $(\pi/2) x)^k f$. This is a good approximation to f for $|x|$ small, but since (sinc $(\pi/2) x)^k$ decays at the boundary of Ω^n, the overall accuracy is poor. This is not helped by increasing the order k of the interpolation. Conversely, looking at (sinc $(\pi/2) x)^k$ suggests that the distortion gets even bigger if k is increased. Of course the interpolation in Fourier reconstruction is different from the simple case of tensor product B-spline interpolation considered here but the artefacts obtained by Fourier reconstruction are similar to those predicted by our simple model.

We shall carry out the error analysis in a Sobolev space framework. From Lemma VII.4.4 we know that the norms

$$\|f\|_{H_0^\alpha(\Omega^n)} = \left(\int_{\mathbb{R}^n} (1+|\xi|^2)^\alpha |\hat{f}(\xi)|^2 \, d\xi\right)^{1/2} \tag{2.2}$$

$$\|f\|_{\tilde{H}_0^\alpha(\Omega^n)} = \pi^{n/2} \left(\sum_k (1+\pi^2|k|^2)^\alpha |\hat{f}(\pi k)|^2\right)^{1/2} \tag{2.3}$$

are equivalent on $H_0^\alpha(\Omega^n)$. This is partially true even if $\hat{f}$ is sampled at points ξ_k close to πk in the following sense:
There is a constant h such that for $k \in \mathbb{Z}^n$
$$|\xi_k - \pi k| \leq h|k|. \tag{2.4}$$

LEMMA 2.1 Let the ξ_k be distributed such that (2.4) holds. Let $\alpha \geq 0$ and $a > 0$. Then, there is a constant $c(\alpha, a, n)$ such that
$$\sum_{|k| \leq a/h} (1+\pi^2|k|^2)^\alpha |\hat{f}(\xi_k)|^2 \leq c(\alpha, a, n) \|f\|^2_{H_0^\alpha(\Omega^n)} \tag{2.5}$$
for $f \in C_0^\infty(\Omega^n)$.

Proof Define a function w by putting $\hat{w} = |\hat{f}|^2$, i.e.
$$w(x) = (2\pi)^{-n/2} \int_{|y| < 1} f(x+y) \overline{f}(y) \, dy$$
by rule R4 of VII.1. Since $f = 0$ outside Ω^n, $w(x) = 0$ for $|x| \geq 2$. Choose $\chi \in C_0^\infty(\mathbb{R}^n)$ such that $\chi = 1$ for $|x| \leq 2$. Then, $w = \chi w$, hence
$$\hat{w} = (2\pi)^{-n/2} \hat{\chi} * \hat{w}$$
or
$$|\hat{f}|^2 = (2\pi)^{-n/2} \hat{\chi} * |\hat{f}|^2.$$

This relation is applied to the left-hand side of (2.5), yielding

$$\sum_{|k| \le a/h} (1+\pi^2|k|^2)^\alpha |\hat{f}(\xi_k)|^2 = (2\pi)^{-n/2} \sum_{|k| \le a/h} (1+\pi^2|k|^2)^\alpha (\hat{\chi} * |\hat{f}|^2)(\xi_k) \quad (2.6)$$

$$= (2\pi)^{-n/2} \int_{\mathbb{R}^n} |\hat{f}(\xi)|^2 \sum_{|k| \le a/h} (1+\pi^2|k|^2)^\alpha \hat{\chi}(\xi_k - \xi) \, d\xi.$$

Since $\chi \in C_0^\infty(\mathbb{R}^n)$ there is a number $c(t) > 0$ for each $t > 0$ such that

$$|\hat{\chi}(\xi)| \le c(t)(1+|\xi|)^{-t}.$$

Now we make use of (2.4). For $\xi \in \mathbb{R}^n$ and $|k| \le a/h$ we have

$$|\xi - \xi_k| = |\xi - \pi k + \pi k - \xi_k| \ge |\xi - \pi k| - |\pi k - \xi_k|$$
$$\ge |\xi - \pi k| - h|k| \ge |\xi - \pi k| - a.$$

Combining the last two estimates with the inequality

$$(1+|\xi|)^{-t} \le (1+a)^t (1+a+|\xi|)^{-t}$$

we obtain for $\xi \in \mathbb{R}^n$, $|k| \le a/h$

$$|\chi(\xi - \xi_k)| \le c(t)(1+|\xi - \xi_k|)^{-t}$$
$$\le c(t)(1+a)^t (1+a+|\xi - \xi_k|)^{-t}$$
$$\le c(t)(1+a)^t (1+|\xi - \pi k|)^{-t}$$
$$\le c(t)(1+a)^t (1+|\xi - \pi k|^2)^{-t/2}.$$

Using this and Peetre's inequality

$$(1+\pi^2|k|^2)^\alpha \le 2^\alpha (1+|\xi - k\pi|^2)^\alpha (1+|\xi|^2)^\alpha$$

we get for the sum in (2.6) the estimate

$$\sum_{|k| \le a/h} (1+\pi^2|k|^2)^\alpha \hat{\chi}(\xi_k - \xi) \le 2^\alpha c(t)(1+a)^t (1+|\xi|^2)^\alpha \sum_k (1+|\xi - \pi k|^2)^{\alpha - t/2}.$$

Now we choose t big enough to make this series converge, e.g. $t = 2\alpha + n + 1$ will do. Then the series is a continuous periodic function of ξ which is bounded, and we conclude that

$$\sum_{|k| \le a/h} (1+\pi^2|k|^2)^\alpha \hat{\chi}(\xi_k - \xi) \le c_1(\alpha, a, n)(1+|\xi|^2)^\alpha$$

with some constant $c_1(\alpha, a, n)$. From (2.6) it now follows that

$$\sum_{|k| \le a/h} (1+\pi^2|k|^2)^\alpha |\hat{f}(\xi_k)|^2 \le (2\pi)^{-n/2} c_1(\alpha, a, n) \int_{\mathbb{R}^n} (1+|\xi|^2)^\alpha |\hat{f}(\xi)|^2 \, d\xi$$

and this is (2.5). □

Now we do Fourier reconstruction with the points ξ_k satisfying (2.4), ignoring the discretizations of step 1, i.e. we compute the (hypothetical) reconstruction

$$f^*(x) = \left(\frac{\pi}{2}\right)^{n/2} \sum_{|k| \leq a/h} e^{i\pi x \cdot k} \hat{f}(\xi_k). \tag{2.7}$$

The following theorem gives our error estimate.

THEOREM 2.2 Let ξ_k be distributed such that (2.4) is satisfied, and let $0 \leq \alpha \leq 1$. Then there is a constant $c(\alpha, a, n)$ such that for $f \in C_0^\infty(\Omega^n)$

$$\|f - f^*\|_{L_2(\Omega^n)} \leq c(\alpha, a, n) h^\alpha \|f\|_{H_0^\alpha(\Omega^n)}.$$

Proof The Fourier series for f in the cube $C = [-1, +1]^n$ reads

$$f(x) = \left(\frac{\pi}{2}\right)^{n/2} \sum_k e^{i\pi x \cdot k} \hat{f}(\pi k).$$

Hence, in C,

$$(f - f^*)(x) = \left(\frac{\pi}{2}\right)^{n/2} \sum_{|k| \leq a/h} e^{i\pi x \cdot k} (\hat{f}(\pi k) - \hat{f}(\xi_k))$$

$$+ \left(\frac{\pi}{2}\right)^{n/2} \sum_{|k| > a/h} e^{i\pi x \cdot k} \hat{f}(\pi k)$$

Parseval's relation yields

$$\|f - f^*\|_{L_2(C)}^2 = \pi^n \sum_{|k| \leq a/h} |\hat{f}(\pi k) - \hat{f}(\xi_k)|^2 + \pi^n \sum_{|k| > a/h} |\hat{f}(\pi k)|^2. \tag{2.8}$$

From the mean value theorem of calculus we find a ξ_k' on the line segment joining πk with ξ_k such that

$$|\hat{f}(\pi k) - \hat{f}(\xi_k)| \leq |\pi k - \xi_k| |\nabla \hat{f}(\xi_k')|$$

were ∇ denotes the gradient. Since ξ_k satisfies (2.4) we obtain

$$|\hat{f}(\pi k) - \hat{f}(\xi_k)| \leq h|k| |\nabla \hat{f}(\xi_k')|. \tag{2.9}$$

The ξ_k' satisfy (2.4) since the ξ_k do, i.e.

$$|\pi k - \xi_k'| \leq h|k|. \tag{2.10}$$

Using (2.9) in (2.8) we obtain

$$\|f - f^*\|_{L_2(C)} \leq \pi^n \sum_{|k| \leq a/h} (h|k|)^2 |\nabla \hat{f}(\xi_k')|^2 + \pi^n \sum_{|k| > a/h} |\hat{f}(\pi k)|^2$$

$$\leq \pi^n \sup_{|k| \leq a/h} \left\{ (h|k|)^2 (1 + \pi^2|k|^2)^{-\alpha} \right\}$$

$$\times \sum_{|k| \leq a/h} (1 + \pi^2|k|^2)^\alpha |\nabla \hat{f}(\xi_k')|^2 \tag{2.11}$$

$$+ \pi^n \sup_{|k| > a/h} (1 + \pi^2|k|^2)^{-\alpha}$$

$$\times \sum_{|k| > a/h} (1 + \pi^2|k|^2)^\alpha |\hat{f}(\pi k)|^2.$$

Since $0 \le \alpha \le 1$ the first sup is bounded by
$$a^{2(1-\alpha)}\pi^{-2\alpha}h^{2\alpha}$$
and the second one by
$$a^{-2\alpha}\pi^{-2\alpha}h^{2\alpha}.$$
Using this in (2.11) yields
$$\|f-f^*\|^2_{L_2(C)} \le \pi^{n-2\alpha}a^{-2\alpha}h^{2\alpha}\Big\{a^2\sum_{|k|\le a/h}(1+\pi^2|k|^2)^\alpha|\nabla\hat{f}(\xi'_k)|^2$$
$$+ \sum_{|k|>a/h}(1+\pi^2|k|^2)^\alpha|\hat{f}(\pi k)|^2\Big\}. \qquad (2.12)$$

Now choose $\chi \in C_0^\infty(\mathbb{R}^n)$ such that $\chi = 1$ on Ω^n. Then, from rule R3 of VII.1,
$$\nabla\hat{f} = -i(x\chi f)\hat{\,}.$$
Because of (2.10) we can apply Lemma 2.1 to the first sum in (2.12), obtaining
$$\sum_{|k|\le a/h}(1+\pi^2|k|^2)^\alpha|\nabla\hat{f}(\xi'_k)|^2 \le c_1(\alpha,a,n)\|x\chi f\|^2_{H_0^\alpha(\Omega^n)} \qquad (2.13)$$
where the norm is to be understood as
$$\|x\chi f\|^2_{H_0^\alpha(\Omega^n)} = \sum_{i=1}^n \|x_i\chi f\|^2_{H_0^\alpha(\Omega^n)}.$$
Since, by Lemma VII.4.5, multiplication with the $C_0^\infty(\mathbb{R}^n)$ function $x_i\chi$ is a continuous operation in $H_0^\alpha(\Omega)$ we have
$$\|x\chi f\|^2_{H_0^\alpha(\Omega^n)} \le c_2(\alpha,n)\|f\|^2_{H_0^\alpha(\Omega^n)}$$
with some constant $c_2(\alpha, n)$. Using this in (2.13) we get the estimate
$$\sum_{|k|\le a/h}(1+\pi^2|k|^2)^\alpha|\nabla\hat{f}(\xi'_k)|^2 \le c_1(\alpha,a,n)c_2(\alpha,n)\|f\|^2_{H_0^\alpha(\Omega^n)}$$
for the first sum in (2.10). The second sum in (2.10) can be bounded in the same way since the norms (2.2), (2.3) are equivalent. Hence, with a new constant $c(\alpha, a, n)$ we finally arrive at
$$\|f-f^*\|^2_{L_2(C)} \le c(\alpha,a,n)h^{2\alpha}\|f\|^2_{H_0^\alpha(\Omega^n)}.$$

This proves the theorem. □

We apply Theorem 2.2 to the reconstruction of a function $f \in C_0^\infty(\Omega^n)$ from the projections $\mathbf{R}_{\theta_j}f, j = 1, \ldots, p$ where the directions θ_j satisfy
$$\sup_{\theta\in S^{n-1}}\inf_{j=1}^p |\theta_j-\theta| \le h/\pi. \qquad (2.14)$$
Choosing $\xi_k = \pi|k|\theta_j$ with j such that θ_j is closest to $k/|k|$, (2.4) is obviously satisfied. It follows that the reconstruction f^* for f has an L_2 error of order

$h^\alpha \|f\|_{H_0^\alpha(\Omega^r)}$. This is precisely what we found out in IV.2 to be the best possible accuracy in the reconstruction of f from $R_{\theta_j} f$, $j = 1, \ldots, p$ with directions θ_j satisfying (2.14). Thus we see that the (hypothetical) Fourier algorithm with points ξ_k satisfying (2.4) is in a sense of optimal accuracy.

Returning to the standard Fourier algorithm we find that the points ξ_k of that algorithm do not satisfy (2.4) with h small, not even if the directions θ_j fulfil (2.14): the radial grid distance is π, independently of h. Thus Theorem 2.2 does not apply, and we do not get an error estimate for the standard Fourier algorithm.

We consider the failure of the standard Fourier algorithm to satisfy (2.4) as an explanation for its poor performance. This seems to be justified since the two improved Fourier algorithms which we describe below and which satisfy (2.4) perform much better.

The improved Fourier algorithms differ from the standard algorithm by the choice of ξ_k and by the way $\hat{g}(\xi_k/|\xi_k|, |\xi_k|)$ is computed. For ease of exposition we restrict ourselves to the case $n = 2$ and we assume that $\theta_j = (\cos \varphi_j, \sin \varphi_j)^T$, $\varphi_j = (j-1)\pi/p$, $j = 1, \ldots, p$. We do not need directions θ_j with $j > p$ since g is even.

The first algorithm simply uses

$$\xi_k = \pi |k| \theta_j \tag{2.15}$$

where θ_j is one of the directions closest to $k/|k|$. Then, (2.4) is satisfied with $h = \pi^2/(2p)$. With this choice the computation of $\hat{g}(\xi_k/|\xi_k|, |\xi_k|)$ calls for the evaluation of $\hat{g}(\theta_j, \sigma)$ for arbitrary real σ which is in no way restricted to a uniform grid. This cannot be done by the ordinary FFT algorithm which gives only the values $\hat{g}(\theta_j, \pi r)$ for $r = -q, \ldots, q-1$. The other values have to be computed by interpolation. The failure of the standard Fourier algorithm taught us that this interpolation is critical. So we choose a rather complicated but accurate and efficient interpolation procedure which combines oversampling of $\hat{g}$ (not of g!) with the generalized sinc series of Theorem III.1.2. The algorithm is as follows.

Step 1: For $j = 1, \ldots, p$, compute approximations $\hat{g}_{jr}$ to $\hat{g}(\theta_j, (\pi/2) r)$ by

$$\hat{g}_{jr} = (2\pi)^{-1/2} h \sum_{l=-q}^{q-1} e^{-i\pi l r/(2q)} g(\theta_j, s_l), \quad r = -2q, \ldots, 2q-1.$$

Since $\hat{g}$ has bandwidth 1, $\hat{g}$ is oversampled by a factor of 2, see III.1.

Step 2: For each $k \in \mathbb{Z}^n$, $|k| < q$, choose θ_j closest to $\pm k/|k|$ and put

$$\hat{f}_k = (2\pi)^{-1/2} \sum_{|\pm|k|-l/2| \leq L/2} \hat{g}_{jl} \, \tilde{\gamma}(\pi(\pm|k|-l/2)) \operatorname{sinc}(2\pi(\pm|k|-l/2)).$$

Here, '+' stands if k is in the upper half-plane and '−' otherwise.

This step deserves some explanations. First, $\tilde{\gamma} \in C^\infty(\mathbb{R}^1)$ is the function in Theorem III.1.2. For $L = \infty$, the series would represent the true value of $\hat{f}(\xi_k)$. As pointed out in the discussion following Theorem III.1.2 the convergence of this series is very fast. So it suffices to retain only a few terms without significant loss in accuracy, i.e. we can choose L relatively small. $\hat{f}_k$ is an approximation to $\hat{f}(\pi k)$

obtained by nearest neighbour interpolation in the angular direction and by generalized sinc interpolation in the radial variable.

Step 3: Compute an approximation f_m to $f(hm)$, $m \in \mathbb{Z}^n$ by

$$f_m = \left(\frac{\pi}{2}\right)^{n/2} \sum_{|k| < q} e^{i\pi m \cdot k/q} \hat{f}_k, \quad |m| < q.$$

This step is identical with step 3 of the standard algorithm.

The work estimate is as follows. In step 1 we have to perform p FFTs of length $4q$ each (put the missing gs to zero) or equivalently, $2p$ FFTs of length $2q$ each, see (VII.5.12–13). This does not change the operation count of $0(pq \log q)$ of the standard algorithm. Step 2 now requires $0(q^2 L)$ operations. Since L can be kept almost constant as $q \to \infty$, this does practically not exceed the $0(q^2 \log q)$ operations of the standard algorithm. Thus we see that the work estimate for the first improved algorithm is practically the same as for the standard algorithm.

In the second improved algorithm (Fig. V.7) which is simpler than the first one we obtain the point ξ_k for $k = (k_1, k_2)^T \geq 0$ in the following way. For $k_1 \geq k_2$ we move πk vertically, for $k_1 < k_2$ horizontally onto the closest ray $\{t\theta_j : t \geq 0\}$. This procedure extends in an obvious way to negative k_1, k_2. The ξ_k satisfy (2.4) with $h = \pi^2/(p\sqrt{2})$. In order to compute $\hat{f}(\xi_k)$ for all such ξ_k it suffices to compute $\hat{g}(\theta_j, \sigma)$ for all σ such that $\sigma\theta_j$ lies on the vertical lines of the cartesian grid $\pi\mathbb{Z}^2$ if $|\cos \varphi_j| \geq |\sin \varphi_j|$ and on the horizontal lines otherwise. The algorithm goes as follows.

Step 1: For $j = 1, \ldots, p$, compute approximations $\hat{g}_{jr}$ to $\hat{g}(\theta_j, \pi r c(j))$, $c(j) = 1/\max\{|\sin \varphi_j|, |\cos \varphi_j|\}$ by

$$\hat{g}_{jr} = (2\pi)^{-1/2} h \sum_{l=-q}^{q-1} e^{-i\pi l c(j) \cdot r/q} g(\theta_j, s_l), \quad r = -q, \ldots, q-1.$$

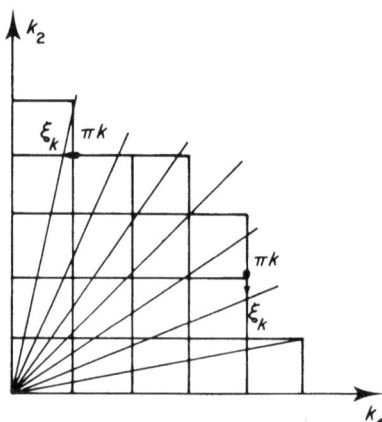

Fig. V.7 Choice of ξ_k in the second improved Fourier algorithm.

This amounts to computing the discrete Fourier transform for arbitrary stepsize in the frequency domain. This can be done by the chirp -z algorithm (VII.5.14).

Step 2: For $k \in \mathbb{Z}^2, |k| \le q$ choose r, j such that $|\pi k - rc(j)\theta_j|$ is as small as possible and put

$$\hat{f}_k = (2\pi)^{-1/2} \hat{g}_{jr}.$$

$\hat{f}_k$ is an approximation to $\hat{f}(\pi k)$ obtained by nearest neighbour interpolation along vertical or horizontal lines. It coincides with $\hat{f}(\xi_k)$, $\xi_k = rc(j)\theta_j$ up to discretization errors made in step 1.

Step 3: Compute approximations f_m to $f(hm)$, $m \in \mathbb{Z}^2$ by

$$f_m = \left(\frac{\pi}{2}\right)^{n/2} \sum_{|k|<q} e^{i\pi m \cdot k/q} \hat{f}_k, \qquad |m| < q.$$

Again the work estimate is $0(q^2 \log q)$.

For further improvement it is advisable to use a filter function F in the computation of f from $\hat{f}$, i.e. to multiply $\hat{f}_k$ by $F(|k|)$. We found that the $\cos^2$ filter

$$F(\sigma) = \begin{cases} \cos^2(\pi\sigma/2q), & |\sigma| < q \\ 0, & |\sigma| > q \end{cases} \qquad (2.16)$$

gave satisfactory results.

We finish this section by showing that the condition (2.4) which looks strange at a first glance since it requires extremely non-uniform sampling of $\hat{f}$ is in fact quite plausible. Suppose we want to reconstruct the approximate δ-function $\delta_{x_0}^b$ with

$$\hat{\delta}_{x_0}^b(\xi) = (2\pi)^{-n/2} \begin{cases} e^{-ix_0 \cdot \xi}, & |\xi| < b, \\ 0, & \text{otherwise,} \end{cases}$$

see (VII.1.3), where $x_0 \in \Omega^n$. Then, for $|\pi k|, |\xi_k| < b$

$$\hat{\delta}_{x_0}^b(\pi k) = \hat{\delta}_{x_0}^b(\xi_k) e^{ix_0 \cdot (\xi_k - \pi k)}.$$

We see that the effect of interpolation can be described by multiplying the Fourier transform by an exponential factor. If the reconstruction is to be reliable this exponential factor has to be close to 1 for πk small and it should not be too far away from 1 as πk approaches b. It is clear that (2.4) guarantees this to be the case for h sufficiently small, $h < \pi^2/(2b)$, say.

The superiority of the improved Fourier algorithms over the standard algorithm is demonstrated by reconstructing the simple test object in Fig. V.8(a) from analytically computed data for $p = 200$ directions and $2q + 1$, $q = 64$ line integrals each. Note that this choice of p, q satisfies approximately the optimality relation $p = \pi q$ of Table III.1. The result of the standard Fourier algorithm is displayed in Fig. V.8(b). We see that the reconstruction shows serious distortions which make it virtually useless. In Fig. V.8(d) we see the result of the second improved Fourier algorithm with the $\cos^2$ filter (2.16). The improvement is obvious. For comparison we displayed in Fig. V.8(c) the reconstruction produced by the filtered backprojection algorithm (1.17) using the filter (1.21) with $\varepsilon = 0$. It differs only slightly from Fig. V.8(d), demonstrating that the second improved Fourier algorithm and the filtered backprojection algorithm are of comparable quality.

V.3 Kaczmarz's Method

Kaczmarz's method is an iterative method for solving linear systems of equations. In this section we give an analysis of this method quite independently of computerized tomography. First we study Kaczmarz's method in a geometrical setting, then we look at it as a variant of the SOR method of numerical analysis. Both approaches provide valuable insights into the application to ART in the next section.

Let $H, H_j, j = 1, \ldots, p$ be (real) Hilbert spaces, and let

$$R_j : H \to H_j, \quad j = 1, \ldots, p$$

be linear continuous maps from H onto H_j. Let $g_j \in H_j$ be given. We want to compute $f \in H$ such that

$$R_j f = g_j, \quad j = 1, \ldots, p. \tag{3.1}$$

We also write $Rf = g$ for (3.1) with

$$R = \begin{pmatrix} R_1 \\ \vdots \\ R_p \end{pmatrix}, \quad g = \begin{pmatrix} g_1 \\ \vdots \\ g_p \end{pmatrix}.$$

Let P_j be the orthogonal projection in H onto the affine subspace $R_j f = g_j$, and let

$$P_j^\omega = (1 - \omega)I + \omega P_j, \tag{3.2}$$
$$P^\omega = P_p^\omega \ldots P_1^\omega$$

where ω is a relaxation parameter. Then, Kaczmarz's method (with relaxation) for the solution of (3.1) reads

$$f^k = P^\omega f^{k-1}, \quad k = 1, 2, \ldots \tag{3.3}$$

with $f^0 \in H$ arbitrary. We shall show that, under certain assumptions, f^k converges to a solution of (3.1) if (3.1) is consistent and to a generalized solution if not.

For $\omega = 1$, (3.3) is the classical Kaczmarz method (without relaxation). Its geometrical interpretation is obvious, see Fig. V.9: Starting out from f^0 we obtain f^1 by successive orthogonal projections onto the affine subspaces $R_j f = g_j$, $j = 1, \ldots, p$.

For the actual computation we need a more explicit form of (3.3). To begin with we compute P_j. Since $P_j f - f \perp \ker(R_j)$ there is $u_j \in H_j$ such that

$$P_j f = f + R_j^* u_j.$$

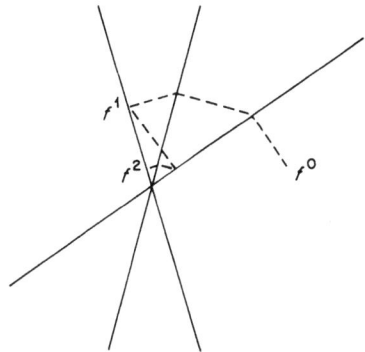

FIG. V.9 Kaczmarz's method for three equations in $\mathbb{R}^2$.

From $R_j P_j f = g_j$ we get

$$R_j R_j^* u_j = g_j - R_j f.$$

Since R_j is surjective, R_j^* and hence $R_j R_j^*$ is injective, and we can write

$$u_j = (R_j R_j^*)^{-1}(g_j - R_j f).$$

Thus we obtain for P_j

$$P_j f = f + R_j^* (R_j R_j^*)^{-1}(g_j - R_j f). \tag{3.4}$$

This leads to the following alternative form of (3.3):

$$\begin{aligned} f_0 &= f^k, \\ f_j &= P_j^\omega f_{j-1} = f_{j-1} + \omega R_j^*(R_j R_j^*)^{-1}(g_j - R_j f_{j-1}), \quad j = 1, \ldots, p, \\ f^{k+1} &= f_p. \end{aligned} \tag{3.5}$$

For the convergence proof we need some lemmas. As a general reference we recommend Yosida (1968).

LEMMA 3.1 Let T be a linear map in H with $\|T\| \leq 1$. Then,

$$H = \ker(I - T) \oplus \overline{\text{range}(I - T)}.$$

Proof For an arbitrary linear bounded map A in H we have

$$H = \ker(A^*) \oplus \overline{\text{range}(A)}.$$

The lemma follows by putting $A = I - T$ and showing that

$$\ker(I - T) = \ker(I - T^*). \tag{3.6}$$

Let $g \in \ker(I - T)$, i.e. $g = Tg$. Then

$$(g, T^* g) = (Tg, g) = (g, g).$$

It follows that
$$\|g - T^*g\|^2 = (g - T^*g, g - T^*g)$$
$$= (g, g) - 2(g, T^*g) + (T^*g, T^*g)$$
$$= -(g, g) + \|T^*g\|^2$$
$$\leq -(g, g) + \|T^*\|^2 \|g\|^2$$
$$\leq 0.$$

Hence $g \in \ker(I - T^*)$. This shows that
$$\ker(I - T) \subseteq \ker(I - T^*)$$
and the opposite inclusion follows by symmetry. This establishes (3.6). □

Rather than dealing with the affine linear orthogonal projections P_j we start with linear orthogonal projections Q_j in H. As in (3.2) we put
$$Q_j^\omega = (1 - \omega)I + \omega Q_j,$$
$$Q^\omega = Q_p^\omega \ldots Q_1^\omega.$$

Since $Q_j = Q_j^2 = Q_j^*$ one verifies easily that
$$\|Q_j^\omega\| \leq 1, \quad 0 < \omega < 2, \tag{3.7}$$
$$\|Q_j^\omega f\|^2 - \|f\|^2 = (2 - \omega)\omega(\|Q_j f\|^2 - \|f\|^2). \tag{3.8}$$

LEMMA 3.2 Let $(f_k)_{k=0, 1, \ldots}$ be a sequence in H such that
$$\|f_k\| \leq 1, \quad \lim_{k \to \infty} \|Q^\omega f_k\| = 1.$$
Then we have for $0 < \omega < 2$
$$\lim_{k \to \infty} (I - Q^\omega) f_k = 0.$$

Proof The proof is by induction with respect to the number p of factors in Q^ω. For $p = 1$ we have
$$\|(I - Q^\omega) f_k\|^2 = \|(I - Q_1^\omega) f_k\|^2 = \omega^2 \|(I - Q_1) f_k\|^2$$
$$= \omega^2 (\|f_k\|^2 + \|Q_1 f_k\|^2 - 2(f_k, Q_1 f_k))$$
$$= \omega^2 (\|f_k\|^2 - \|Q_1 f_k\|^2)$$
$$= \frac{\omega}{2 - \omega} (\|f_k\|^2 - \|Q_1^\omega f_k\|^2)$$

where we have used (3.8). If $\|f_k\| \leq 1$, $\|Q_1^\omega f_k\| \to 1$ it follows that, for $0 < \omega < 2$, $\|(I - Q^\omega) f_k\| \to 0$, hence the lemma for $p = 1$. Now assume the lemma to be correct for $p - 1$ factors. We put
$$Q^\omega = Q_p^\omega S^\omega, \quad S^\omega = Q_{p-1}^\omega \ldots Q_1^\omega.$$

We then have
$$(I - Q^\omega)f_k = (I - S^\omega)f_k + (S^\omega - Q^\omega)f_k \qquad (3.9)$$
$$= (I - S^\omega)f_k + (I - Q_p^\omega)S^\omega f_k.$$

Now let $\|f_k\| \leq 1$, $\|Q^\omega f_k\| \to 1$. Because of (3.7) we have
$$\|Q^\omega f_k\| = \|Q_p^\omega S^\omega f_k\| \leq \|S^\omega f_k\| \leq \|f_k\|,$$
hence $\|S^\omega f_k\| \to 1$ and, of course, $\|S^\omega f_k\| \leq 1$. Since the lemma is correct for $p - 1$ factors, $(I - S^\omega)f_k \to 0$. Applying the lemma for the single factor Q_p^ω to the sequence $f'_k = S^\omega f_k$ we also obtain $(I - Q_p^\omega)S^\omega f_k \to 0$. Hence, from (3.9), it follows that $(I - Q^\omega)f_k \to 0$. This is the lemma for p factors, and the proof is finished. □

LEMMA 3.3 For $0 < \omega < 2$, $(Q^\omega)^k$ converges, as $k \to \infty$, strongly to the orthogonal projection onto $\ker(I - Q^\omega)$.

Proof Let T be the orthogonal projection onto $\ker(I - Q^\omega)$. From Lemma 3.1 and (3.7) we know that
$$H = \ker(I - Q^\omega) \oplus \overline{\text{range}(I - Q^\omega)}, \qquad (3.10)$$
hence $I - T$ is the orthogonal projection onto $\overline{\text{range}(I - Q^\omega)}$. Thus,
$$(I - T)(I - Q^\omega) = I - Q^\omega,$$
$$(I - Q^\omega)T = 0.$$

From the first equation we get $T = TQ^\omega$, from the second one $T = Q^\omega T$. In particular, T and Q^ω commute.

Now let $f \in H$. The sequence $(\|(Q^\omega)^k f\|)_{k = 0, 1, \ldots}$ is decreasing, hence its limit c exists. If $c = 0$ we get from $T = Q^\omega T = TQ^\omega$
$$Tf = (Q^\omega)^k Tf = T(Q^\omega)^k f \to 0$$
as $k \to \infty$, hence
$$Tf = 0, \lim_{k \to \infty} (Q^\omega)^k f = 0,$$
i.e. $(Q^\omega)^k f \to Tf$. If $c > 0$ we put
$$g_k = \|(Q^\omega)^k f\|^{-1} (Q^\omega)^k f.$$
Then we have
$$\|g_k\| = 1, \lim_{k \to \infty} \|Q^\omega g_k\| = 1,$$
hence we obtain from Lemma 3.2
$$\lim_{k \to \infty} (I - Q^\omega)g_k = 0$$
or
$$\lim_{k \to \infty} (I - Q^\omega)(Q^\omega)^k f = 0.$$

It follows that $(Q^\omega)^k$ converges strongly to 0 on range $(I - Q^\omega)$, and this extends to the closure since the $(Q^\omega)^k$ are uniformly bounded. On $\ker(I - Q^\omega)$, $(Q^\omega)^k$ converges trivially to I. The lemma follows from (3.10). □

LEMMA 3.4 For $0 < \omega < 2$ we have
$$\ker(I - Q^\omega) = \bigcap_{j=1}^{p} \ker(I - Q_j).$$

Proof A fixed point of Q_j is also a fixed point of Q_j^ω. This settles the inclusion '⊃'.

On the other hand, If $f = Q^\omega f$, then, from (3.7),
$$\|f\| = \|Q_p^\omega \ldots Q_2^\omega Q_1^\omega f\| = \|Q^\omega f\| \le \|f\|.$$

Hence, $\|Q^\omega f\| = \|f\|$, and from (3.8), $\|Q_1 f\| = \|f\|$. Since Q_1 is a projection, $Q_1 f = f$. Since now
$$f = Q_p^\omega \ldots Q_2^\omega f$$
we can show in the same way that $Q_2 f = f$ and so forth, $Q_3 f = \ldots = Q_p f = f$. This settles the inclusion '⊂'. □

LEMMA 3.5 For $0 < \omega < 2$, $(Q^\omega)^k$ converges strongly, as $k \to \infty$, to the orthogonal projection onto
$$\bigcap_{j=1}^{p} \ker(I - Q_j).$$

Proof This follows immediately from the two preceding lemmas. □

Now we can state the convergence theorem of the geometric theory.

THEOREM 3.6 Assume that (3.1) has a solution. Then, if $0 < \omega < 2$ and $f^0 \in \text{range}(R^*)$ (e.g. $f^0 = 0$), f^k converges, as $k \to \infty$, to the solution of (3.1) with minimal norm.

Proof Let Q_j be the orthogonal projection onto $\ker(R_j)$, and let f be any solution of (3.1). Then, for $h \in H$,
$$P_j h = f + Q_j(h - f),$$
$$P_j^\omega h = f + Q_j^\omega(h - f),$$
$$P^\omega h = f + Q^\omega(h - f),$$
$$(P^\omega)^k h = f + (Q^\omega)^k(h - f).$$

According to Lemma 3.5,
$$f^k = (P^\omega)^k f^0 \to f + T(f^0 - f) = (I - T)f + Tf^0$$
as $k \to \infty$ where T is the orthogonal projection onto
$$\ker(R) = \bigcap_{j=1}^{p} \ker(R_j).$$

If $f^0 \in \text{range}(R^*) = \text{range}(R_1^*) + \ldots + \text{range}(R_p^*)$, then $Tf^0 = 0$ and $(I-T)f$ is the solution of (3.1) with minimal norm, see IV.1. □

So far we have considered the geometrical theory of Kaczmarz's method. We obtain an entirely different view if we resolve the recursion (3.5). Putting

$$f_j = f_0 + \sum_{k=1}^{j} R_k^* u_k, \quad j = 1, \ldots, p$$

in (3.5) we get

$$f_0 + \sum_{k=1}^{j} R_k^* u_k = f_0 + \sum_{k=1}^{j-1} R_k^* u_k + \omega R_j^* (R_j R_j^*)^{-1} \left(g_j - R_j f_0 - \sum_{k=1}^{j-1} R_j R_k^* u_k \right).$$

Using the injectivity of R_j^* we solve for u_j, obtaining

$$R_j R_j^* u_j = \omega \left(g_j - R_j f_0 - \sum_{k=1}^{j-1} R_j R_k^* u_k \right). \tag{3.11}$$

Now let

$$u = \begin{pmatrix} u_1 \\ \vdots \\ u_p \end{pmatrix}.$$

If we decompose

$$RR^* = \begin{pmatrix} R_1 R_1^* & \ldots & R_1 R_p^* \\ \vdots & & \vdots \\ R_p R_1^* & \ldots & R_p R_p^* \end{pmatrix} = D + L + L^*,$$

$$D = \begin{pmatrix} R_1 R_1^* & & 0 \\ & \ddots & \\ 0 & & R_p R_p^* \end{pmatrix}, \quad L = \begin{pmatrix} 0 & & & \\ R_2 R_1^* & 0 & & \\ \vdots & & \ddots & \\ R_p R_1^* & \ldots & R_p R_{p-1}^* & 0 \end{pmatrix}$$

then we can rewrite (3.11) as

$$Du = \omega(g - Rf_0 - Lu).$$

Solving for u we obtain

$$u = \omega(D + \omega L)^{-1}(g - Rf_0),$$

hence

$$f_p = f_0 + \sum_{k=0}^{p-1} R_k^* u_k$$

$$= f_0 + R^* u$$

$$= f_0 + \omega R^*(D + \omega L)^{-1}(g - Rf_0)$$

$$= B_\omega f_0 + b_\omega,$$

$$B_\omega = I - \omega R^*(D + \omega L)^{-1} R, \quad b_\omega = \omega R^*(D + \omega L)^{-1} g. \tag{3.12}$$

The Kaczmarz method for solving

$$Rf = g \qquad (3.13)$$

now simply reads

$$f^{k+1} = B_\omega f^k + b_\omega \qquad (3.14)$$

with $f^0 \in H$ arbitrary.

If (3.13) has a solution, the solution with minimal norm is $f = R^* u$ where

$$RR^* u = g, \qquad (3.15)$$

see IV.1. We want to relate (3.14) to the SOR method (successive over-relaxation, Young (1971)) for (3.15) which reads

$$u^{k+1} = (1 - \omega) u^k + \omega D^{-1} (g - L u^{k+1} - L^* u^k).$$

After some algebra this can be written as

$$u^{k+1} = C_\omega u^k + c_\omega, \qquad (3.16)$$

$$C_\omega = I - \omega (D + \omega L)^{-1} RR^*, \qquad c_\omega = \omega (D + \omega L)^{-1} g.$$

Note that $R^* C_\omega = B_\omega R^*$ and $R^* c_\omega = b_\omega$. Hence, carrying out the SOR method (3.16) with $f^k = R^* u^k$ leads precisely to the Kaczmarz method (3.14). This makes it possible to analyse Kaczmarz's method in the framework of SOR. In order to avoid purely technical difficulties we assume in the following that H and H_j are finite dimensional.

LEMMA 3.7 Let $0 < \omega < 2$. Then, range (R^*) is an invariant subspace and $\ker(R)$ the eigenspace for the eigenvalue 1 of B_ω. The eigenvalues of the restriction B'_ω of B_ω to range (R^*) are precisely the eigenvalues $\neq 1$ of C_ω.

Proof From the explicit expressions for B_ω, C_ω it is obvious that range (R^*), $\ker(R)$ are invariant subspaces of B_ω and range $((D + \omega L)^{-1} R)$, $\ker(R^*)$ are invariant subspaces of C_ω. For the latter ones we have

$$\text{range}((D + \omega L)^{-1} R) \cap \ker(R^*) = \langle 0 \rangle. \qquad (3.17)$$

For if

$$y = (D + \omega L)^{-1} Rz, \qquad R^* y = 0$$

with some $z \in H$, then

$$((D + \omega L) y, y) = (Rz, y) = (z, R^* y) = 0.$$

Hence

$$((2D + \omega L + \omega L^*) y, y) = ((D + \omega L) y, y) + ((D + \omega L^*) y, y) = 0.$$

Since $2D + \omega L + \omega L^*$ is positive definite for $0 < \omega < 2$ it follows that $y = 0$.

Now let λ be an eigenvalue of B'_ω, i.e.

$$(1 - \lambda) f = \omega R^* (D + \omega L)^{-1} Rf, \qquad f \in \text{range}(R^*)$$

and $f \neq 0$. Because of (3.17) we must have $\lambda \neq 1$. It follows that

$$f = R^* (D + \omega L)^{-1} Rg$$

with some $g \neq 0$, and
$$B_\omega f - \lambda f = (B_\omega R^* - \lambda R^*)(D + \omega L)^{-1} Rg = 0.$$
Because of $B_\omega R^* = R^* C_\omega$ this can be rewritten as
$$R^*(C_\omega - \lambda I)(D + \omega L)^{-1} Rg = 0.$$
Since range $(D + \omega L)^{-1} R$ is an invariant subspace of C_ω satisfying (3.17) it follows that
$$(C_\omega - \lambda I)(D + \omega L)^{-1} Rg = 0,$$
hence λ is eigenvalue of C_ω.

Conversely, if $C_\omega u = \lambda u$ with $\lambda \neq 1$, $u \neq 0$, then
$$(1 - \lambda)u = \omega(D + \omega L)^{-1} RR^* u,$$
hence $u \in$ range $(D + \omega L)^{-1} R$ and therefore, because of (3.17), $f = R^* u \neq 0$. It follows that
$$\begin{aligned} B_\omega f - \lambda f &= B_\omega R^* u - \lambda R^* u \\ &= R^* C_\omega u - \lambda R^* u \\ &= R^*(C_\omega u - \lambda u) \\ &= 0, \end{aligned}$$
i.e. λ is eigenvalue of B'_ω.

It remains to show that ker (R) is the eigenspace for the eigenvalue 1 of B_ω. Let $u \neq 0$ and $B_\omega u = u$. Then,
$$R^*(D + \omega L)^{-1} Ru = 0$$
and (3.17) implies $u \in \ker(R)$. Since $B_\omega u = u$ for $u \in \ker(R)$ is obvious the proof is complete. □

The spectral radius $\rho(B)$ of a matrix B is the maximum of the absolute values of the eigenvalues of B. The following lemma uses standard arguments of numerical analysis.

LEMMA 3.8 Let $0 < \omega < 2$. Then, the restriction B'_ω of B_ω to range (R^*) satisfies
$$\rho(B'_\omega) < 1.$$

Proof According to Lemma 3.7 it suffices to show that the eigenvalues $\neq 1$ of C_ω are < 1 in absolute value. Let $C_\omega u = \lambda u$ with $\lambda \neq 1$ and $u \neq 0$, Then,
$$((1 - \omega)D - \omega L^*)u = \lambda(D + \omega L)u. \tag{3.18}$$
We normalize u such that $(u, Du) = 1$ and we put $(Lu, u) = a = \alpha + i\beta$ with α, β real. Forming the inner product of (3.18) with u we obtain
$$1 - \omega - \omega \bar{a} = \lambda(1 + \omega a),$$

hence
$$|\lambda|^2 = \frac{(1-\omega-\omega\alpha)^2 + \omega^2\beta^2}{(1+\omega\alpha)^2 + \omega^2\beta^2}. \tag{3.19}$$

Since $RR^* = D + L + L^*$ is positive semi-definite we have $1 + a + \bar{a} = 1 + 2\alpha \geq 0$, hence $\alpha \geq -1/2$. We can exclude $\alpha = -1/2$ since in that case $|\lambda| = 1$. For $\alpha > -1/2$ we have $|1-\omega-\alpha\omega| < |1+\alpha\omega|$ as long as $0 < \omega < 2$, and (3.19) implies that $|\lambda| < 1$. □

Now we come to the main result of the SOR theory of Kaczmarz's method.

THEOREM 3.9   Let $0 < \omega < 2$. Then, for $f^0 \in \text{range}(R^*)$, e.g. $f_0 = 0$, the Kaczmarz method (3.14) converges to the unique solution $f_\omega \in \text{range}(R^*)$ of
$$R^*(D+\omega L)^{-1}(g - Rf_\omega) = 0. \tag{3.20}$$

If (3.13) has a solution, then f_ω is the solution of (3.13) with minimal norm. Otherwise,
$$f_\omega = f_M + 0(\omega) \tag{3.21}$$
where f_M minimizes
$$(D^{-1}(g - Rf), g - Rf) \tag{3.22}$$
in H.

Proof   Since $f^0, b_\omega \in \text{range}(R^*)$ the iteration takes place in $\text{range}(R^*)$ where B_ω is a contraction, see Lemma 3.8. Hence the convergence of f^k to the unique solution $f_\omega \in \text{range}(R^*)$ of
$$f_\omega = B_\omega f_\omega + b_\omega \tag{3.23}$$
follows from the elementary theory of iterative methods, see e.g. Young (1971), equation (3.23) is equivalent to (3.20). For the proof of (3.21) it suffices to remark that f_M is determined uniquely by
$$R^*D^{-1}(g - Rf_M) = 0, \quad f_M \in \text{range}(R^*), \tag{3.24}$$
see Theorem IV.1.1 with $A = D^{-1/2}R$ and that (3.23) differs from (3.24) only by $0(\omega)$. □

We want to make a few comments.

(1) The convergence rate in Theorem 3.9 is geometrical.
(2) Even though the treatment of Kaczmarz's method in Lemma 3.8 is quite analogous to the usual proofs for SOR, there are some striking differences between Theorem 3.9 and the classical SOR convergence results. In the latter ones, the parameter ω is used only to speed up convergence. In Theorem 3.9, ω not only has an effect on the convergence behaviour (see the next section) but it also determines, at least in the inconsistent case, what the method converges to. All we know from (3.21) is that for ω small, f_ω is close to the Moore–Penrose

generalized solution of $Rf = g$ with respect to the inner product $(f, g)_D = (D^{-1}f, g)$. Furthermore, the limit f_ω not only depends on ω but also on the arrangement of the equations $R_j f = g_j$ in the system $Rf = g$.

V.4 Algebraic Reconstruction Technique (ART)

By ART we mean the application of Kaczmarz's method to Radon's integral equation. Depending on how the discretization is carried out we come to different versions of ART.

V.4.1. *The Fully Discrete Case*

Here, Radon's integral equation is turned into a linear system of equations by what is called a collocation method with piecewise constant trial functions in numerical analysis. We consider only the two-dimensional case, the extension to higher dimensions being obvious.

Suppose we want to solve the equations

$$\int_{L_j} f(x)\,dx = g_j, \qquad j = 1, \ldots, N \tag{4.1}$$

with straight lines L_j for the function f which is concentrated in Ω^2. First we discretize the function f by decomposing it into pixels (= picture elements), i.e. we cover Ω^2 by little squares S_m, $m = 1, \ldots, M$ and assume f to be constant in each square. This amounts to replacing the function f by a vector $F \in \mathbb{R}^M$ whose mth component is the value of f in S_m. Now let

$$a_{jm} = \text{length of } (L_j \cap S_m) \tag{4.2}$$

Since L_j meets only a small fraction ($\sqrt{M}$, roughly) of the pixels, most of the a_{jm} are zero. Putting

$$a_j = (a_{j1}, \ldots, a_{jM})^\top,$$

(4.1) can be rewritten as

$$a_j^\top F = g_j, \qquad j = 1, \ldots, N. \tag{4.3}$$

It is to this linear system that we apply Kaczmarz's method with

$$R_j F = a_j^\top F, \qquad H = \mathbb{R}^M, \qquad H_j = \mathbb{R}^1.$$

Since for $\alpha \in \mathbb{R}^1$

$$R_j^* \alpha = \alpha a_j, \qquad R_j R_j^* \alpha = \alpha |a_j|^2$$

with the euclidean norm, the iteration (3.5) reads

$$F_j = F_{j-1} + \frac{\omega}{|a_j|^2}(g_j - a_j^\top F_{j-1})a_j, \qquad j = 1, \ldots, N. \tag{4.4}$$

This describes one step of the ART iteration, transforming the kth iterate $F^k = F_0$ into the $(k+1)$st iterate $F^{k+1} = F_N$.

The implementation of (4.4) requires a subroutine returning for each j a list of pixels which are hit by L_j and the non-zero components a_{jl} of a_j. Since there are only $O(\sqrt{M})$ such pixels, each step of (4.4) changes only $O(\sqrt{M})$ pixel values and needs only $O(\sqrt{M})$ operations. Thus, one step of the ART iteration requires $O(N\sqrt{M})$ operations. For the parallel scanning geometry with p directions and $2q+1$ readings each we have $M = (2q+1)^2$, $N = (2q+1)p$. If $p = \pi q$ we obtain $O(p^3)$ operations per step. This is the number of operations of the complete filtered backprojection algorithm (1.17). We see that ART is competitive—for the parallel geometry—only if the number of steps is small.

A definite advantage of ART lies in its versatility. It can be carried out for any scanning geometry and even for incomplete data problems. This does not say that the results of ART are satisfactory for such problems, see Chapter VI.

The convergence of ART follows from Theorem 3.9: if F^0 is in $\langle a_1, \ldots, a_N \rangle$ (e.g. $F^0 = 0$), then F^k converges to a generalized solution (in the sense of (3.20)) F_ω of (4.3) if $0 < \omega < 2$. If (4.3) is consistent (which is unlikely in view of the discretization errors) then F_ω is the solution of least norm, otherwise F_ω converges to the minimizer of

$$\sum_{j=1}^{N} \frac{1}{|a_j|^2} (g_j - a_j^T F)^2$$

as $\omega \to 0$.

V.4.2. The Semidiscrete Case

Here we use a moment type discretization of the Radon integral equation. Again we restrict ourselves to the plane. Let $L_{jl}, j = 1, \ldots, p, l = 1, \ldots, q$ be subdomains of Ω^2 (e.g. strips, cones, ...) and let χ_{jl} be a positive weight function on L_{jl}. We assume that $L_{jl} \cap L_{jk} = 0$ if $l \neq k$. As an example, $L_{jl}, l = 1, \ldots, q$ may be parallel non-overlapping thin strips orthogonal to the direction θ_j. This is a model for parallel scanning in CT, allowing for finite width of the rays and detector inhomogeneities. It is clear that other scanning modes can also be modelled in this way, see Section V.5.

The system of equations we want to solve is

$$\int_{L_{jl}} \chi_{jl}(x) f(x) \, dx = g_{jl}, \quad j = 1, \ldots, p, \quad l = 1, \ldots, q. \tag{4.5}$$

Putting, with $(,)$ the inner product in $L_2(\Omega^2)$,

$$R_j f = \begin{pmatrix} (\chi_{j1}, f) \\ \vdots \\ (\chi_{jq}, f) \end{pmatrix}, \quad g_j = \begin{pmatrix} g_{j1} \\ \vdots \\ g_{jq} \end{pmatrix}$$

we can apply Kaczmarz's method to (4.5) with $H = L_2(\Omega)$, $H_j = \mathbb{R}^q$. We have for $h \in \mathbb{R}^q$

$$R_j^* h = \sum_{l=1}^{q} h_l \chi_{jl}$$

$$(R_j R_j^* h)_k = \sum_{l=1}^{q} h_l (\chi_{jl}, \chi_{jk}).$$

Because of our assumption on L_{jl}, this reduces to

$$(R_j R_j^* h)_k = (\chi_{jk}, \chi_{jk}) h_k.$$

Thus the iteration (3.5) reads

$$f_j = f_{j-1} + \omega \sum_{l=1}^{q} \frac{1}{\|\chi_{jl}\|^2} (g_{jl} - (\chi_{jl}, f_{j-1})) \chi_{jl}$$

or

$$f_j(x) = f_{j-1}(x) + \frac{\omega}{\|\chi_{jl}\|^2} (g_{jl} - (\chi_{jl}, f_{j-1})) \chi_{jl}(x) \quad (4.6)$$

where $l = l(j, x)$ is the unique index for which $x \in L_{jl}$. With j running from 1 to p, (4.6) describes a complete step of the semi-continuous ART algorithm with $f^k = f_0$, $f^{k+1} = f_p$. An application of Theorem 3.6 shows that the method converges for $0 < \omega < 2$ to the solution of least norm of (4.5), provided $f^0 \in \langle \chi_{11}, \ldots, \chi_{pq} \rangle$, e.g. $f^0 = 0$. Since in that case all the iterates are in the finite dimensional space $\langle \chi_{11}, \ldots, \chi_{pq} \rangle$, (4.6) can in principle be executed without further discretizations. However, the computational cost is clearly prohibitive. Therefore we use a pixel decomposition of f as above, resulting in an algorithm very similar to (4.4).

V.4.3. Complete Projections

Here we solve the system

$$R_{\theta_j} f = g_j, \quad j = 1, \ldots, p, \quad \text{or } Rf = g \quad (4.7)$$

where $\theta_j \in S^{n-1}$ are such that $\theta_j \neq \pm \theta_i$ for $i \neq j$ and f is a function on Ω^n. From Theorem II.1.6 we know that $\mathbf{R}_\theta: L_2(\Omega^n) \to L_2([-1, +1], w^{1-n})$, $w(s) = (1-s^2)^{1/2}$ is bounded. It is also surjective since

$$f(x) = \frac{1}{|S^{n-2}|} (w(x \cdot \theta))^{1-n} g(x \cdot \theta), \quad x \in \Omega^n$$

is a solution of $\mathbf{R}_\theta f = g$. Therefore we can apply Kaczmarz's method (3.3) to (4.1) with

$$H = L_2(\Omega^n), \quad H_j = L_2([-1, +1], w^{1-n}), \quad R_j = \mathbf{R}_{\theta_j}$$

From II.1 we obtain for the adjoint $\mathbf{R}_{\theta_j}^*$ of $\mathbf{R}_{\theta_j}$ as an operator from H onto H_j:

$$\mathbf{R}_{\theta_j}^* g(x) = \mathbf{R}_{\theta_j}^\# w^{1-n} g(x) = (w^{1-n} g)(x \cdot \theta_j) \tag{4.8}$$

$$\mathbf{R}_{\theta_j} \mathbf{R}_{\theta_j}^* g(s) = \int_{\theta_j^\perp \cap \Omega^n} (w^{1-n} g)((s\theta_j + y)\theta_j) \, dy$$

$$= \int_{|y| < w(s)} (w^{1-n} g)(s) \, dy$$

$$= \frac{1}{n-1} |S^{n-2}| g(s).$$

According to (3.4) the orthogonal projection P_j is

$$P_j f(x) = f(x) + \frac{n-1}{|S^{n-2}|} (w^{1-n} (g_j - \mathbf{R}_{\theta_j} f))(x \cdot \theta_j), \tag{4.9}$$

and the iteration in (3.5) assumes the form

$$f_j(x) = f_{j-1}(x) + \omega' (w^{1-n} (g_j - \mathbf{R}_{\theta_j} f_{j-1}))(x \cdot \theta_j), \tag{4.10}$$

$$j = 1, \ldots, p, \qquad \omega' = \omega \frac{n-1}{|S^{n-2}|}.$$

From Theorem (3.6) we know that, if (4.1) is consistent and if $f^0 \in \text{range}(R^*)$, i.e. if

$$f^0(x) = \sum_{j=1}^p h_j(x \cdot \theta_j), \qquad h_j \in L_2([-1, +1], w^{n-1})$$

(e.g. $f^0 = 0$), then Kaczmarz's method (3.3) or (3.5) converges to a solution of (4.1) with minimal norm.

Thus, in principle, the question of convergence (at least in the consistent case) is settled. However, this result is not very satisfactory from a practical point of view. It does not say anything about the speed of convergence, nor does it give any hint as to how to choose the relaxation parameter ω to speed up convergence. In order to deal with such questions we shall give a deeper convergence analysis by making full use of the specific properties of the operators $\mathbf{R}_{\theta_j}$.

As in IV.3 we introduce the functions

$$C_{m,j}(x) = C_m^{n/2}(x \cdot \theta_j)$$

in Ω^n. We show that $C_{m,1}, \ldots, C_{m,p}$ are linearly independent for $m \geq p-1$. For, assume that

$$\alpha_1 C_{m,1} + \ldots + \alpha_p C_{m,p} = 0 \tag{4.11}$$

in Ω^n, Consider the differential operator

$$D = \frac{\partial}{\partial x_{l_2}} \cdots \frac{\partial}{\partial x_{l_p}}$$

of order $p-1$. Since $\theta_1 \neq \pm \theta_j$ for $j \neq 1$ we have $\theta_1^\perp + \theta_j^\perp = \mathbb{R}^n$ for $j = 2, \ldots, p$. Thus, each derivative in D can be written as

$$\frac{\partial}{\partial x_{l_j}} = a_j D'_j + b_j D''_j, \quad j = 2, \ldots, p$$

where D'_j, D''_j are derivatives in directions perpendicular to θ_1, θ_j, respectively. Now we write $D = D' + D''$ with

$$D'' = b_2 \ldots b_p D''_2 \ldots D''_p,$$

and D' is a sum of differential operators each of which contains a derivative D'_j. Hence

$$D' C_{m,1} = 0,$$
$$D'' C_{m,j} = 0, \quad j = 2, \ldots, p$$

and (4.11) implies that

$$\alpha_1 D C_{m,1} = \alpha_1 D'' C_{m,1} = D'' (\alpha_1 C_{m,1} + \ldots + \alpha_p C_{m,p}) = 0$$

in Ω^n. Without loss of generality we may assume that the components θ_l^1 of θ^1 do not vanish. If this should be violated we rotate the coordinate system a little. Since

$$D C_{m,1}(x) = \theta_{l_2}^1 \ldots \theta_{l_p}^1 (C_m^{n/2})^{(p-1)} (x \cdot \theta_1)$$

it follows that $C_m^{n/2}$ is a polynomial of degree $< p-1$, unless $\alpha_1 = 0$. Hence, for $m \geq p-1$, we must have $\alpha_1 = 0$. In the same way, we show that $\alpha_j = 0$, $j = 2, \ldots, p$. This establishes our claim that $C_{m,1}, \ldots, C_{m,p}$ are linearly independent for $m \geq p-1$.

Now we define

$$\mathscr{C}_m = \langle C_{m,1}, \ldots, C_{m,p} \rangle.$$

Note that because of (IV.3.7), $\mathscr{C}_m \perp \mathscr{C}_k$ for $m \neq k$ in $L_2(\Omega^n)$. Because of (4.8) and since the Gegenbauer polynomials form a complete orthogonal set in $L_2([-1, +1], w^{n-1})$ we have

$$\text{range}(\mathbf{R}_{\theta_j}^*) = \langle C_{0,j}, C_{1,j}, \ldots \rangle$$

hence

$$\text{range}(R^*) = \text{range}(\mathbf{R}_{\theta_1}^*) + \ldots + \text{range}(\mathbf{R}_{\theta_p}^*) \quad (4.12)$$

$$= \bigoplus_{m=0}^{\infty} \mathscr{C}_m.$$

Incidentally, (4.12) implies that R^* has closed range.

Let f_M be the minimal norm solution of (4.1), i.e. the solution of (4.7) in range (R^*), see IV.1. The errors

$$e^k = f_M - f^k$$

satisfy

$$e^{k+1} = Q^\omega e^k, \quad Q^\omega = Q_p^\omega \ldots Q_1^\omega, \quad Q_j^\omega = (1-\omega)I + \omega Q_j$$

where Q_j is the orthogonal projection on ker $(\mathbf{R}_{\theta_j})$, compare the proof of Theorem 3.6. Q_j can be obtained from (4.10) by putting $g_j = 0$, i.e.

$$Q_j f(x) = f(x) - \frac{n-1}{|S^{n-2}|} (w^{1-n} \mathbf{R}_{\theta_j} f)(x \cdot \theta_j).$$

We can rewrite (IV.3.4) in the form

$$\mathbf{R}_{\theta_1} C_{m,2} = \alpha_m (\theta_1 \cdot \theta_2) w^{n-1} C_m^{n/2}, \qquad \alpha_m(t) = \frac{\pi^{(n-1)/2}}{\Gamma\left(\frac{n+1}{2}\right)} C_m^{n/2}(t)$$

hence

$$Q_j C_{m,i} = C_{m,i} - \frac{n-1}{|S^{n-2}|} \alpha_m (\theta_i \cdot \theta_j) C_{m,j}. \qquad (4.13)$$

This means that $\mathscr{C}_m$ is an invariant subspace of Q_j, hence of Q_j^ω and of Q^ω. In order to compute the norm $\rho_m(\omega)$ of Q^ω in $\mathscr{C}_m$ we use a matrix representation of Q^ω in $\mathscr{C}_m$. Let $m < p$. Then, the $C_{m,1}, \ldots, C_{m,m+1}$ form a basis of $\mathscr{C}_m$, and we have for each $f \in \mathscr{C}_m$

$$f = \sum_{i=1}^{m+1} a_i C_{m,i}, \qquad Q_j^\omega f = \sum_{i=1}^{m+1} a_i' C_{m,i}$$

for suitable numbers a_i, a_i'. Equation (4.13) translates into

$$a_i' = a_i, \quad i \neq j$$

$$a_j' = a_j - \omega \sum_{k \neq j} \alpha_{m,k,j} a_k,$$

$$\alpha_{m,k,j} = \frac{n-1}{|S^{n-2}|} \alpha_m (\theta_k \cdot \theta_j).$$

Introducing the $m+1 \times m+1$ matrices

$$A_{m,j}^\omega = \begin{pmatrix} 1 & & & & & \\ & 1 & & & & \\ & & \ddots & & & \\ -\omega \alpha_{m,1,j} & \ldots & 1-\omega & \ldots & -\omega \alpha_{m,m+1,j} \\ & & & \ddots & & \\ & & & & & 1 \end{pmatrix}$$

which coincide, except for the jth row, with the unit matrix, we obtain the matrix representation of Q^ω in $\mathscr{C}_m$ in the product form

$$A_m(\omega) = A_{m,m+1}^\omega \ldots A_{m,1}^\omega.$$

From (IV.3.7) we obtain

$$\|f\|_{L_2(\Omega^*)}^2 = c(m,n) a^\mathsf{T} \alpha_m a$$

where $a = (a_1, \ldots, a_{m+1})^T$, $c(m, n)$ is some constant, and

$$(\alpha_m)_{k,j} = \alpha_{m,k,j}.$$

It follows that

$$\rho_m^2(\omega) = \sup_{f \in \mathscr{C}_m} \frac{\|Q^\omega f\|_{L_2(\Omega^n)}}{\|f\|_{L_2(\Omega^n)}}$$

$$= \sup_{a \in \mathbb{R}^{m+1}} \frac{(A_m(\omega)a)^T \alpha_m (A_m(\omega)a)}{a^T \alpha_m a}$$

i.e. $\rho_m^2(\omega)$ is the largest eigenvalue of the $m+1 \times m+1$ eigenvalue problem

$$(A_m(\omega))^T \alpha_m A_m(\omega) a = \rho_m^2(\omega) \alpha_m a. \tag{4.14}$$

Note that α_m, being the Gram matrix of the linearly independent functions $C_{m,1}, \ldots, C_{m,m+1}$ in $L_2(\Omega^n)$, is non-singular.

Now let $f^0 \in$ range (R^*). Since $f_M \in$ range (R^*) and since range (R^*) is an invariant subspace of Q^ω, all errors e^k are in range (R^*). Because of (4.12) we can write

$$e^k = \sum_{m=0}^{\infty} d_{km} e_m^k, \quad e_m^k \in \mathscr{C}_m$$

and

$$e_m^k = (Q^\omega)^k e_m^0.$$

It follows that

$$\|e_m^k\| \leq \rho_m^k(\omega) \|e_m^0\|.$$

We see that $\rho_m^k(\omega)$ determines the rate of decay of that part of e^k which is in $\mathscr{C}_m$. This holds for $m < p$. There is no point in studying the contribution of $\mathscr{C}_m$ with $m \geq p$. The reason is simply that the part of f in $\mathscr{C}_p, \mathscr{C}_{p+1}, \ldots$ is not determined by the data. From our results on resolution in III.2 we know that f can be determined reliably from an m-resolving set of directions if f is essentially b-bandlimited with bandwidth ϑm, $0 < \vartheta < 1$. According to (III.2.2) the number p of directions of an m-resolving set is at least

$$p \geq \binom{m+n-1}{n-1} \geq m+1$$

with equality for $n = 2$. Hence we cannot expect p directions to resolve functions of essential bandwidth p or larger. The Fourier transform of $C_{m,i}$ can be computed from Theorem II.1.1, (IV.3.4) and (VII.3.18): we obtain with some constant $c(n)$

$$\hat{C}_{m,i}(\sigma\theta) = (2\pi)^{(1-n)/2} (\mathbf{R}_\theta U_{m,i})\hat{\,}(\sigma)$$

$$= (2\pi)^{(1-n)/2} \alpha_m(\theta \cdot \theta_i)(w^{n-1} C_m^{n/2})\hat{\,}(\sigma)$$

$$= c(n) i^{-m} \alpha_m(\theta \cdot \theta_i) \sigma^{-n/2} J_{m+n/2}(\sigma).$$

From Debye's formula in the form of (VII.3.20) we see that this assumes values significantly different from zero for $|\sigma| \geq \theta(m+n/2)$ only. It follows that the functions in $\mathscr{C}_m$ cannot be recovered from p projections if $m \geq p$. We also note that, in the language of II.1, the subspaces $\mathscr{C}_m$ do not represent details of size approximately $2\pi/m$ or larger. Hence the $\mathscr{C}_m$ with m small are responsible for the overall features of f while the $\mathscr{C}_m$ with m large contribute to the small details.

The numbers $\rho_m(\omega)$ can easily be computed numerically by solving the eigenvalue problem (4.14) on a computer. We did some calculations in the two-dimensional case. Figure V.10 shows a plot of $\rho_m(\omega)$ for $p = 32$ equally spaced angles φ_j and for $\omega = 1, 0.5$ and 0.1. The angles are arranged in natural order, i.e. $\varphi_j = (j-1)\pi/p, j = 1, \ldots, p$. We see that the behaviour of $\rho_m(\omega)$ depends in a decisive way on the choice of ω. For ω large (e.g. $\omega = 1$), ρ_m decreases from $\rho_0 = 0.86$ to ρ_{p-1} virtually zero, while for ω small (e.g. $\omega = 0.1$), ρ_m increases from the small value $\rho_0 = 0.26$ to $\rho_{p-1} = 0.90$. This has the following practical consequence for the iterates f^k: for ω large, the small details in f are picked up quickly, while the smooth parts of f (e.g. the mean value) converge only slowly. For ω small, the opposite is the case. Thus, choosing ω small has an effect similar to digital filtering (see IV.1) on the early iterates. This may account for the surprisingly small values of ω which are being used in practice. The situation changes drastically if the angles φ_j are permuted in a random way, see Fig. V.11. Now the $\rho_m(\omega)$ are much more favourable for ω large, with values virtually 0 on the first few $\mathscr{C}_m$, and with maximum significantly smaller than for the natural order in Fig. V.10. In fact it is observed in practice that ART performs much better for orderings other than the natural one.

From the point of view of numerical analysis one might want to choose ω such that the largest ρ_m is as small as possible. In Fig. V.10 this is the case for ω close to 0.5. One could also work with different values of ω at each step, mimicking the non-stationary methods of numerical analysis, see Young (1971).

As has been pointed out in IV.1, an iterative method such as ART can only be semiconvergent when applied to an ill-posed problem. An example for this semiconvergence is given in Fig. V.12. The original in Fig. V.12(a), a brain phantom created by Shepp and Logan (1974), has been reconstructed from $p = 256$ projections with $2q+1$, $q = 75$ line integrals each using ART with relaxation parameter $\omega = 0.05$. The data have been contaminated by adding random errors. Figure V.12(b)–(d) show the iterates 2, 4, 40. Obviously, the reconstruction deteriorates after step 4.

V.5 Direct Algebraic Methods

These methods assume a certain rotational invariance of the scanning geometry. They reduce Radon's integral equation to a huge linear system which, due to the rotational invariance, is block Toeplitz or even block cyclic what makes it amenable to the methods of VII.5.

Again let f be supported in the unit ball Ω^n of $\mathbb{R}^n$. We assume the data to come in p groups numbered 0 to $p-1$, the jth group containing q measurements g_{jl},

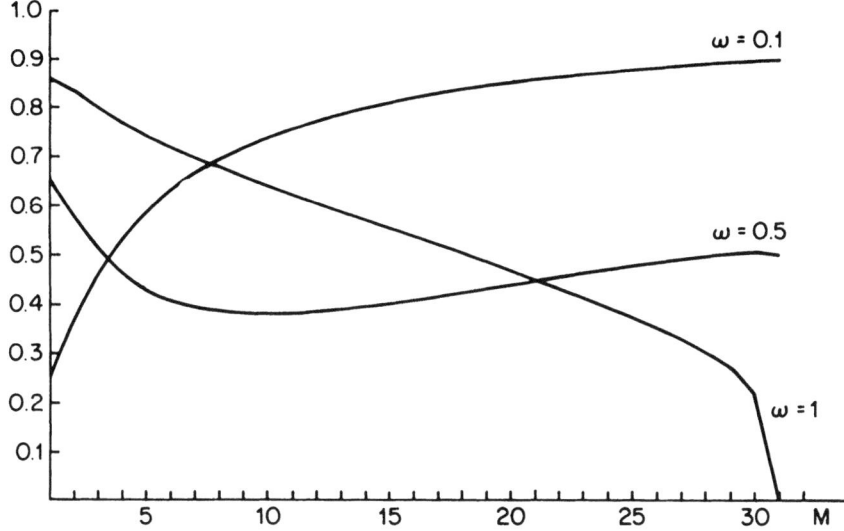

FIG. V.10 The norms $\rho_m(\omega)$ of Q^ω in $\mathscr{C}_m$, $m = 0, \ldots, 31$ for $p = 32$ equally distributed angles in natural order.

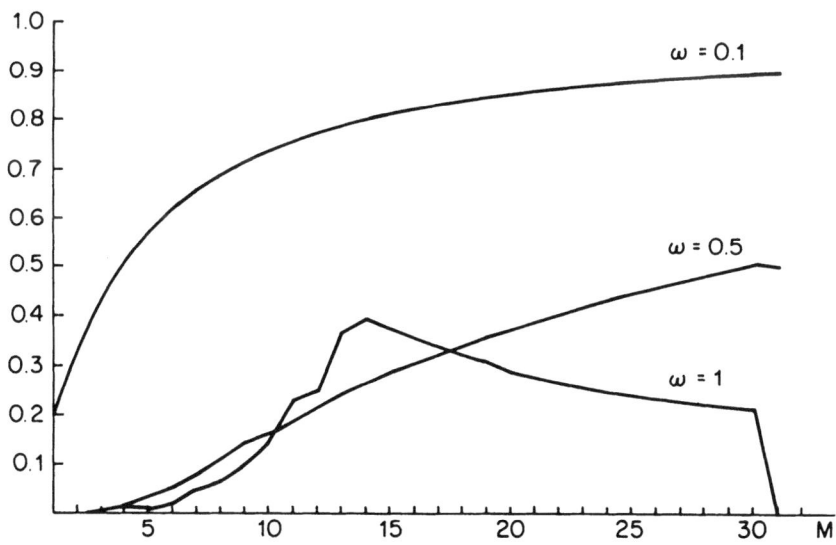

FIG. V.11 Same as Fig. V.10, but with random ordering of the angles.

$l = 1, \ldots, q$. The measurements are assumed to be

$$g_{jl} = (\chi_{jl}, f)_{L_2(\Omega^n)} = R_{jl} f.$$

As in Section V.4 the functions χ_{jl} model the scanning geometry. The supports L_{jl} of χ_{jl} are the rays of the scanning geometry and may be thought of as narrow strips or cones. Such a scanning geometry is called rotational invariant if there is a rotation U such that, for $j = 0, \ldots, p-1$,

$$\chi_{jl} = \chi_{0l} \circ U^{-j}, \qquad l = 1, \ldots, q \tag{5.1}$$

where $\circ$ means composition. If, in addition, $U^p = I$ then the geometry is called cyclic.

We give a few examples of rotational invariant scanning geometries.

V.5.1. Parallel Geometry in the Plane

Let $\theta_j, j = 0, \ldots, p-1$ be p equally spaced directions, i.e. $\theta_j = (\cos \varphi_j, \sin \varphi_j)^T$, $\varphi_j = j\Delta\varphi$ with the angular increment $\Delta\varphi$. Let $w_l, l = 1, \ldots, q$ be some weight functions in $C[-1, +1]$. Put

$$R_{jl} f = \int_{-1}^{+1} w_l(s) \, \mathbf{R}_{\theta_j} f(s) \, ds.$$

From the explicit form of $\mathbf{R}_\theta^\#$ in II.1 we get

$$R_{jl} f = \int_{\Omega^2} w_l(x \cdot \theta_j) f(x) \, dx$$

i.e. we have

$$\chi_{jl}(x) = w_l(x \cdot \theta_j). \tag{5.2}$$

The scanning geometry is obviously rotational invariant, U being the rotation by an angle of $\Delta\varphi$. This is true even in the limited angle case, see VI.2. Typically, the functions w_l have small support, modelling thin beams. Since the supports of the functions w_l are not required to cover all of $[-1, +1]$, we can deal with the exterior and the interior problem, see VI.3 and VI.4. If $\Delta\varphi = 2\pi/p$, then the scanning geometry is cyclic.

V.5.2. Fan Beam and Cone Beam Geometries

Let $a_j, j = 0, \ldots, p-1$ be equally spaced sources on a circle surrounding Ω^n, e.g. in $\mathbb{R}^2$ $a_j = r(\cos \varphi_j, \sin \varphi_j)^T$, $\beta_j = j\Delta\beta$, $\Delta\beta$ the angular increment. Let w_l be some weight function in $C(S^{n-1})$. Put

$$R_{jl}f = \int_{S^{n-1}} w_l(U^{-j}\theta) D_{a_j} f(\theta) \, d\theta$$

where U is the rotation in the plane of the circle of sources around the origin by an angle of $\Delta\beta$. On introducing $x = a_j + t\theta$ we get

$$R_{jl}f = \int_{S^{n-1}} w_l(U^{-j}\theta) \int_0^\infty f(a_j + t\theta) \, dt \, d\theta$$

$$= \int_{\Omega^n} w_l\left(U^{-j} \frac{x - a_j}{|x - a_j|}\right) |x - a_j|^{1-n} f(x) \, dx$$

i.e. we have

$$\chi_{jl}(x) = w_l\left(U^{-j} \frac{x - a_j}{|x - a_j|}\right) |x - a_j|^{1-n}. \tag{5.3}$$

The scanning geometry is obviously rotational invariant and even cyclic if $\Delta\beta = 2\pi/p$. Note that this geometry comprises the majority of the incomplete data problems in Chapter VI.

Rather than solving Radon's integral equation we now solve the linear system

$$R_{jl}f = g_{jl}, \quad j = 0, \ldots, p-1, \quad l = 1, \ldots, q. \tag{5.4}$$

Arranging into groups yields the system

$$R_j f = g_j, \quad j = 0, \ldots, p-1$$

$$R_j = \begin{pmatrix} R_{j1} \\ \vdots \\ R_{jq} \end{pmatrix}, \quad g_j = \begin{pmatrix} g_{j1} \\ \vdots \\ g_{jq} \end{pmatrix}$$

and this in turn is written as

$$Rf = g,$$

$$R = \begin{pmatrix} R_0 \\ \vdots \\ R_{p-1} \end{pmatrix}, \quad g = \begin{pmatrix} g_0 \\ \vdots \\ g_{p-1} \end{pmatrix}.$$

Here, $R: L_2(\Omega^n) \to \mathbb{R}^{pq}$ is a discrete version of the Radon transform.

For solving the underdetermined system (5.4) we can use the

Tikhonov–Phillips method of IV.1; for other methods see the end of this section. This amounts to compute the minimizer f_γ of

$$\|Rf - g\|^2 + \gamma \|f\|^2$$

with the euclidean norm in $\mathbb{R}^{pq}$ and the L_2-norm in $L_2(\Omega^n)$. From (IV.1.6) we get

$$f_\gamma = R^* h, \quad h = (RR^* + \gamma I)^{-1} g. \tag{5.5}$$

The adjoint R^* of R is computed as in Section V.4 to yield

$$R^* h = \sum_{j=0}^{p-1} R_j^* h_j, \quad R_j^* h_j = \sum_{l=1}^{q} h_{jl} \chi_{jl} \tag{5.6}$$

where $h = (h_0, \ldots, h_{p-1})^T$, $h_j = (h_{j1}, \ldots, h_{jq})^T$. Recalling that the χ_{jl} are supported by narrow strips or cones defining the rays we see that (5.6) is basically a discrete backprojection.

The computation of the vector h to be backprojected calls for the solution of the $qp \times qp$ linear system

$$(RR^* + \gamma I)h = g. \tag{5.7}$$

In general, this system is far too large for being solved directly on a computer. However, we shall see that, due to the rotational invariance, (5.7) can be solved quite efficiently by FFT techniques.

The operator RR^* in (5.7) is a $p \times p$ matrix of $q \times q$ blocks $R_i R_j^*$ whose k, l element is

$$(R_i R_j^*)_{kl} = (\chi_{ik}, \chi_{jl})_{L_2(\Omega^n)}.$$

From (5.1) we see that

$$(\chi_{ik}, \chi_{jl})_{L_2(\Omega^n)} = (\chi_{0k} \circ U^{-i}, \chi_{0l} \circ U^{-j})_{L_2(\Omega^n)}$$
$$= (\chi_{0k}, \chi_{0l} \circ U^{i-j})_{L_2(\Omega^n)}$$

depends on $j - i$ only, i.e. we can write

$$R_i R_j^* = S_{j-1}$$
$$(S_j)_{kl} = (\chi_{0k}, \chi_{0l} \circ U^{-j})_{L_2(\Omega^n)} \tag{5.8}$$
$$= (\chi_{0k}, \chi_{jl})_{L_2(\Omega^n)}.$$

Note that $S_{-j} = S_j^T$. With this notation, (5.7) assumes the form

$$\begin{pmatrix} S_0 + \gamma I & S_1 & \cdots & S_{p-1} \\ S_{-1} & S_0 + \gamma I & S_1 \cdots & S_{p-2} \\ & \cdots & & \\ S_{1-p} & \cdots & S_{-1} & S_0 + \gamma I \end{pmatrix} \begin{pmatrix} h_0 \\ \vdots \\ h_{p-1} \end{pmatrix} = \begin{pmatrix} g_0 \\ \vdots \\ g_{p-1} \end{pmatrix}. \tag{5.9}$$

We see that we end up with a system whose matrix is block Toeplitz, and, if the geometry is cyclic, even with a block cyclic convolution, since in that case $S_{p-j} = S_{-j}$. In either case, (5.9) can be solved with $0(pq^2 + pq \log p)$ operations by the methods in VII.5.

We work out the details of the direct algebraic algorithm for a simple parallel scanning geometry in $\mathbb{R}^2$ in which the functions w_l in (5.2) are simply

$$w_l(s) = \begin{cases} 1, & |s - s_l| \leq d/2, \\ 0, & \text{otherwise} \end{cases} \tag{5.10}$$

where s_l, $l = 1, \ldots, q$, are arbitrary numbers in $[-1, +1]$. This means that our data are

$$g_{jl} = \int_{L_{jl}} f(x) \, dx, \quad j = 1, \ldots, p, \quad l = 1, \ldots, q$$

where L_{jl} is the strip of width d perpendicular to θ_j whose axis goes through the point $s_l \theta_j$, i.e.

$$L_{jl} = \{x \in \mathbb{R}^2 : |x \cdot \theta_j - s_l| \leq d/2\}$$

In practice the strips L_{jl} for fixed j will be non-overlapping but this is not necessary for our approach.

The (k, l) element of the matrix S_j is now simply

$$(S_j)_{kl} = \text{area}\,(\Omega^2 \cap L_{0k} \cap L_{jl}) \tag{5.11}$$

and this is $d^2/\sin^2(\theta_j \cdot \theta_0)$ if $L_{0k} \cap L_{jl}$ is inside Ω^2, 0 if $L_{0k} \cap L_{jl}$ is outside Ω^2 and something in between if $L_{0k} \cap L_{jl}$ meets the circumference on Ω^2. Numerical experiments show that the method is quite sensitive with respect to changes in these latter entries of S_j. So these entries have to be carefully computed.

In the cyclic case, i.e. if $\Delta\varphi = 2\pi/p$, the direct algebraic algorithm goes as follows:

Step 1: Compute the matrices S_j from (5.11) and carry out the Fourier transform

$$\hat{S}_k = \frac{1}{p} \sum_{j=0}^{p-1} e^{-2\pi i k j/p} S_j + \frac{\gamma}{p} I, \quad k = 0, \ldots, p-1.$$

Compute and store the matrices $\hat{S}_k^{-1}$, $k = 0, \ldots, p-1$.

Step 2: Carry out the Fourier transform

$$\hat{g}_k = \frac{1}{p} \sum_{j=0}^{p-1} e^{-2\pi i k j/p} g_j, \quad k = 0, \ldots, p-1,$$

compute the vectors

$$\hat{h}_k = \frac{1}{p} (\hat{S}_k)^{-1} \hat{g}_k, \quad k = 0, \ldots, p-1 \tag{5.12}$$

and do the inverse Fourier transform

$$h_j = \sum_{k=0}^{p-1} e^{2\pi i k j/p} \hat{h}_k, \quad j = 0, \ldots, p-1.$$

Step 3: Perform the 'backprojection'

$$f_\gamma(x) = \sum_{\substack{j,l \\ x \in L_{jl}}} h_{jl}.$$

Note that step 1 is preparatory and can be done once and for all as soon as the specifications of a certain CT machine (including a good value for the regularization parameter γ) are known. For each set of data, only steps 2 and 3 must be carried out.

The number of operations is as follows. In step 1 we have to compute a Fourier transform of length p on $q \times q$ matrices. This can be done with $O(q^2 p \log p)$ operations if FFT is used. The Fourier transforms of length p on q—dimensional vectors in step 2 require $O(qp \log p)$ operations while (5.12) needs $O(pq^2)$ operations. The backprojection in step 3 on a $q \times q$ grid can be done with $O(pq^2)$ operations. Thus the total number of operations for step 2 and 3 is $O(pq^2 + pq \log p)$ which is essentially what we found for the filtered backprojection algorithm (1.17).

We conclude this section by pointing out that direct methods are in no way restricted to the computation of the Tikhonov–Phillips regularized solution f_γ. For instance, we may compute the estimate (IV.1.16) for f very much in the same way. In this case we have to replace (5.5) by

$$f_B = \overline{f} + FR^*h, \qquad h = (RFR^* + \Sigma)^{-1}(g - R\overline{f}), \qquad (5.13)$$

see (IV.1.16). Here, F is to be interpreted as integral operator with kernel $F(x, x')$, i.e.

$$Ff(x) = \int_{\Omega^n} F(x, x') f(x') \, dx'.$$

If F is a radial function such as (IV.1.17), then

$$(R_i F R_j^*)_{kl} = \int_{\Omega^n} \int_{\Omega^n} \chi_{ik}(x) F(x, x') \chi_{jl}(x') \, dx \, dx'$$

depends only on $j - i$ provided (5.1) is satisfied. Thus RFR^* is Toeplitz as well as RR^*, and (5.13) can be dealt with, up to an additional smoothing by the integral operator F, exactly in the same way as (5.5). A further possibility is to compute the minimum norm solution of the system (5.4).

Actual reconstructions done with the direct algebraic algorithm can be found in Chapter VI.

V.6 Other Reconstruction Methods

Many other types of algorithms have been suggested. We mention only a few.

V.6.1. The Davison–Grünbaum Method (Davison and Grünbaum, 1981)

Again we take Ω^n to be the reconstruction region. Assume that the projections $g_j = \mathbf{R}_{\theta_j} f$ are available for p directions $\theta_1, \ldots, \theta_p$. Then, the form of Radon's inversion formula suggests to try a reconstruction f_{DG} to f in the form

$$f_{\text{DG}}(x) = \sum_{j=1}^{p} v_j(x \cdot \theta_j), \qquad v_j = w_j * g_j.$$

This is basically what we did in the filtered backprojection algorithm. But now we disregard everything we know about Radon's inversion formula, determining the functions w_j so as to make f_{DG} a good approximation to f.

To begin with we compute

$$\begin{aligned}
f_{\text{DG}}(x) &= \sum_{j=1}^{p} (w_j * g_j)(x \cdot \theta_j) \\
&= \sum_{j=1}^{p} \int_{\mathbb{R}^1} w_j(x \cdot \theta_j - s) g_j(s) \, ds \\
&= \sum_{j=1}^{p} \int_{\mathbb{R}^1} w_j(x \cdot \theta_j - s) \mathbf{R}_{\theta_j} f(s) \, ds \\
&= \sum_{j=1}^{p} \int_{\mathbb{R}^1} \int_{\theta_j^\perp} w_j(x \cdot \theta_j - s) f(s\theta_j + t) \, dt \, ds \\
&= \sum_{j=1}^{p} \int_{\mathbb{R}^n} w_j((x-y) \cdot \theta_j) f(y) \, dy
\end{aligned}$$

where we have put $y = s\theta_j + t$. Thus,

$$f_{\text{DG}} = W * f, \qquad W(x) = \sum_{j=1}^{p} w_j(x \cdot \theta_j). \tag{6.1}$$

Now we try to determine W, i.e. the functions w_j, such that W approximates the δ-function. The basic difference to the approach in the filtered backprojection algorithm in Section V.1 is that the function w_j in (6.1) depends on the direction θ_j, allowing for arbitrary spacing of the angles.

Now we have to determine the functions w_j. Davison and Grünbaum suggest to choose a 'point spread function' Φ freely and to find functions w_j such that

$$\|\Phi - W\|_{L_2(\Omega^n)} \tag{6.2}$$

is as small as possible. For $x \in \tfrac{1}{2}\Omega^n$ we then have the error estimate

$$\begin{aligned}
|(f_{\text{DG}} - \Phi * f)(x)| &= |(W - \Phi) * f(x)| \\
&\leq \|W - \Phi\|_{L_2(\Omega^n)} \|f\|_{L_\infty(\tfrac{1}{2}\Omega^n)}
\end{aligned} \tag{6.3}$$

provided that f is supported in $\frac{1}{2}\Omega^n$. Thus, making $\|W - \Phi\|_{L_2(\Omega^n)}$ small guarantees that f_{DG} is close to $\Phi * f$ which is a smoothed version of f.

In order to solve the minimization problem (6.2) we use the machinery developed in IV.3. There we have seen that $\mathbf{R}_{\theta_j}$ is a bounded operator from $L_2(\Omega^n)$ into $L_2([-1, +1], w^{1-n})$, $w(s) = (1 - s^2)^{1/2}$ with adjoint

$$\mathbf{R}_{\theta_j}^* g(x) = (w^{1-n} g)(x \cdot \theta_j).$$

Formula (IV.3.4) reads

$$\mathbf{R}_{\theta_i} \mathbf{R}_{\theta_j}^* u_m = \alpha_m(\theta_i \cdot \theta_j) u_m, \qquad u_m = w^{n-1} C_m^{n/2}. \tag{6.4}$$

Putting

$$R = \begin{pmatrix} \mathbf{R}_{\theta_1} \\ \vdots \\ \mathbf{R}_{\theta_p} \end{pmatrix}, \qquad U = w^{n-1} \begin{pmatrix} w_1 \\ \vdots \\ w_p \end{pmatrix}$$

we obtain $W = R^*U$ and we have to minimize

$$\|\Phi - R^*U\|_{L_2(\Omega^n)}.$$

The normal equations for this minimization problem are

$$RR^*U = R\Phi, \tag{6.5}$$

see Theorem IV.1.1. From (6.4) we get for each $c \in \mathbb{R}^p$

$$RR^*(u_m c) = A_m(u_m c),$$

$$(A_m)_{ij} = \alpha_m(\theta_i \cdot \theta_j).$$

Thus RR^* is a bounded operator in $(L_2([-1, +1], w^{1-n})^p$ with invariant subspaces $\mathcal{U}_m = u_m \mathbb{R}^p$ whose matrix representation on $\mathcal{U}_m$ is A_m. Writing

$$U = \sum_{m=0}^{\infty} u_m c_m$$

$$R\Phi = \sum_{m=0}^{\infty} u_m b_m,$$

$$b_m = \frac{1}{\beta_m} \int_{-1}^{+1} w^{1-n} u_m R\Phi \, ds = \frac{1}{\beta_m} \int_{-1}^{+1} C_m^{n/2} R\Phi \, ds,$$

$$\beta_m = \int_{-1}^{+1} w^{1-n} u_m^2 \, ds = \int_{-1}^{+1} w^{n-1} (C_m^{n/2})^2 \, ds,$$

see (VII.3.1), (6.5) reduces to

$$A_m c_m = b_m, \qquad m = 0, 1, \ldots. \tag{6.6}$$

These $p \times p$ systems have to be solved numerically to obtain the functions w_j. Once these functions have been determined the Davison–Grünbaum algorithm can be set up.

V.6.2. The Algorithm of Madych and Nelson (Madych and Nelson, 1983, 1984)

This algorithm differs from the Davison–Grünbaum algorithm only in the way the functions w_j are chosen. Let $n = 2$. We assume Φ to be a polynomial of degree $p - 1$. Such a polynomial can be written as

$$\Phi(x) = \sum_{j=1}^{p} w_j(x \cdot \theta_j) \tag{6.7}$$

with (one-dimensional) polynomials w_j, provided the directions $\pm \theta_1, \ldots, \pm \theta_p$ are different. This follows from the fact that the polynomials $C_{m,j}, j = 1, \ldots, p$, in V.4 are linearly independent for $n \geq p - 1$. Again the idea is to choose a polynomial Φ which is a reasonable point spread function, i.e. which resembles the δ-function, and to solve (6.7) for the functions w_j.

V.6.3. The ρ-filtered Layergram Method (Bates and Peters, 1971)

This is an implementation of the inversion formula (II.2.10). In terms of Fourier transforms it reads

$$f = \tfrac{1}{2}(2\pi)^{1-n}(|\xi|^{n-1}(\mathbf{R}^\# g)\hat{\ })\check{\ }, \quad g = \mathbf{R}f.$$

Thus we have to do a backprojection, followed by n-dimensional Fourier transforms.

The discrete implementation of this formula is by no means obvious. There are two difficulties. First, in orter to compute $(\mathbf{R}^\# g)\hat{\ }$ one needs $\mathbf{R}^\# g$ on all of $\mathbb{R}^n$, not only in the reconstruction region. Second, it is clear from Theorem II.1.4 that $(\mathbf{R}^\# g)\hat{\ }(\xi)$ has a singularity at $\xi = 0$. See Rowland (1979) for details. Because of these difficulties, the ρ-filtered layergram method has not been used much.

V.6.4. Marr's Algorithm (Marr, 1974a)

This is an implementation of the inversion formula (IV.3.14) for the PET geometry, see III.3. This means that we work in two dimensions with Ω^2 the reconstruction region, and $g = \mathbf{R}f$ is measured for the $p(p-1)/2$ lines joining p sources which are uniformly distributed on the circumference of Ω^2. Equivalently we may say that $g(\theta, s)$ is sampled at the points (θ_j, s_l) where, for p even,

$$s_k = \cos k\pi/p, \quad k = 1, \ldots, p-1$$

$$\theta_j = (\cos \varphi_j, \sin \varphi_j)^\mathsf{T}, \quad \varphi_j = \pi j/p, \quad j = 0, \ldots, 2p - 1$$

with $j + k$ even, compare Fig. III.5. Note that each of the $p(p-1)/2$ lines is represented twice by these $p(p-1)$ points.

We use the inversion formula (IV.3.14) for $n = 2$ in a slightly different notation. Putting

$$g_{ml}(\theta, s) = \frac{1}{\pi} w(s) U_m(s) e^{il\varphi}, \quad \theta = (\cos \varphi, \sin \varphi)^\mathsf{T}$$

$$f_{ml}(s\theta) = 2^{1/2} P_{(m-l)/2, l}(s^2) s^l e^{il\varphi}$$

where $w(s) = (1-s^2)^{1/2}$, U_m is the Chebyshev polynomial of the second kind, and $P_{k,l}$, $k = 0, 1, \ldots$ are the normalized orthogonal polynomials in $[0, 1]$ with weight function t^l. Then, (IV.3.14) reads (the dash stands for $l+m$ even)

$$f = \sum_{m=0}^{\infty} \sideset{}{'}\sum_{|l| \le m} \sigma_m^{-1} (g, g_{ml})_{L_2(Z, 1/w)} f_{ml}. \tag{6.8}$$

We remark that $\sigma_{ml}^2 = \sigma_m^2 = 4\pi/(m+1)$ in the case $n = 2$, see (IV.3.15).

For the approximate evaluation of the inner product we use a discrete version of this inner product which is adapted to the sampling of g, namely

$$(g, h)_p = \frac{2\pi^2}{p^2} \sum_{k=1}^{p-1} \sideset{}{'}\sum_{j=0}^{2p-1} g(\theta_j, s_k) \overline{h}(\theta_j, s_k)$$

where the dash indicates that j assumes only values for which $j + k$ even. Putting

$$\gamma_{ml}^* = \sigma_m^{-1} (g, g_{ml})_p \tag{6.9}$$

and truncating (6.8) at $m = M$ we obtain Marr's reconstruction formula

$$f_M^* = \sum_{m=0}^{M} \sideset{}{'}\sum_{|l| \le m} \gamma_{ml}^* f_{ml}. \tag{6.10}$$

As it happens the functions g_{ml} are not only orthogonal with respect to the inner product in $L_2(Z, 1/w)$ but also with respect to the inner product $(\cdot, \cdot)_p$:

$$(g_{ml}, g_{m'l'})_p = \begin{cases} 1, & m = m', l = l', \\ 0, & \text{otherwise} \end{cases} \tag{6.11}$$

whenever $m, m' < p - 1$. Equation (6.11) is established as follows. We have

$$(g_{ml}, g_{m'l'})_p = \frac{2\pi^2}{p^2} \sum_{k=1}^{p-1} \sideset{}{'}\sum_{j=0}^{2p-1} \frac{1}{\pi^2} w^2(s_k) U_m(s_k) U_{m'}(s_k) e^{i(l-l')\pi j/p}$$

$$= \frac{2}{p^2} \sum_{k=1}^{p-1} \sin((m+1)k\pi/p) \sin((m'+1)k\pi/p) \sideset{}{'}\sum_{j=0}^{2p-1} e^{i(l-l')\pi j/p}.$$

In the j-sum we put $j = 2j'$ for k even and $j = 2j'+1$ for k odd, obtaining

$$\sideset{}{'}\sum_{j=0}^{2p-1} e^{i(l-l')\pi j/p} = \sum_{j'=0}^{p-1} e^{2i(l-l')\pi j'/p} \cdot \begin{cases} 1, & k \text{ even,} \\ e^{i(l-l')/\pi/p}, & k \text{ odd.} \end{cases}$$

By the usual orthogonality relation for the exponential function this vanishes for $|l - l'| < 2p$ except $l = l'$ and $|l - l'| = p$. In the latter case,

$$\sideset{}{'}\sum_{j=0}^{2p-1} e^{i(l-l')\pi j/p} = (-1)^k p,$$

and

$$(g_{ml}, g_{m'l'})_p = \frac{2}{p} \sum_{k=1}^{p-1} (-1)^k \sin(m+1)k\pi/p \sin(m'+1)k\pi/p. \tag{6.12}$$

If $l = l'$ then we have the same result without the factor $(-1)^k$. In either case, l and

l' hence m and m' have the same parity. Thus (6.11) follows from (6.12) and

$$\sum_{k=1}^{p-1} \varepsilon_k \sin(m+1)k\pi/p \sin(m'+1)k\pi/p = \begin{cases} p/2, & m = m', \\ 0, & \text{otherwise} \end{cases}$$

for $m+m'$ even and $m, m' < p-1$ where $\varepsilon_k = 1$ or $\varepsilon_k = (-1)^k$.

The discrete orthogonality relation (6.11) permits an interesting interpretation of Marr's formula (6.10): assume we want to compute among all functions of the form

$$f_M = \sum_{m=0}^{M} {\sum_{|l| \le m}}' \gamma_{ml} f_{ml}$$

that one which minimizes

$$\|Rf_M - g\|_p \tag{6.13}$$

where $\|\cdot\|_p$ is the norm derived from the inner product $(\cdot,\cdot)_p$, then $f_M = f_M^*$ as long as $M < p-1$. This follows immediately from (6.11) and

$$\|Rf_M - g\|_p = \left\|\sum_{m=0}^{M} {\sum_{|l| \le m}}' \gamma_{ml} Rf_{ml} - g\right\|_p$$

$$= \left\|\sum_{m=0}^{M} {\sum_{|l| \le m}}' \sigma_{ml} \gamma_{ml} g_{ml} - g\right\|_p$$

since this is minimal for $\sigma_{ml}\gamma_{ml} = (g, g_{ml})_p$, hence $\gamma_{ml} = \gamma_{ml}^*$. Thus Marr's reconstruction formula provides a polynomial minimizing the discrete residual (6.13).

V.6.5. Methods based on Cormack's Inversion Formula

In its original form, Cormack's formula (II.2.18) is virtually useless due to severe numerical instabilities, compare the discussion in VI.3. However, the modified form (II.2.20) does not suffer from instabilities. In fact, successful reconstructions have been done with (II.2.20), see Cormack (1964), Hansen (1981) and Perry (1975).

V.7 Bibliographical Notes

The filtered backprojection algorithm has been introduced in the medical field by Shepp and Logan (1974) and Ramachandran and Lakshminarayanan (1971), but it has been applied in radio astronomy by Bracewell and Riddle (1967) as early as 1967. They gave the following alternative form for the filter w_b of (1.20) for $\varepsilon = 0$:

$$w_b(s) = \frac{b}{4\pi} \delta^b(s) - \frac{b^2}{8\pi^2} \operatorname{sinc}\left(\frac{bs}{2}\right)^2 \tag{7.1}$$

with δ^b the approximate δ-function (VII.1.2). For the reconstruction of essentially b-band-limited functions δ^b can be replaced by δ. This leads to a slightly different algorithm where the filter involves only the sinc function. The investigation of the resolution achieved by the filtered backprojection algorithm goes back to Bracewell and Riddle (1967) and Tretiak (1975); our proof of Theorem 1.1 is based on Lewitt et al. (1978a). Filtered backprojection algorithms for fan-beam data have been given by Lakshminarayanan (1975), Herman and Naparstek (1977) and others. Our treatment is based on Horn (1973). The idea of using (1.2) as starting point for reconstruction algorithms is due to K. T. Smith and others who systematically investigated the interplay between the filters w_b, w_b in a series of papers, see Leahy et al. (1979) (which paper contains the n-dimensional analogue of (1.25)), Smith (1983, 1984), Smith and Keinert (1985), see also Chang and Herman (1980). The material on three-dimensional filtered backprojection algorithms has been taken from Marr, et al. (1981). An error estimate for the three-dimensional problem has been given by Louis (1983).

Fourier reconstruction in $\mathbb{R}^2$ has been suggested by Bracewell (1979) in radio astronomy and by Crowther et al. (1970) in electron microscopy. Both papers contain a heuristic derivation of the relation $p = \pi q$ by a loose application of the sampling theorem to the polar coordinate grid. Bracewell (1979) observed that the failure of the standard Fourier algorithm comes from the interpolation. He also showed that interpolation which is correct in the sense of the sampling theorem requires a huge number of operations. Condition (2.4) for the distribution of the interpolation points ξ_k has been introduced in Löw and Natterer (1981), see also Natterer (1985). Stark et al. (1981) replaced nearest neighbour interpolation by a more sophisticated interpolation procedure and found experimentally that radial interpolation is far more critical than angular interpolation. Since (2.4) puts a severe restriction on radial interpolation, these experiments confirm (2.4). Of course, one can avoid interpolation altogether by introducing polar coordinates. This leads to the filtered backprojection algorithm.

ART has been introduced by Gordon et al. (1970) independently of G. Hounsfield (1973) who built the first commercially available CT scanner for which he received the 1979 Nobel prize for medicine, jointly with A. Cormack. The connection of ART with the Kaczmarz method has been discovered by Guenther et al. (1974). This paper gives also a convergence estimate for Kaczmarz's method in the case $\omega = 1$ in terms of the angles between ker (R_j) and $\bigcap_{i > j}$ ker (R_i); for the derivation see Smith et al. (1977). Our proof of Theorem 3.6 is based on Amemiya and Ando (1965).

The connection between Kaczmarz's method and the successive over-relaxation method (SOR) has first been seen by Björck and Elving (1979); our proof of Theorem 3.9 is based on this fact. The observation that $f_\omega \to f_M$ as $\omega \to 0$ has been made by Censor et al. (1983). The rediscovery of Kaczmarz's method and its obvious usefulness in CT has led to a vast number of publications on this and related methods. We mention only Herman and Lent (1976), ch. 11 of Herman (1980) and the survey articles of Censor (1981, 1983). The convergence analysis for Kaczmarz's method applied to complete projections in Section V.4 is based on Hamaker and Solmon (1978) and on unpublished lecture notes of D. Solmon.

The basic idea of the direct algebraic algorithm is due to Lent (1975). First numerical experiments have been reported in Natterer (1980b). The algorithm suggested by Buonocore *et al.* (1981) is essentially a direct algebraic algorithm for (5.12), the 'natural pixels' of that paper being the supports of our functions χ_{jl} which in fact come into play quite naturally in our framework without any discretization of the image. A different kind of direct algebraic methods is obtained by representing the image by trial functions with rotational symmetry which also results in a block-cyclic structure of the relevant matrix. Such algorithms have been suggested by Altschuler and Perry (1972) (see also Altschuler (1979) and chs 13–14 of Herman (1980), Pasedach (1977), and Ham (1975)). An explicit representation of the minimum norm solution for a finite number of equally spaced directions in $\mathbb{R}^2$ has been given by Logan and Shepp (1975); this corresponds to a direct algebraic algorithm in the limit case of an infinite number of strip integrals in each direction. We remark that the probabilistic approach based on (5.13) has been suggested by Hurwitz (1975) and Tasto (1977). For an iterative implementation see Herman *et al.* (1979).

VI
Incomplete Data

The relevance of incomplete data problems has already been pointed out in Chapter I. In Section VI.1 we discuss some features which are shared by all incomplete data problems, such as the nature of the artefacts, the degree of ill-posedness, and data completion. In Sections VI.2–5 we work out the details for specific problems. In Section VI.5 an inversion formula which is adapted to a special three-dimensional scanning mode is given. In Section VI.6 we demonstrate that homogeneous objects can be recovered from very few data.

VI.1 General Remarks

Let f be a function with support in Ω^n. If $g = \mathbf{R}f$ is given (possibly in discretized form) on all of $S^{n-1} \times [-1, +1]$ we call the data complete, otherwise incomplete. Analogous definitions apply to the other integral transforms introduced in II.1. Typical examples of incomplete data problems are:

(i) The limited angle problem. Here, $\mathbf{R}_\theta f$ is given only for θ in a subset of some half-sphere.
(ii) The exterior problem. Here, $\mathbf{R}f(\theta, s)$ is given only for $|s| \geq a$ where $0 < a < 1$. Of course, $f(x)$ is to be determined for $|x| \geq a$ only.
(iii) The interior problem. Here, $\mathbf{R}f(\theta, s)$ is given only for $|s| \leq a$, where $0 < a < 1$. Of course, $f(x)$ is to be determined for $|x| \leq a$ only.
(iv) The restricted source problem. Here, $\mathbf{D}_a f$ is given only for a on a curve surrounding Ω^n.

In I.1 we have seen that these problems arise quite naturally in practical applications.

For incomplete data problems only a few of the results from Chapter II remain valid. For (i), (ii) the stability estimates of II.5 do not hold, (iii) is uniquely solvable for n odd only, and in (iv) we have stability only under serious restrictions on the curve on which the sources run. In contrast to the mild ill-posedness of the problems with complete data (see IV.2), incomplete data problems tend to be severely ill-posed. This ill-posedness is the most serious difficulty in dealing with incomplete data problems.

The structure of Radon's inversion formula (II.2.5) gives considerable insight into the nature of the ill-posedness. For $n = 3$ it reads

$$f(x) = \frac{1}{8\pi^2} \int_{S^{n-1}} g''(\theta, x \cdot \theta) d\theta, \qquad g = \mathbf{R}f. \tag{1.1}$$

It averages over the planes through x. The biggest contributions come from the planes in whose neighbourhood g varies strongly. This is the case for those planes which are tangent to surfaces of discontinuity of f. If the integrals over such planes are missing, then (1.1) cannot even approximately be evaluated on such planes. In two dimensions the same argument applies except that the effect undergoes some blurring due to the presence of the non-local Hilbert transform. Thus we come to the following rule of thumb.

In incomplete data problems, artefacts show up mainly in the vicinity of lines (planes) which are tangent to curves (surfaces) of discontinuity of f and for which the value of $\mathbf{R}f$ is missing.

In order to illustrate this rule we reconstructed the phantom of Fig. VI.1(a) from limited angle data. We used a parallel scanning geometry, leaving out lines which make an angle $\leq 15°$ with the vertical axes. We did the reconstruction using the filtered backprojection algorithm (V.1.17), (V.1.21) with $\varepsilon = 0$, putting the data in the missing angular range to zero. The artefacts in the reconstruction in Fig. VI.1(b) are precisely as predicted by our rule. Note that the artefacts extend up to the boundary, indicating that the reconstructed function does not even have compact support. This is not surprising since the filtered backprojection algorithm computes, apart from discretization and filtering, a reconstruction f^E satisfying

$$\hat{f}^E(\sigma\theta) = (2\pi)^{(1-n)/2} \hat{g}^E(\theta, \sigma) \tag{1.2}$$

where g^E is the function g extended by zero in the missing angular range. g^E is not likely to be in the range of $\mathbf{R}$, hence f^E does not decay fast at infinity. Remember that the crucial point in the proof of Theorem II.4.2 was to show that the consistency conditions for g imply that $f \in \mathcal{S}$.

Figure VI.1(c) shows the reconstruction from lines outside the black hole. The artefacts are much less pronounced since all tangents to curves of discontinuity are available.

In order to avoid the severe artefacts caused by inconsistent data we do the extension in a consistent way. Let I be the subset of $S^{n-1} \times [-1, +1]$ on which $g^I = \mathbf{R}f$ is given. We want to find a function g^c in range $(\mathbf{R})$ such that $g^c = g^I$ on I. In case there is more than one solution to this extrapolation problem we choose the solution of minimal norm. This leads to the definition of g^c as the solution of the minimization problem

$$\text{Minimize } \|g\|_{L_2(Z,w)} \text{ in } \overline{\text{range}(\mathbf{R})} \text{ subject to } g = g^I \text{ on } I. \tag{1.3}$$

Here, $\mathbf{R}$ is considered as operator on $C_0^\infty(\Omega^n)$ and the closure is in $L_2(Z, w)$. We choose the solution of least norm to make the extension as stable as possible. w is a suitable weight function. We shall compute g^c in the following sections, and it will turn out that consistent completion of data significantly reduces the artefacts.

Methods such as ART or the direct algebraic methods (if applicable) do not need any preprocessing of the incomplete data. This does not mean that these methods produce always good reconstructions, but in favourable cases they may be useful.

In the following sections we discuss the peculiarities of the incomplete data problems mentioned above.

VI.2 The Limited Angle Problem

We consider only the plane problem. We assume $g = \mathbf{R}f$ to be given on $I = S_\Phi^1 \times [-1, +1]$ where $S_\Phi^1 = \{\theta: \theta = (\cos\varphi, \sin\varphi)^\mathsf{T}, |\varphi| \leq \Phi\}$. The data are incomplete if $\Phi < \pi/2$.

From Theorem II.3.4 we know that f is uniquely determined as long as $\Phi > 0$. However, the stability estimate from Theorem II.5.1 does not hold for $\Phi < \pi/2$. More precisely we can show that an estimate of the form

$$\|f\|_{H_0^s(\Omega^2)} \leq C(s, t)\|\mathbf{R}f\|_{H^{s+t}(S_\Phi^1 \times \mathbf{R}^1)} \tag{2.1}$$

cannot hold for arbitrary $s \in \mathbf{R}^1$, not even if t is arbitrarily large. For the proof we produce a function f_+ with support in Ω^2 which is not continuous but $\mathbf{R}f_+ \in C^\infty(S_\Phi^1 \times \mathbf{R}^1)$. With $f \in C_0^\infty(\Omega^2)$ a radial function such that $f(0) \neq 0$ we may define

$$f_+(x) = \begin{cases} f(x) & \text{in the upper half-plane,} \\ 0 & \text{in the lower half-plane.} \end{cases}$$

Then $\mathbf{R}f_+$ is a smooth function of the straight lines as long as the straight lines are not parallel to the x_1-axes for which $\varphi = \pi/2$. Thus $\mathbf{R}f_+ \in C^\infty(S_\Phi^1 \times [-1, +1])$ but f is not continuous. This shows that (2.1) cannot hold for $s > 1$ because of Lemma VII.4.6.

In the terminology of IV.1 the failure of (2.1) to hold means that the limited angle problem is severely ill-posed. To confirm this we compute the singular values of the operator

$$\mathbf{R}: L_2(\Omega^2) \to L_2\left(I, \frac{1}{w}\right), \quad w = (1 - s^2)^{1/2}.$$

For $n = 2$, (IV.3.4–5) read

$$\mathbf{R}_{\theta_1}\mathbf{R}_{\theta_2}^\# U_m = \alpha_m(\theta_1 \cdot \theta_2) w U_m,$$

$$\alpha_m(t) = \frac{2}{m+1} U_m(t)$$

with U_m the Chebyshev polynomials of the second kind (VII.3.3). Putting $u_m = w U_m$ this leads precisely as in IV.3 to

$$\mathbf{R}\mathbf{R}^*(h u_m)(\omega, s) = A_m(\Phi) h(\omega) u_m(s)$$

where, for each $h \in L_2(S_\Phi^1)$

$$A_m(\Phi)h(\omega) = \int_{S_\Phi^1} \alpha_m(\omega \cdot \theta) h(\theta)\,d\theta.$$

Hence **RR*** has the invariant subspace $L_2(S_\Phi^1)u_m$ and coincides with the operator $A_m(\Phi)$ on this subspace. Putting $\omega = (\cos\psi, \sin\psi)^T$, $\theta = (\cos\varphi, \sin\varphi)^T$ we get

$$\alpha_m(\omega \cdot \theta) = \frac{2}{m+1} U_m(\cos(\varphi-\psi))$$

$$= \frac{2}{m+1} \frac{\sin(m+1)(\varphi-\psi)}{\sin(\varphi-\psi)}$$

with the usual modification for $\varphi = \psi$. Since

$$\frac{\sin(m+1)\varphi}{\sin\varphi} = e^{im\varphi} + e^{i(m-2)\varphi} + \ldots + e^{-im\varphi}$$

we find that

$$\text{range}(A_m(\Phi)) = \langle e^{im\varphi}, e^{i(m-2)\varphi}, \ldots, e^{-im\varphi} \rangle.$$

Hence $A_m(\Phi)$ has the eigenvalue 0 with multiplicity ∞, plus the eigenvalues of the matrix $(2\pi/m+1)A'_m(\Phi)$ where $A'_m(\Phi)$ is the Toeplitz matrix

$$A'_m(\Phi) = \begin{pmatrix} a_0 & a_2 & \cdots & a_{2m} \\ a_2 & a_0 & \cdots & a_{2m-2} \\ & & \cdots & \\ a_{2m} & a_{2m-2} & \cdots & a_0 \end{pmatrix},$$

(2.2)

$$a_l = a_l(\Phi) = \frac{1}{\pi} \int_{-\Phi}^{\Phi} e^{il\varphi} d\varphi = \frac{2}{\pi} \begin{cases} \Phi, & l = 0, \\ \dfrac{\sin l\Phi}{l}, & l \neq 0. \end{cases}$$

The eigenvalues of the matrix $A'_m(\Phi)$ have been studied by Slepian (1978). They are denoted (p. 1376) by $\lambda_l(m+1, \Phi/\pi)$, $l = 0, \ldots, m$. This means that the non-zero eigenvalues of the operator **RR*** are $(2\pi/m+1)\lambda_l(m+1, \Phi/\pi)$, and the sought-for singular values of **R** are

$$\sigma_{ml} = \left(\frac{2\pi}{m+1} \lambda_l(m+1, \Phi/\pi)\right)^{1/2}, \quad m = 0, 1, \ldots, l = 0, 1, \ldots, m. \quad (2.3)$$

For $\Phi = \pi/2$, $\lambda_l(m+1, \Phi/\pi) = 1$, i.e. $\sigma_{ml}^2 = 2\pi/(m+1)$. This agrees with (IV.3.15) since we worked in IV.3 with $L_2(S^1 \times \mathbb{R}^1)$ rather than with $L_2(S^1_{\pi/2} \times \mathbb{R}^1)$ as we did in the derivation of (2.3) for $\Phi = \pi/2$.

We are interested in the asymptotic behaviour of the singular values. Making use of the η-notation in (III.2.4) we can express the basic result of Slepian (1978) as follows:

$$\lambda_l(m+1, \Phi/\pi) = \begin{cases} 1 - \eta(\vartheta, m), & l \leq \vartheta\, \dfrac{2\Phi}{\pi}\, m, \\ \eta(\vartheta, m), & l \geq \vartheta^{-1}\, \dfrac{2\Phi}{\pi}\, m. \end{cases} \quad (2.4)$$

This means that for m large, a fraction slightly smaller than $2\Phi/\pi$ of the eigenvalues is close to 1, a fraction slightly smaller than $1 - (2\Phi/\pi)$ is close to zero, with a very small transition region in between. For a plot of the eigenvalues see

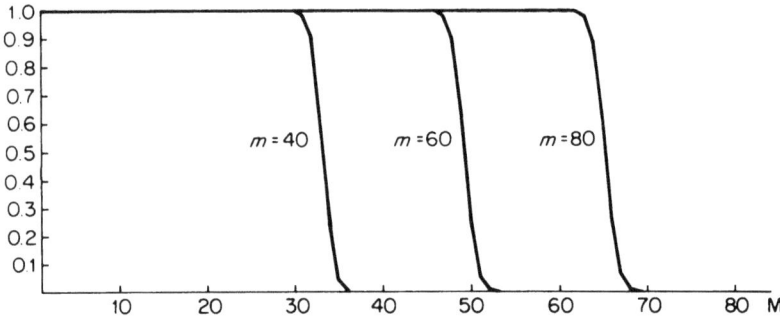

FIG. VI.2. Eigenvalues $\lambda_l(m+1, 0.4)$, $l = 0, \ldots, m$ of the matrix $A'_m(0.4\pi)$ from (2.2) for $m = 40$, $m = 60$ and $m = 80$. The dichotomy expressed by (2.4) is apparent.

Fig. VI.2. We conclude that the singular values σ_{ml} with $l \geq \theta^{-1}(2\Phi/\pi)m$ decay exponentially as $m \to \infty$, and this confirms that the limited angle problem is severely ill-posed.

Now we compute the complete data g^c defined in (1.3). The expansion (II.4.2) for g^c in the case $\lambda = 1$ reads with $w = (1-j^2)^{1/2}$

$$g^c(\theta, s) = w \sum_{m=0}^{\infty} U_m(s) g^c_m(\varphi), \quad \theta = \begin{pmatrix} \cos \varphi \\ \sin \varphi \end{pmatrix}, \tag{2.5}$$

$$g^c_m(\varphi) = \frac{2}{\pi} \int_{-1}^{+1} g^c(\theta, s) U_m(s) \, ds. \tag{2.6}$$

g^c_m is a trigonometric polynomial of degree m of the form

$$g^c_m(\varphi) = \sum_{|l| \leq m}{}' \hat{g}^c_{m,l} e^{il\varphi} \tag{2.7}$$

where the dash indicates that the sum extends only over l with $l+m$ even. Since $g^c = g^I$ on I we must have

$$g^c_m(\varphi) = g^I_m(\varphi) \quad \text{for } |\varphi| \leq \Phi, \tag{2.8}$$

$$g^I_m(\varphi) = \frac{2}{\pi} \int_{-1}^{+1} g^I(\theta, s) U_m(s) \, ds. \tag{2.9}$$

Of course the polynomials g^c_m are uniquely determined by (2.8) provided that $\Phi > 0$. Thus its coefficients $\hat{g}^c_{m,l}$ can be computed from the incomplete data via (2.8).

We outline the procedure for discrete data. We assume $g^I = Rf$ to be given for the $2r+1$ directions $\theta_j = (\cos \varphi_j, \sin \varphi_j)^T$, $\varphi_j = \pi j/(2p)$, $j = -r, \ldots, r$ where $r \leq (2/\pi)\Phi p$ at the equidistant points $s_l = lh$, $l = -q, \ldots, q$.

Step 1: For $m = 0, \ldots, M$ compute approximations $g_{m,j}^l$ to $g_m^l(\varphi_j)$ by

$$g_{m,j}^l = \frac{2h}{\pi} \sum_{l=-q}^{q} g^l(\theta_j, s_l) U_m(s_l), \quad j = -r, \ldots, r.$$

This is a discrete version of (2.9).

Step 2: From $m = 0, \ldots, M$, solve the over-determined (for $m < 2r$) linear system

$$\sum_{|l| \leq m}{}' \hat{g}_{m,l}^c e^{i\pi l j/(2p)} = g_{m,j}^l, \quad j = -r, \ldots, r. \tag{2.10}$$

Step 3: For $m = 0, \ldots, M$, compute approximations $g_{m,j}^c$ to $g_m^c(\varphi_j)$ by

$$g_{m,j}^c = \sum_{|l| \leq m}{}' \hat{g}_{m,l}^c e^{il\varphi_j}, \quad j = -p, \ldots, -r-1, r+1, \ldots, p-1.$$

Step 4: Approximate the data in the missing range by

$$g^c(\theta_j, s_l) \sim w(s_l) \sum_{m=0}^{M} U_m(s_l) g_{m,j}^c,$$

$$j = -p, \ldots, -r-1, r+1, \ldots, p-1, \quad l = -q, \ldots, q.$$

This is obtained by truncating (2.5) at $m = M$.

Step 2 is the crucial step of the algorithm. The reason is that (2.10) is highly ill-conditioned. This is to be expected since the limited angle problem is severely ill-posed. It is also plausible because we perform an extrapolation for trigonometric polynomials, and extrapolation is notoriously unstable. We want to investigate the nature of this ill-conditioning. Let us write

$$B_m \hat{g}_m^c = g_m^l \tag{2.11}$$

for (2.10) where $\hat{g}_m^c$ contains the $m+1$ unknowns $\hat{g}_{m,l}^c$ and g_m^l the $2r+1$ right-hand sides of (2.10). B_m is the $(2r+1) \times (m+1)$ matrix with j, l element $e^{i\pi l j/(2p)}$. The components of $\hat{g}_m^c$ are numbered $m, m-2, \ldots, -m$ and so are the columns of B_m. The $(m+1) \times (m+1)$ matrix $C_m = B_m^* B_m$, with rows and columns numbered $m, m-2, \ldots, -m$ has k, l element $C_{m,l-k}$ with

$$C_{m,l} = \sum_{j=-r}^{r} e^{i\pi l j/(2p)} = \begin{cases} 2r+1, & l = 0, \\ \dfrac{\sin l \dfrac{\pi(r+1/2)}{2p}}{\sin \dfrac{l\pi/2}{2p}}, & l \neq 0. \end{cases} \tag{2.12}$$

C_m is the discrete analog of $A_m'(\Phi)$. In fact, if r, p tend to infinity in such a way that $r/p \to (2/\pi) \Phi$, then

$$\frac{1}{2p} C_m \to A_m'(\Phi)$$

as is easily verified by comparing (2.12) with (2.2). This means that for r, p large, the singular values of B_m, i.e. the square roots of the eigenvalues of C_m are approximately $(2p\,\lambda_l\,(m+1,\Phi/\pi))^{1/2}$, $l = 0, 1, \ldots, m$. In view of the behaviour of the $\lambda_l\,(m+1, \Phi/\pi)$ for m large, see (2.4), B_m is highly ill-conditioned for m large.

In order to solve (2.10) or (2.11) we have to resort to the methods of IV.1 1 for the solution of ill-posed problems. In principle we could work with the truncated singular value decomposition. However it is simpler and computationally much more efficient to use Tikhonov–Phillips regularization. This amounts to solving

$$(B_m^* B_m + \gamma I)\hat{g}_m^c = B_m^* g_m^l$$

or

$$(C_m + \gamma I)\hat{g}_m^c = \hat{g}_m^l, \qquad (2.13)$$

$$\hat{g}_{m,l}^l = \sum_{j=-r}^{r} e^{-il\pi j/(2p)}\, g_{m,j}^l, \quad |l| \leq m,\, l+m \text{ even.} \qquad (2.14)$$

Since C_m is a Toeplitz matrix, (2.13) can be solved efficiently even for m large using FFT techniques, see VII.5. FFT techniques can be employed in the other steps too.

This means that the computing time for the completion procedure is small compared with the time needed for doing the reconstruction from the completed data.

In the application of the algorithm we have to make two decisions: we have to choose M and γ. We found that $M = q$ is a good choice, γ has to be chosen by trial and error. If γ is too large, then the reconstruction is too smooth and lacks small details. For γ too small the reconstruction contains rapid oscillations.

In order to see what can be achieved by the completion procedure we reconstructed the object in Fig. VI.3(a) from line integrals making an angle less than 75° with the horizontal axes. In this range we used 215 equally spaced directions and 161 line integrals for each direction. This amounts to running our completion algorithm with $p = 128$, $r = 107$, $q = 80$ and to rotate the object by an angle of $\pi/2$. In Fig. VI.3(c) we display the reconstruction done by applying the filtered backprojection algorithm to the incomplete data. Except for a different scaling, this picture is identical to Fig. V.1(b). In Fig. VI.3(b), the result of the filtered backprojection algorithm for the completed data set is shown. We see that the strong artefacts outside the object are reduced by the completion procedure, but new artefacts are added in the interior. The cross-sections in Fig. VI.3(c) reveal that the completion procedure also corrects the severe damping of the function values within the annulus. In total, the completion procedure corrects the most apparent distortions but it tends to introduce new artefacts which are comparatively small but nevertheless quite disturbing.

Now we turn to the reconstruction techniques for the limited angle problem which do not need a complete data set. From a computational point of view, ART can be used without any changes, and even the convergence analysis of V.4 can be carried out as in the full angle case. However, the norms $\rho_m(\omega)$ of Q^ω behave quite differently in the limited angle case. We computed $\rho_m(\omega), m = 0, \ldots, 31$ for

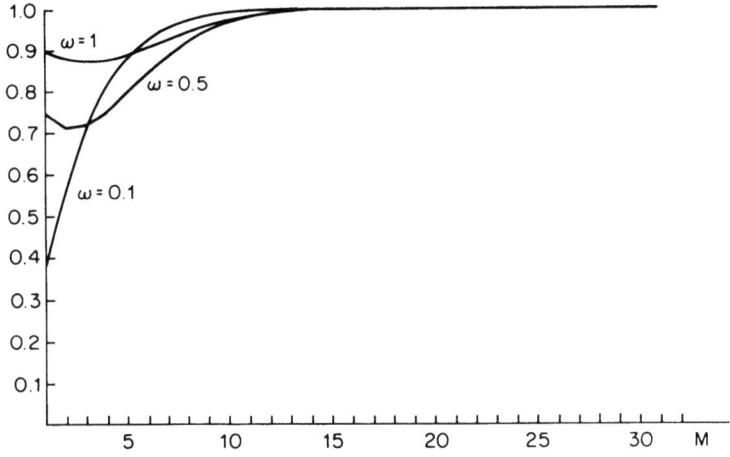

FIG. VI.4 The norms $\rho_m(\omega)$ of Q^ω in $\mathscr{C}_m, m = 0, \ldots, 31$ for $p = 32$ equally distributed angles in an angular range of 150° in natural order.

$p = 32$ equally distributed angles in an angular range of 150°, $\varphi_j = (j-1)\,150/180\,\pi, j = 1, \ldots, 32$. In Fig. VI.4 we used the natural order, in Fig. VI.5 a random arrangement of the φ_j. In both cases, and irrespective of the value of ω, most of the $\rho_m(\omega)$ are virtually 1. However, those first few $\rho_m(\omega)$ which are significantly less than 1 do depend on ω and on the ordering, qualitatively in the same way as in the full angle case. That means that choosing a small ω and arranging the angles in a clever way improves convergence only on

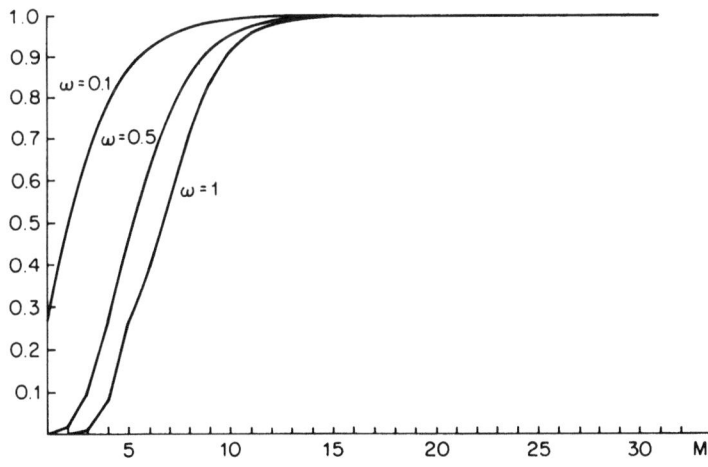

FIG. VI.5 Same as Fig. VI.3, but with random ordering of the angles.

the first few subspaces $\mathscr{C}_m$, while nothing can be achieved on the remaining $\mathscr{C}_m$s. This again reflects the inherent ill-posedness of the limited angle problem.

VI.3 The Exterior Problem

The exterior problem is uniquely solvable. This follows from Theorem II.3.1. However, uniqueness hinges on the fast decay of f at infinity, as is shown by the example following that theorem. Again we restrict ourselves to the plane problem. We assume that $g^I = \mathbf{R}f$ is given on $I = \{(\theta, s): \theta \in S^1, a \leq |s| \leq 1\}$.

As in the limited angle case we can show that the exterior problem is severely ill-posed. It suffices to produce a function f_+ in Ω^2 which is not continuous in $|x| > a$ but for which $\mathbf{R}f_+$ is smooth outside $S^1 \times [-a, a]$. With $f \in C_0^\infty(\Omega^2)$ a radial function such that $f \neq 0$ in a neighbourhood of $\{x: |x| < a\}$, the function f_+ which agrees with f in the upper half-plane and is zero elsewhere is obviously such a function.

In principle, the exterior problem can be solved by Cormack's inversion formula (II.2.18) which expresses the Fourier coefficients f_l of f in terms of the Fourier coefficients g_l of g:

$$f_l(r) = -\frac{1}{\pi} \int_r^\infty (s^2 - r^2)^{-1/2} T_{|l|}\left(\frac{s}{r}\right) g_l'(s)\, ds. \tag{3.1}$$

It permits to compute $f_l(r), r \geq a$ from the values of $g_l(s)$ for $|s| \geq a$. Since, for $u \geq 1$,

$$T_l(u) \geq \tfrac{1}{2}(u + \sqrt{(u^2 - 1)})^l,$$

see (VII.3.5), the kernel $T_{|l|}(s/r)$ in (3.1) increases exponentially as $|l| \to \infty$. On the other hand, we derive from Theorem II.4.1

$$\int_{\mathbf{R}^1} s^m g_l(s)\, ds = 0, \quad m < |l| \tag{3.2}$$

which means that g_l is strongly oscillating for $|l|$ large. Hence in (3.1) a function assuming large positive values is integrated against a rapidly oscillating function. This causes intolerable cancellations and reflects the severe ill-posedness of the exterior problem. The formula (II.2.20) does not suffer from this instability but it is clearly not a solution to the exterior problem.

In order to carry out the data completion procedure of Section VI.1 we need range (**R**) in the sense of (1.3). By Theorem II.4.2, a function $g \in \mathscr{S}(Z)$ which vanishes for $|s| \geq 1$ is in range (**R**) if and only if

$$\int_{S^1} \int_{-1}^{+1} P_m(s) e^{-il\varphi} g(\theta, s)\, ds\, d\theta = 0, \quad |l| > m \tag{3.3}$$

g even

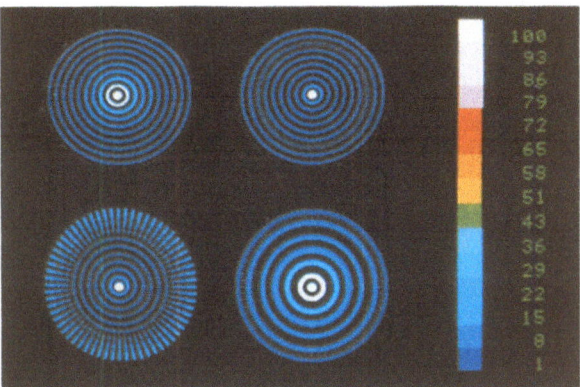

Figure V. 5: Filtered backprojection. a(top left): Original, given by a function with maximal function value 900. b(top right): Reconstruction from correctly sampled data. c(bottom left): Reconstruction from too few directions. d(bottom right): Reconstruction from undersampled projections.

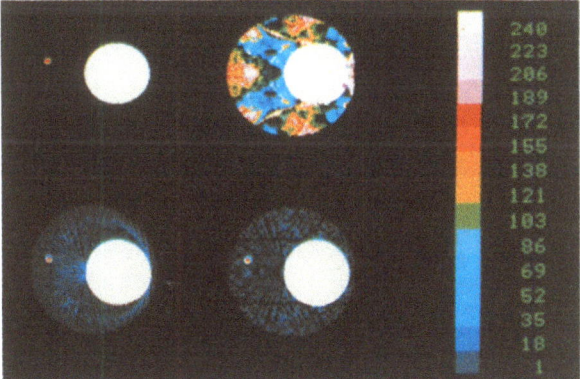

Figure V. 8: Fourier reconstruction. a(top left): Original, consisting of two circles. Function value within the large circle is 900. b(top right): Standard Fourier algorithm. c(bottom left): Filtered backprojection. d(bottom right): Second improved Fourier algorithm.

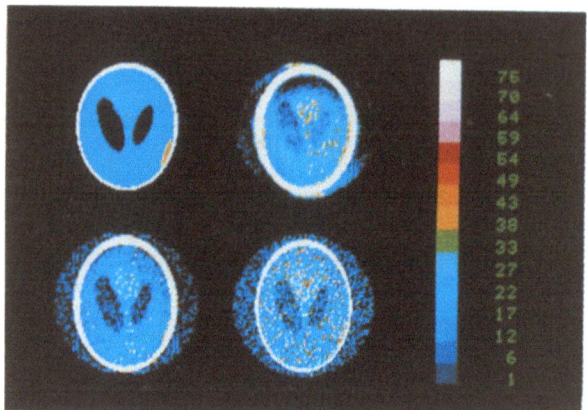

Figure V. 12: Semiconvergence phenomenon of ART. a(top left): Original. b(top right): Step 2. c(bottom left): Step 4. d(bottom right): Step 40.

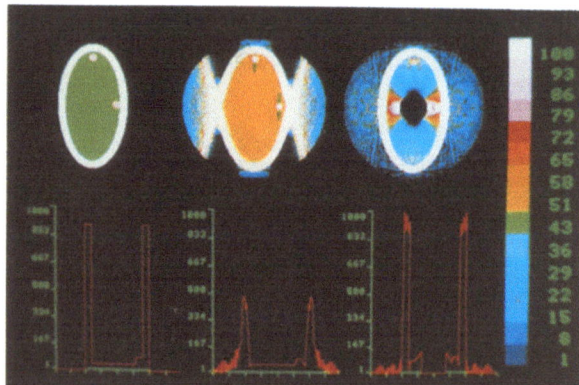

Figure VI. 1: Artifacts in the reconstruction from incomplete data. a(left): Original. b(middle): Reconstruction from limited angle. c(right): Reconstruction from exterior data. The lower row shows horizontal cross-sections through the middle of the object. The reconstructions have been done with the filtered backprojection algorithm, putting the data in the missing range 0.

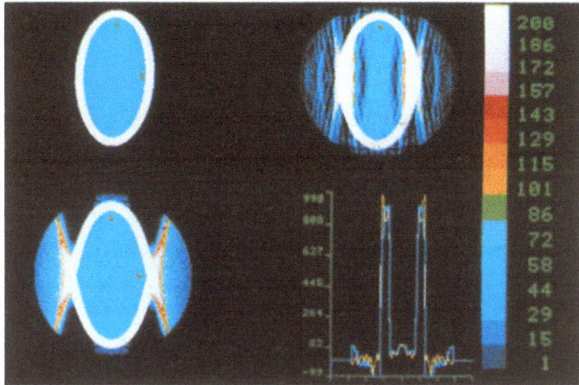

Figure VI. 3: Reconstruction from limited angle data. a(top left): Original. Function value in the ellipsoidal annulus is 900. b(top right): Reconstruction from completed data. c(bottom left): Reconstruction from incomplete data. d(bottom right): Horizontal cross section through the upper green spot of b(yellow) and c(blue).

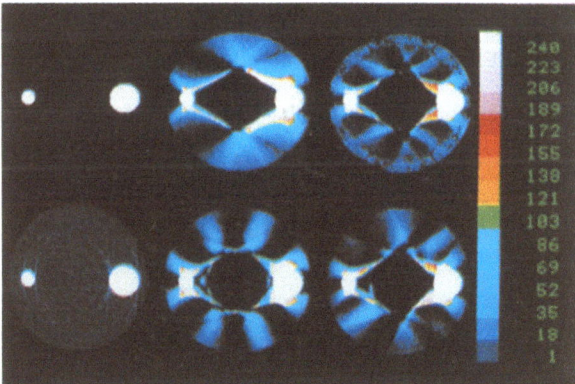

Figure VI. 6: Reconstruction from exterior data. a(top left): Original, consisting of two circles. Function value in the bigger circle is 900. b(top middle): Filtered backprojection algorithm, putting the missing data 0. c(top right): Direct algebraic method. d(bottom left): Filtered backprojection with the full data set. e(bottom middle): Filtered backprojection with completed data. f(bottom right): ART.

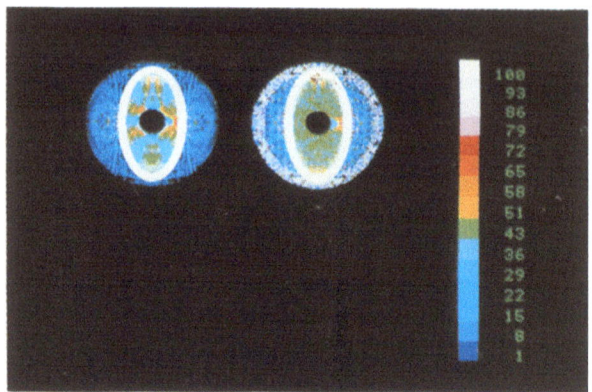

Figure VI. 7: Reconstruction of the original in fig. 1.1a from exterior data. a(left): Filtered backprojection with completed data. b(right): Direct algebraic method.

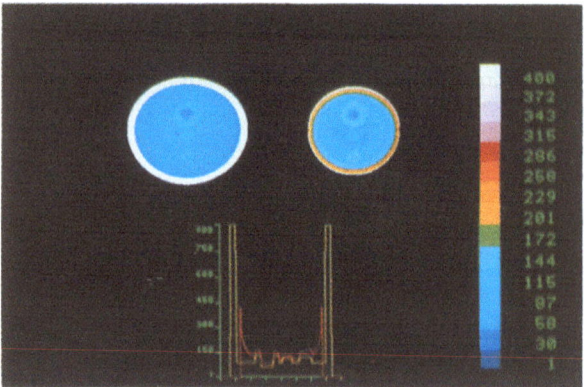

Figure VI. 8: Reconstruction from interior data by the direct algebraic algorithm. a(top left): Original. Function value in the ellipsoidal annulus is 900. b(top right): Reconstruction by the direct algebraic algorithm within $|x| \leq 0.7$ c(bottom): Cross section through original (yellow) and reconstruction (red).

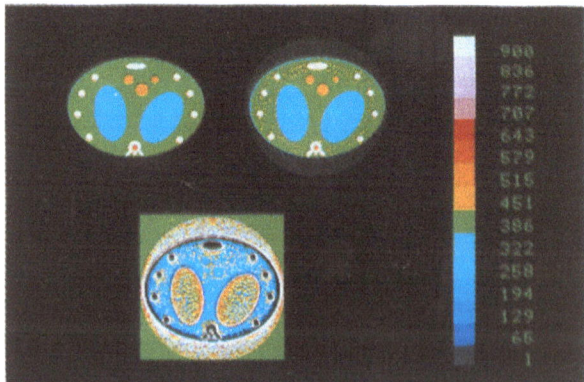

Figure VI. 9: Reconstruction of $I^{-1}f$. a(top left): Original. b(top right): Reconstruction with the filtered backprojection algorithm. c(bottom): Reconstruction of $I^{-1}f$.

where $\theta = (\cos \varphi, \sin \varphi)^T$ and P_m are the Legendre polynomials (VII.3.6). If we choose $w = 1$, then $\overline{\text{range}(\mathbf{R})}$ consists of those functions g in $L_2(Z)$ which satisfy (3.3). In terms of the Fourier coefficients $\hat{g}_l$ of g this means that

$$\int_{-1}^{+1} P_m(s) \hat{g}_l(s) \, ds = 0, \qquad |l| > m,$$

$$\hat{g}_l(-s) = (-1)^l \hat{g}_l(s).$$

In view of the orthogonality properties of P_m we finally get

$$\overline{\text{range}(\mathbf{R})} = \bigoplus_{l=-\infty}^{\infty} e^{il\varphi} \, \mathcal{U}_l \tag{3.4}$$

where

$$\mathcal{U}_l = \langle P_{|l|}, P_{|l|+2}, \ldots \rangle.$$

Now we want to compute the completed data g^c from (1.3). Let $\hat{g}_l^c, \hat{g}_l^I$ be the Fourier coefficients of g^c, g^I, respectively. In view of (3.4), $\hat{g}_l^c$ is the solution of the minimization problem

Minimize $\|g_l\|$ in $\mathcal{U}_l$ subject to $g_l = \hat{g}_l^I$ on $\{s : a < |s| < 1\}$, (3.5)

$\|\cdot\|$ being the norm in $L_2([-1, +1])$. (3.5) has the solution

$$\hat{g}_l^c(s) = \begin{cases} \hat{g}_l^I(s), & a \le |s| \le 1, \\ v_l(s), & |s| \le a, \end{cases} \tag{3.6}$$

$$v_l = \sum_{m < |l|}' v_{lm} P_{m,a}, \quad P_{m,a}(x) = P_m(x/a)$$

where the dash indicates that $m + |l|$ even, and the v_{lm} are given by

$$v_{lm} = -\frac{2m+1}{2a} \int_{1 \ge |s| \ge a} \hat{g}_l^I(s) P_{m,a}(s) \, ds \tag{3.7}$$

for $m < |l|$ and $m + |l|$ even. To verify this it suffices to remark that (3.7) implies $\hat{g}_l^c \in \mathcal{U}_l$ and $v_l \perp \mathcal{U}_l$ in $L_2(-1, +1)$, hence, for any $z \in \mathcal{U}_l$ with $z = 0$ for $a \le |s| \le 1$,

$$\|\hat{g}_l^c + z\|^2 = \|\hat{g}_l^c\|^2 + 2 \int_{-a}^{a} v_l \bar{z} \, ds + \|z\|^2$$

$$= \|\hat{g}_l^c\|^2 + 2 \int_{-1}^{+1} v_l \bar{z} \, ds + \|z\|^2$$

$$= \|\hat{g}_l^c\|^2 + \|z\|^2 \ge \|\hat{g}_l^c\|^2.$$

In (3.7), the Legendre polynomials with argument > 1 show up. Since the Legendre polynomials—as the Chebyshev polynomials—increase exponentially outside their interval of orthogonality the determination of v_{lm} is highly unstable for l large. This means that v_l can be computed reliably for moderate values of l only, $|l| \leq L$, say. In view of the ill-posedness of the exterior problem this is not surprising. In order to find a good value for L and to decide what to do for $|l| > L$ we remind ourselves that our main concern is consistency of the data. Therefore we introduce a measure of consistency

$$C_l(\hat{g}) = \sum_{m < |l|}{}' \left(m + \frac{1}{2}\right) |(\hat{g}, P_m)_{L_2(-1, +1)}|^2$$

and choose L such that this measure of consistency is reduced by the completion process. This means that we use (3.7) only as long as, for the actually computed v_l,

$$C_l(\hat{g}_l^c) \ll C_l(\hat{g}_l^F) \tag{3.8}$$

where $\hat{g}_l^F$ is obtained by extending $\hat{g}_l$ by zero in $|s| \leq a$. L is taken to be the maximal index for which (3.8) holds for $|l| \leq L$. For $|l| > L$, v_l is replaced by 0.

The implementation of the completion procedure for a parallel scanning geometry is obvious. Since a linear map takes straight lines into straight lines we can use any algorithm for circular holes for ellipsoidal holes after a suitable linear transformation.

Apart from the completion procedure we have two further methods for dealing with the exterior problem: ART and the direct algebraic method. In Fig. VI.6 we compare these methods. The original in Fig. VI.6(a) is simple enough: it consists of two circles with midpoints at a distance 0.7 from the origin and with radius 0.1, 0.2, respectively. In Fig. VI.6(d) we show the reconstruction with the filtered backprojection algorithm from $p = 256$ projections with $2q + 1, q = 80$ line integrals each. Figure VI.6(b) gives the reconstruction by the same algorithm, with the integrals along lines hitting the circular hole of radius $a = 0.4$ put equal to zero. The strong artefacts are precisely as we expect from our rule of thumb in Section VI.1: artefacts show up mainly along those tangents to the circles which hit the black hole $|x| < 0.4$. In Fig. VI.6(e) the reconstruction from completed data ($L = 6$) with filtered backprojection is displayed. The typical artefacts are still there, but they are much weaker. They same applies to Fig. VI.6(c) (direct algebraic method, the line integrals being replaced by strip integrals) and to Fig. VI.6(f) (ART, 15 iterations, $\omega = 0.1$). We conclude that for an object such as Fig. VI.6(a), all three methods improve the 'brute force approach' of simply ignoring the missing data, but they do not give results comparable to the case of complete data.

The object displayed in Fig. VI.1(a) is much easier to reconstruct from exterior data. This is demonstrated in Fig. VI.7. Figure VI.7(a) gives the result of the completion procedure ($L = 5$), followed by the ordinary filtered backprojection algorithm. In Fig. VI.7(b) we display the reconstruction using the direct algebraic algorithm. In both cases we used $p = 256$ (hollow) projections consisting of 129 line or strip integrals outside the black hole. We see that the results are much better than the reconstruction of Fig. VI.1(c) obtained by ignoring the missing data, and they are quite close to the original in Fig. VI.1(a).

We remark that failure and success in the exterior problem are in full agreement with our rule of thumb in Section VI.1.

VI.4 The Interior Problem

The interior problem in two dimensions, in which $g^I = \mathbf{R}f$ is given on $I = S^1 \times [-a, a]$, is not uniquely solvable, as can be seen from the following radially symmetric two-dimensional example: let $h \in C^\infty(\mathbb{R}^1)$ be an even function which vanishes outside $[a, 1]$. Then, $g(\theta, s) = h(|s|)$ satisfies the hypothesis of Theorem II.4.2, hence there is $u \in C_0^\infty(\Omega^2)$ such that $\mathbf{R}u = g$. The inversion formula (II.2.15) for radial functions yields for $l = 0$, $n = 2$ the solution

$$u(x) = -\frac{1}{\pi} \int_{|x|}^{\infty} (s^2 - |x|^2)^{-1/2} h'(s) \, ds$$

of $\mathbf{R}u = g$. Obviously, $\mathbf{R}u(\theta, s) = 0$ for $|s| \leq a$, and u does not vanish in $|x| < a$ for h suitably chosen. On the other hand, the interior problem is uniquely solvable in odd dimensions. This follows from the local character of Radon's inversion formula (II.2.5).

However, we shall see that functions u with $\mathbf{R}u$ vanishing on I do not vary much for x well in the interior of $|x| < a$. By Radon's inversion formula in the form of (II.2.7) we obtain for such a function u by an integration by parts

$$u(x) = \frac{1}{4\pi^2} \int_{S^1} \int_{|s| \geq a} \frac{(\mathbf{R}u(\theta, s))'}{s - x \cdot \theta} \, ds \, d\theta$$

$$= \frac{1}{4\pi^2} \int_{S^1} \int_{|s| \geq a} \frac{\mathbf{R}u(\theta, s)}{(s - x \cdot \theta)^2} \, ds \, d\theta.$$

It follows that for $|x| \leq b < a$

$$|u(x) - u(0)| = \frac{1}{4\pi^2} \int_{S^1} \int_{|s| \geq a} \left| \frac{1}{(s - x \cdot \theta)^2} - \frac{1}{s^2} \right| |\mathbf{R}u(\theta, s)| \, ds \, d\theta$$

$$\leq C_1(a, b) \|\mathbf{R}u\|_{L_2(Z)} \tag{4.1}$$

$$C_1(a, b) = \frac{1}{4\pi^2} \left(\int_0^{2\pi} \int_{|s| \geq a} \left(\frac{1}{(s - b \cos \varphi)^2} - \frac{1}{s^2} \right)^2 ds \, d\varphi \right)^{1/2}.$$

The values of $C_1(a, b)$ are surprisingly low, as can be seen from Table 4.1 which has been obtained by numerical integration.

TABLE 4.1 Values of $C_1(a, b)$.

b	a		
	0.4	0.6	0.8
0.2	0.13	0.039	0.016
0.4		0.11	0.039
0.6			0.078

Equation (4.1) is applied as follows. Suppose a complete data set g^c has been found such that $g^c \in \text{range}(\mathbf{R})$ and $g^c = g^I$ on I, e.g. the function g^c from (1.3) for $w = 1$, and $\mathbf{R}f^c = g^c$ has been solved. Then, $u = f - f^c$ has the property that $\mathbf{R}u = 0$ on I, and we obtain from (4.1) with M an unknown constant ($M = (f - f^c)(0)$)

$$|(f - f^c)(x) - M| \leq C_1(a, b)\|g - g^c\|_{L_2(Z-I)} \tag{4.2}$$

for $|x| \leq b$. In view of the smallness of $C_1(a, b)$, a crude approximation to the missing part of g suffices to determine f accurately for $|x| \leq b$ up to an additive constant. In spite of the non-uniqueness we thus can compute a solution to the interior problem which is satisfactory if only changes in the values of f are sought.

The computation of the completed data g^c is quite analogous to Section VI.3.

Now we turn to algorithms which do not need completed data. ART and the direct algebraic methods of V.4 and V.5 can be used without any changes on these data. In the (hypothetical) consistent case, ART converges to the solution with minimal norm of a discretized version of $g^I = \mathbf{R}f$ on I (compare Theorems V.3.9 and V.3.6) if properly initialized. The same is true for the direct algebraic method in the limit $\gamma \to 0$ (compare IV.1). Thus, both methods provide us with an approximation to the minimal norm solution f_M of the equation $\mathbf{R}f = g$ on I and it is interesting to know something about the variation of $u = f - f_M$. From (4.1) we get for $|x| \leq b$

$$|u(x) - u(0)| \leq C_1(a, b)\|\mathbf{R}u\|_{L_2(Z)}.$$

On the other hand, we have because of $\mathbf{R}u = 0$ in $|s| \leq a$

$$\|\mathbf{R}u\|_{L_2(Z)} \leq 2\sqrt{\pi}(1 - a^2)^{1/4}\|u\|_{L_2(\Omega^2)}.$$

Since $u = f - f_M \perp f_M$ in $L_2(\Omega^2)$ we also have in $L_2(\Omega^2)$

$$\|u\|^2 \leq \|u\|^2 + \|f_M\|^2 = \|u + f_M\|^2 = \|f\|^2.$$

Combining the last three estimates we obtain for $|x| \leq b$

$$|u(x) - u(0)| \leq C_2(a, b)\|f\|_{L_2(\Omega^2)},$$
$$C_2(a, b) = 2\sqrt{\pi}(1 - a^2)^{1/4}C_1(a, b). \tag{4.4}$$

If $C_2(a, b)$ is sufficiently small, then (4.4) states that f_M differs only little from f, except for an additive constant.

As an example we reconstructed the phantom in Fig. VI.8(a) from $p = 256$ projections consisting of $2q + 1$, $q = 56$, strip integrals all of which meet the circle of radius $a = 0.7$. In particular we did not use strips lying entirely outside the blue ellipse which has half-axes 0.74 and 0.8. We used strip integrals rather than line integrals because we did the reconstruction with the direct algebraic algorithm of V.5. The reconstruction is displayed in Fig. VI.8(b). We see that the small circles and the annulus in the 'region of interest' $|x| < 0.7$ are clearly visible, but the colours are shifted towards white. This becomes even more obvious in the cross-section through the original and the reconstruction shown in Fig. VI.8(c).

An alternative method which reconstructs density differences but not the absolute values is as follows. The inversion formula (II.2.1) for $n = 2$, $\alpha = -1$ reads

$$\mathbf{I}^{-1}f = \frac{1}{4\pi}\mathbf{R}^*I^{-2}g.$$

By R3 from VII.1, $-I^{-2}g$ is simply the second derivative of g. Hence,

$$\mathbf{I}^{-1}f = -\frac{1}{4\pi}\mathbf{R}^*g''. \tag{4.5}$$

What is important here is that the operator on the right-hand side is local. This means that $\mathbf{I}^{-1}f(x)$ can be computed from integrals along lines which meet an arbitrarily small neighbourhood of x. In particular we can reconstruct $\mathbf{I}^{-1}f$ in $|x| < a$ from the data of the interior problem.

Of course what one wants to reconstruct is f, not $\mathbf{I}^{-1}f$. But we shall show that there is an interesting relation between f and $\mathbf{I}^{-1}f$: $\mathbf{I}^{-1}f$ is smooth where f is, and vice versa. Thus, f or its derivatives have discontinuities precisely where $\mathbf{I}^{-1}f$ or its derivatives have. Practically, this means that $\mathbf{I}^{-1}f$ gives the same information as f if only rapid changes in f, such as edges, are sought for.

The fact about the smoothness of $\mathbf{I}^{-1}f$ we referred to above is essentially the pseudo-local property of pseudo-differential operators, see Treves (1980), Theorem 2.2. We give a version of that theorem which suits our purpose.

THEOREM 4.1 Let $f \in L_1(\mathbb{R}^n)$, and let $f \in C^\infty(U)$ for some open set $U \subseteq \mathbb{R}^n$. Then, for k an integer with $|k| < n$, $I^{-k}f \in C^\infty(U)$.

Proof In terms of Fourier transforms we have in the sense of distributions

$$\mathbf{I}^{-k}f(x) = (2\pi)^{-n/2}\int_{\mathbb{R}^n} e^{ix\cdot\xi}|\xi|^k\hat{f}(\xi)\,d\xi.$$

Let $a_k(\xi) = |\xi|^k$ for $|\xi| \geq 1$, say, and $a_k \in C^\infty(\mathbb{R}^n)$. It suffices to prove the theorem for the operator

$$J^{-k}f(x) = (2\pi)^{-n/2} \int_{\mathbb{R}^n} e^{ix\cdot\xi} a_k(\xi) \hat{f}(\xi) \,d\xi$$

since $J^{-k}f - I^{-k}f \in C^\infty$.

Let V be an open bounded set in U such that $\bar{V} \subseteq U$, and let $\Psi \in C_0^\infty(U)$ be 1 in V. Then

$$J^{-k}f = J^{-k}(\Psi f) + J^{-k}((1-\Psi)f).$$

Since $\Psi f \in C_0^\infty(U)$, $J^{-k}(\Psi f) \in C^\infty(\mathbb{R}^n)$. We show that

$$J^{-k}((1-\Psi)f)(x) = (2\pi)^{-n} \int_{\mathbb{R}^n}\int_{\mathbb{R}^n} e^{i(x-y)\cdot\xi} a_k(\xi) ((1-\Psi)f)(y) \,dy\,d\xi$$

is in $C^\infty(V)$. With Δ_ξ the Laplacian acting on the variable ξ we have for any integer p

$$(-\Delta_\xi)^p e^{i(x-y)\cdot\xi} = |x-y|^{2p} e^{i(x-y)\cdot\xi},$$

hence

$$J^{-k}((1-\Psi)f)(x) = (2\pi)^{-n} \int_{\mathbb{R}^n}\int_{\mathbb{R}^n} \{(-\Delta_\xi)^p e^{i(x-y)\cdot\xi}\} a_k(\xi) \frac{((1-\Psi)f)(y)}{|x-y|^{2p}} \,dy\,d\xi.$$

Note that the integral makes sense for $x \in V$ since $(1-\Psi)f = 0$ in a neighbourhood of x. By an integration by parts we get

$$J^{-k}((1-\Psi)f)(x) = (2\pi)^{-n} \int_{\mathbb{R}^n}\int_{\mathbb{R}^n} e^{i(x-y)\cdot\xi} b_k(\xi) \frac{((1-\Psi)f)(y)}{|x-y|^{2p}} \,dy\,d\xi$$

where

$$b_k(\xi) = (-\Delta_\xi)^p a_k(\xi) = O(|\xi|^{k-2p})$$

as $|\xi| \to \infty$. For $2p - k > n$ we can interchange the order of integration, obtaining

$$J^{-k}((1-\Psi)f)(x) = (2\pi)^{-n} \int_{\mathbb{R}^n} |x-y|^{-2p} K(x,y) ((1-\Psi)f)(y) \,dy,$$

$$K(x,y) = \int_{\mathbb{R}^n} b_k(\xi) e^{i(x-y)\cdot\xi} \,d\xi.$$

Since $K \in C^\infty(\mathbb{R}^n \times \mathbb{R}^n)$, $J^{-k}((1-\Psi)f) \in C^\infty(V)$. This holds for any open bounded $V \subset U$ with $\bar{V} \subseteq U$, i.e. $J^{-k}((1-\Psi)f) \in C^\infty(U)$. This proves the theorem. □

In order to demonstrate the method of reconstructing $I^{-1}f$ we created the thorax phantom in Fig. VI.9(a). The reconstruction of this phantom from parallel data with $p = 500$, $q = 160$ using our standard filtered backprojection algorithm (V.1.17) with w_b from (V.1.21) and $\varepsilon = 0$ is displayed in Fig. VI.9(b). In Fig. VI.9(c) we show the reconstruction of $\mathbf{I}^{-1}f$ by an algorithm very similar to (V.1.17), replacing the convolution in step 1 by taking central second differences. We see that the colours are different from the original, but the geometry of the phantom comes out clearly. Remember that the latter reconstruction is purely local.

Summing up we come to the conclusion that in the interior problem it is possible to reconstruct features which are characterized by rapid changes in the density function. If only such features are sought for, the reconstruction suffers only little from the non-uniqueness of the interior problem.

VI.5 The Restricted Source Problem

In a typical three-dimensional reconstruction problem, the sources are restricted to a curve A surrounding Ω^3, i.e. $g = \mathbf{D}f$ is given on $A \times S^2$. From Theorem II.3.6 we know that f is uniquely determined by these data.

However, a stability estimate corresponding to Theorem II.5.1 does not hold in general. To see this we assume that there is a plane E which meets Ω^3 but misses the curve A which we assume to be smooth and of finite length. Then we shall show that there is a function f_+ which is not continuous in Ω^3 but for which $\mathbf{D}f_+ \in C^\infty(A \times S^2)$. For this purpose we choose a function $f \in C_0^\infty(\Omega^3)$ which does not vanish on all of $\Omega^3 \cap E$. Let E_+ be one of the half-spaces generated by E, and let

$$f_+(x) = \begin{cases} f(x), & x \in E_+, \\ 0, & \text{otherwise.} \end{cases}$$

Since the distance between A and E is positive, straight lines through A can meet E only transversally, hence $\mathbf{D}f_+ \in C^\infty(A \times S^2)$. It follows that a stability estimate cannot hold whenever there exists such a plane E. Unfortunately, this is the case for the practically used source curves which consist of a circle surrounding Ω^3 as in Wood et al. (1979) or two parallel circles as in Kowalski (1979) and Hamaker (1980).

In order to obtain a stability estimate we have to exclude planes E meeting Ω^3 but missing A. Let $x = a(\lambda)$, $\lambda \in \Lambda \subseteq \mathbb{R}^1$ be a parametric representation of A with $a \in C^1(\Lambda)$. A is said to satisfy Tuy's condition if for each $x \in \Omega^3$ and $\theta \in S^2$ there is $\lambda = \lambda(x, \theta) \in \Lambda$ such that

$$(a(\lambda) - x) \cdot \theta = 0, \quad a'(\lambda) \cdot \theta \neq 0. \tag{5.1}$$

The first condition requires that for each x in Ω^3 and for each plane containing x this plane contains also some point of A, and the second condition says that the curve intersects the plane transversally in that point. We remark that Tuy's condition is satisfied, for example, by two orthogonal circles surrounding Ω^3 but not for one circle or two parallel circles.

Below we shall give an inversion formula for $\mathbf{D}$ using only data on I provided A

fulfils Tuy's condition. In this formula we extend $\mathbf{D}_a f$ to a function on $\mathbb{R}^3$ by putting

$$\mathbf{D}_a f(y) = \int_0^\infty f(a + ty)\, dt.$$

This is equivalent to extending $\mathbf{D}_a f$ as a function homogeneous of degree -1. Such a function is locally integrable and it makes sense to compute its Fourier transform $(\mathbf{D}_a f)\hat{\,}$, see (VII.1).

THEOREM 5.1 If A satisfies Tuy's condition (5.1), then, for $f \in C_0^\infty(\Omega^3)$,

$$f(x) = (2\pi)^{-3/2} i^{-1} \int_{S^2} (a'(\lambda) \cdot \theta)^{-1} \frac{d}{d\lambda} (\mathbf{D}_{a(\lambda)} f)\hat{\,}(\theta)\, d\theta$$

where $\lambda = \lambda(x, \theta)$ as in (5.1).

Proof From VII.1 we have with convergence in $\mathscr{S}$

$$(\mathbf{D}_a f)\hat{\,}(\eta) = \lim_{r \to \infty} (2\pi)^{-3/2} \int_{|y| < r} e^{-i\eta \cdot y} \mathbf{D}_a f(y)\, dy$$

$$= \lim_{r \to \infty} (2\pi)^{-3/2} \int_{|y| < r} e^{-i\eta \cdot y} \int_0^\infty f(a + ty)\, dt\, dy$$

$$= \lim_{r \to \infty} (2\pi)^{-3/2} \int_0^\infty \int_{|y| < r} e^{-i\eta \cdot y} f(a + ty)\, dy\, dt.$$

In the inner integral we introduce $x = a + ty$, obtaining

$$(\mathbf{D}_a f)\hat{\,}(\eta) = \lim_{r \to \infty} (2\pi)^{-3/2} \int_0^\infty t^{-3} \int_{|x - a| \le tr} e^{-i\eta \cdot (x - a)/t} f(x)\, dx\, dt$$

$$= \lim_{r \to \infty} (2\pi)^{-3/2} \int_0^\infty t^{-3} e^{i\eta \cdot a/t} \int_{|x - a| \le tr} e^{-i\eta \cdot x/t} f(x)\, dx\, dt$$

$$= \int_0^\infty t^{-3} e^{i\eta \cdot a/t} \hat{f}\left(\frac{1}{t}\eta\right) dt.$$

For $\eta = \theta \in S^2$ we get on putting $t = 1/\rho$

$$(\mathbf{D}_a f)\hat{\,}(\theta) = \int_0^\infty \rho^3 e^{i\rho\theta \cdot a} \hat{f}(\rho\theta)\, d\rho. \tag{5.2}$$

We compare this with the Fourier inversion formula in polar coordinates which reads

$$f(x) = (2\pi)^{-3/2} \int_{S^2} \int_0^\infty \rho^2 e^{i\rho\theta \cdot x} \hat{f}(\rho\theta) \, d\rho \, d\theta.$$

We see that the inner integral is similar to the inner integral in (5.2). To enhance this similarity we put in (5.2) $a = a(\lambda)$ and differentiate with respect to λ. This yields

$$\frac{d}{d\lambda} (\mathbf{D}_{a(\lambda)} f)\,\hat{}\,(\theta) = ia'(\lambda) \cdot \theta \int_0^\infty \rho^2 e^{i\rho\theta \cdot a(\lambda)} \hat{f}(\rho\theta) \, d\rho. \tag{5.3}$$

Now we make use of Tuy's condition. For each $x \in \Omega^3$ and $\theta \in S^2$ we can find $\lambda = \lambda(x, \theta)$ such that (5.1) holds. Thus, in (5.3), we can replace $\theta \cdot a(\lambda)$ by $\theta \cdot x$, yielding

$$\frac{d}{d\lambda} (\mathbf{D}_{a(\lambda)} f)\,\hat{}\,(\theta) = ia'(\lambda) \cdot \theta \int_0^\infty \rho^2 e^{i\rho\theta \cdot x} \hat{f}(\rho\theta) \, d\rho.$$

The integral on the right-hand side is now precisely the inner integral in the Fourier inversion formula. Since, also by (5.1), $a'(\lambda) \cdot \theta \neq 0$, we finally obtain

$$f(x) = (2\pi)^{-3/2} i^{-1} \int_{S^2} (a'(\lambda) \cdot \theta)^{-1} \frac{d}{d\lambda} (\mathbf{D}_{a(\lambda)} f)\,\hat{}\,(\theta) \, d\theta$$

where $\lambda = \lambda(x, \theta)$. □

The formula of Theorem 5.1 is called Tuy's inversion formula. It is not clear if it can be turned into an efficient reconstruction algorithm, and even if this were possible it would not help much because Tuy's formula requires $\mathbf{D}_a f$ on all of S^2, while in practice $\mathbf{D}_a f$ can be measured only in a cone.

What is more important is that Tuy's formula makes one expect a certain degree of stability if the curve of sources meets Tuy's condition. The reason is that no highly unstable operations show up in Tuy's formula. In fact Finch (1985) proved a stability estimate in a Sobolev space framework.

Not much can be said about algorithms at present. Direct algebraic methods are applicable for source curves with circular symmetry such as a circle or two parallel circles, but we know that such source curves lead to severely ill-posed reconstruction problems. We do not know of possibilities to use direct algebraic methods for curves satisfying Tuy's condition.

VI.6 Reconstruction of Homogeneous Objects

If only very few projections of an object are available, then even approximate reconstruction is impossible. However, if the class of objects is suitably restricted it may be possible to restore uniqueness. As an example we consider convex homogeneous objects in the plane, i.e. we assume that the function f we are looking for is the characteristic function of a convex set Ω in $\mathbb{R}^2$. Two typical uniqueness theorems read as follows:

THEOREM 6.1 There are four directions $\theta_1, \ldots, \theta_4$ such that for each convex Ω, f is determined uniquely by $\mathbf{R}_{\theta_j} f, j = 1, \ldots, 4$.

THEOREM 6.2 Let a_1, a_2, a_3 be not collinear and let Ω be a convex set which does not contain either of the a_j. Then f is uniquely determined by $\mathbf{D}_{a_j} f$, $j = 1, 2, 3$.

For the proofs—which are entirely different from what we did in II.3—see Gardner and McMullen (1980) and Falconer (1983). For more results in this direction see Volčič (1984).

These positive results encourage to think about numerical methods for reconstructing characteristic functions for very few, say three to four, projections. An approach entirely within discrete mathematics has been proposed by Kuba (1984). We shall describe a method based on Theorem II.1.1 which works well in practice but which lacks theoretical justification.

We consider a domain Ω which is starlike with respect to the origin, i.e. each half-line starting out from 0 meets the boundary of Ω precisely once. The boundary of Ω can therefore be represented in the polar coordinate form

$$x = F(\omega)\omega, \quad \omega \in S^1 \tag{6.1}$$

where $F(\omega) > 0$. The Fourier transform of the characteristic function f of Ω can be computed as follows:

$$\hat{f}(\sigma\theta) = \frac{1}{2\pi} \int_\Omega e^{-i\sigma\theta \cdot x} dx$$

$$= \frac{1}{2\pi} \int_{S^1} \int_0^{F(\omega)} r e^{-i\sigma\theta \cdot \omega} dr\, d\omega.$$

Using the formula

$$\int_0^F r e^{-ira} dr = F^2 K(aF),$$

$$K(u) = \begin{cases} u^{-2}((1+iu)e^{-iu} - 1), & u \neq 0, \\ \frac{1}{2}, & u = 0 \end{cases} \tag{6.1}$$

which is easily verified by an integration by parts, we obtain

$$\hat{f}(\sigma\theta) = \frac{1}{2\pi} \int_{S^1} F^2(\omega) K(\sigma\theta \cdot \omega F(\omega)) \, d\omega.$$

Now let $g = \mathbf{R}f$. Theorem II.1.1 holds for f, hence

$$\hat{g}(\theta, \sigma) = (2\pi)^{1/2} \hat{f}(\sigma\theta).$$

Combining the last two relations we obtain

$$\hat{g}(\theta, \sigma) = (A_\theta F)(\sigma),$$
$$(A_\theta F)(\sigma) = (2\pi)^{-1/2} \int_{S^1} F^2(\omega) K(\sigma\theta \cdot \omega F(\omega)) \, d\omega. \tag{6.2}$$

For each direction θ, A_θ is a nonlinear integral operator mapping functions on S^1 into functions on $\mathbb{R}^1$. If g is available for p directions $\theta_1, \ldots, \theta_p$, we have the system

$$\hat{g}_{\theta_j} = A_{\theta_j} F, \quad \hat{g}_{\theta_j}(\sigma) = \hat{g}(\theta_j, \sigma), \quad j = 1, \ldots, p \tag{6.3}$$

for the unknown function F. Equation (6.3) is a system of nonlinear first kind integral equations.

In general, we cannot expect (6.3) to be uniquely solvable. However, we know from Theorem 6.1 that there are four directions $\theta_1, \ldots, \theta_p$ such that (6.3) for these directions is uniquely solvable within the class of functions F representing convex objects. In this case we even have a result on continuous dependence, see Volčič (1983), but nevertheless we expect (6.3) to be severely ill-posed in the terminology of IV.1. Thus, solving (6.3) requires some kind of regularization. The following variant of the Tikhonov–Phillips method has proven to be successful: determine an approximation F_γ to F by minimizing

$$\frac{1}{p} \sum_{j=1}^{p} \|\hat{g}_{\theta_j} - A_{\theta_j} F\|^2_{L_2(\mathbb{R}^1)} + \gamma \|F\|^2_{H^1(S^1)}. \tag{6.4}$$

Here, γ is the regularization parameter which has to be chosen carefully.

In our numerical experiments we used a straightforward discretization of (6.4) by the trapezoidal rule and a standard minimization subroutine. The results are shown in Fig. VI.10. The original (a) has been reconstructed from the directions $\varphi_j = (\cos \varphi_j, \sin \varphi_j)^T$ with the angles φ_j

0°	45°	90°	135°	for reconstruction (b),
0°	30°	60°		for reconstruction (c),
0°	10°	20°		for reconstruction (d).

We see that even in the case of only three directions in an angular range as small as 20° there is some similarity between the reconstructed object and the original.

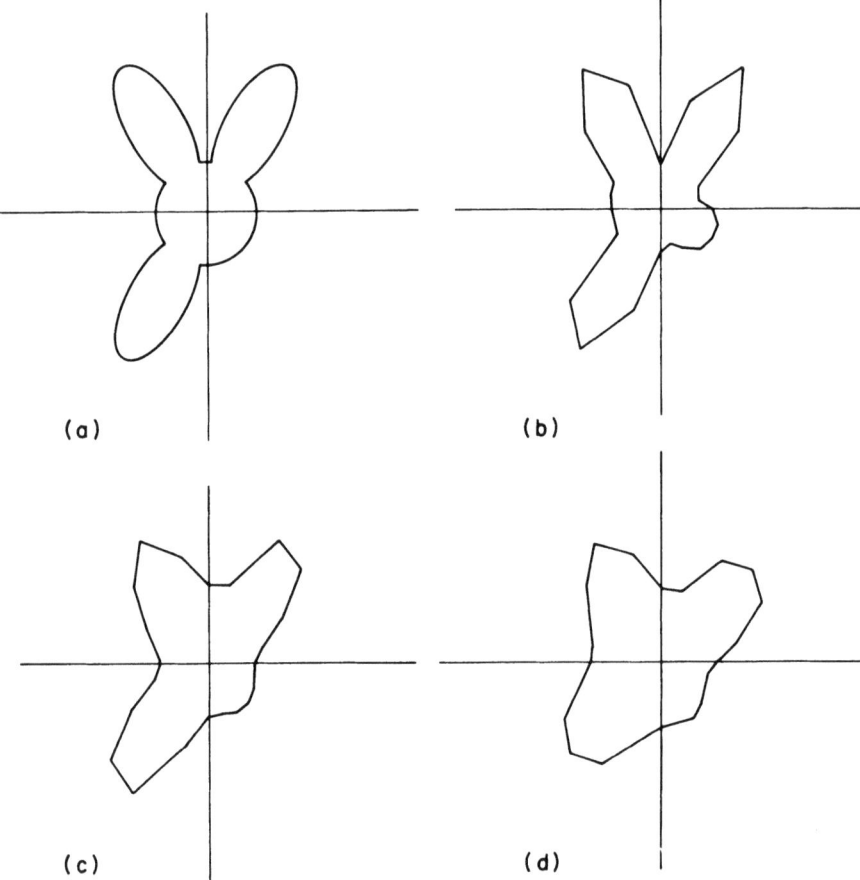

FIG. VI.10 Reconstruction of a homogeneous object in the plane. (a, top left): Original. (b, top right): Reconstruction from the directions 0°, 45°, 90°, 135°. (c, bottom left): Reconstruction from the directions 0°, 30°, 60°. (d, bottom right): Reconstruction from the directions 0°, 10°, 20°.

VI.7 Bibliographical Notes

Consistent completion of data as a means to reduce artefacts in incomplete data problems was first suggested by Lewitt *et al.* (1978b).

Our treatment of the limited angle problem is based on Louis (1980), see also Peres (1979). For a different approach to the limited angle problem based on extrapolation of band-limited functions see Tuy (1981), Lent and Tuy (1981), and Tam *et al.* (1980). For a numerical method based on the Davison–Grünbaum algorithm in V.6 see Davison (1983).

The singular value decomposition for the exterior problem has been given by Quinto (1985). This paper also contains a characterization of the null space of the exterior problem considered in the whole space. Quinto (1986) gives an exterior inversion method. A reconstruction formula for the exterior problem along the lines of Marr (1974) has been given by Perry (1977).

The idea of reconstructing $\mathbf{I}^{-1}f$ rather than f for the interior problem is due to Smith (1984), also the observations based on (4.1), see Hamaker *et al.* (1980).

Tuy's inversion formula has been published in Tuy (1983). The method of proving that the restricted source problem is severely ill-posed in the absence of Tuy's condition is due to Finch (1985). We used this method throughout the chapter.

VII
Mathematical Tools

In this chapter we collect some well-known results for easy reference. We give proofs only for less accessible results and in cases where the proof serves as a motivation. Most of the time we simply refer to the literature.

VII.1 Fourier Analysis

The Fourier transform plays an important role throughout the book, particularly in the theory of the integral transforms in Chapter II and in the sampling theorem in Chapter III. For our purpose it suffices to study the Fourier transform in the Schwartz space $\mathscr{S}(\mathbb{R}^n)$ and in its dual $\mathscr{S}'(\mathbb{R}^n)$. This theory is easily accessible in textbooks (Yosida, 1968), so we restrict ourselves to the basic facts and concentrate on some less well known examples which we have used in the preceding chapters.

$\mathscr{S}(\mathbb{R}^n)$, or $\mathscr{S}$, is the linear space of those C^∞ functions f on $\mathbb{R}^n$ for which

$$|f|_{k,l} = \sup_{x \in \mathbb{R}^n} |x^k D^l f(x)|$$

is finite for all multi-indices $k, l \in \mathbb{Z}_+^n$. For $f \in L_1(\mathbb{R}^n)$, the Fourier transform $\hat{f}$ and the inverse Fourier transform $\check{f}$ are defined by

$$\hat{f}(\xi) = (2\pi)^{-n/2} \int_{\mathbb{R}^n} e^{-ix\cdot\xi} f(x)\,dx,$$

$$\check{f}(\xi) = (2\pi)^{-n/2} \int_{\mathbb{R}^n} e^{ix\cdot\xi} f(x)\,dx.$$

The Fourier inversion formula reads

$$\check{\hat{f}} = \hat{\check{f}} = f, \quad f \in \mathscr{S},$$

i.e. the transforms are inverses to each other and map $\mathscr{S}$ in a one-to-one manner onto itself. If f has compact support, then $\hat{f}$ extends to an analytic function in $\mathbb{C}^n$.

If not stated otherwise the following rules hold in $L_1(\mathbb{R}^n)$. Later on in this section they will be generalized.

R1: For $r > 0$ let $f_r(x) = f(rx)$. Then
$$\hat{f}_r(\xi) = r^{-n}\hat{f}(r^{-1}\xi).$$

R2: For $y \in \mathbb{R}^n$ let $f_y(x) = f(x+y)$. Then
$$\hat{f}_y(\xi) = e^{i\xi \cdot y}\hat{f}(\xi).$$

R3: For $k \in \mathbb{Z}_+^n$ we have for $f \in \mathscr{S}$
$$(D^k f)^\wedge = i^{|k|}\xi^k \hat{f}, \quad (x^k f)^\wedge = i^{|k|} D^k \hat{f}.$$

R4: We have for $g \in \mathscr{S}$
$$(f*g)^\wedge = (2\pi)^{n/2}\hat{f}\hat{g}, \quad (fg)^\wedge = (2\pi)^{-n/2}\hat{f}*\hat{g}$$

where the convolution $f*g$ is defined by
$$(f*g)(x) = \int_{\mathbb{R}^n} f(x-y)g(y)\,dy.$$

R5: We have Parseval's relation
$$\int_{\mathbb{R}^n} f\hat{g}\,dx = \int_{\mathbb{R}^n} \hat{f}g\,dx.$$

For the inverse Fourier transform we obtain the corresponding rules from $\check{f} = \tilde{\hat{f}}$.

$\mathscr{S}'$ is the space of linear functionals T over $\mathscr{S}$ which are continuous in the following sense: there are $k, l \in \mathbb{Z}_+^n$ and $c < \infty$ such that
$$|Tf| \le c \sum_{k' \le k} |f|_{k',l}$$

for $f \in \mathscr{S}$. The elements of $\mathscr{S}'$ are called (tempered) distributions. Distributions are differentiated according to
$$D^k Tf = (-1)^{|k|} T D^k f.$$

If $g \in C^\infty$ and all of its derivatives increase only polynomially, then the product $gT = Tg$ is the distribution
$$gT(f) = T(gf).$$

Finally, if $g \in \mathscr{S}$, then we define the convolution
$$(T*g)(x) = Tg_x$$

where $g_x(y) = g(x-y)$.

If g is a measurable function on $\mathbb{R}^n$ such that
$$\int |g(x)|(1+|x|)^q\,dx < \infty$$

for a suitable q, then we can define the distribution T_g by
$$T_g f = \int_{\mathbb{R}^n} gf\,dx.$$

We say that T_g is represented by g. Integration by parts yields

$$D^k T_g = T_{D^k g}$$

if $D^k g$ satisfies the same growth condition as g. This relation suggests to identify T_g with g and to write simply g for T_g.

Now we extend the Fourier transform to $\mathscr{S}'$ by defining

$$\hat{T}f = T\hat{f}$$

and correspondingly for $\check{T}$. Because of R3, $\hat{T}$ is in $\mathscr{S}'$ if T is. If $g \in L_1(\mathbb{R}^n)$ we have by R5

$$\hat{T}_g f = T_g \hat{f} = \int g\hat{f}\,dx = \int \hat{g}f\,dx = T_{\hat{g}}f,$$

hence $\hat{T}_g = T_{\hat{g}}$, i.e. the distributional Fourier transform and the Fourier transform in the sense $L_1(\mathbb{R}^n)$ coincide. If f is locally integrable and $f_r = f$ in $|x| < r$ but 0 otherwise, then $\hat{f}_r \to \hat{f}$ pointwise in $\mathscr{S}'$ as $r \to \infty$. Similarly, if $g \in L_2(\mathbb{R}^n)$, then Plancherel's theorem states that $\hat{T}_g = T_{\hat{g}}$ with some L_2 function $\hat{g}$ which we call the Fourier transform of g. One can show that

$$\hat{g}(\xi) = (2\pi)^{-n/2} \lim_{r \to \infty} \int_{|x| < r} e^{-ix\cdot\xi} g(x)\,dx$$

the limit being understood in the sense of convergence in $L_2(\mathbb{R}^n)$. The extension of rule R3 to $\mathscr{S}'$ is obvious. Rule R4 holds if $f \in \mathscr{S}'$ and $g \in \mathscr{S}$. R5 holds in $L_2(\mathbb{R}^n)$ as well, and it readily follows that

$$(f, g) = (\hat{f}, \hat{g})$$

with the inner product in $L_2(\mathbb{R}^n)$, i.e. the Fourier transform is an isometry in $L_2(\mathbb{R}^n)$.

Now let $f \in L_2([-a, a]^n)$. The functions

$$u_k(x) = (2a)^{-n/2} e^{i\pi x \cdot k/a}, \quad k \in \mathbb{Z}^n$$

constitute a complete orthogonal system in $L_2([-a, a]^n)$, hence with the inner product in $L_2([-a, a]^n)$,

$$f = \sum_k (f, u_k) u_k$$

converges in $L_2([-a, a]^n)$. Written out this gives the Fourier series

$$f(x) = \sum_k \hat{f}_k e^{i\pi x \cdot k/a}, \quad \hat{f}_k = (2a)^{-n} \int_{[-a, a]^n} f(x) e^{-i\pi x \cdot k/a}\,dx.$$

$\hat{f}_k$ are the Fourier coefficients of f. If $f = 0$ outside $[-a, a]^n$, then we can write

$$f(x) = \left(\frac{\pi}{2}\right)^{n/2} a^{-n} \sum_k \hat{f}\left(\frac{\pi}{a}k\right) e^{i\pi x \cdot k/a},$$

and we have Parseval's relation

$$(f, g) = \left(\frac{\pi}{a}\right)^n \sum_k \hat{f}\left(\frac{\pi}{a}k\right) \overline{\hat{g}\left(\frac{\pi}{a}k\right)}$$

if $g = 0$ outside $[-a, a]^n$.

In the following we compute the Fourier transforms of some special distributions. To begin with we consider Dirac's δ-function

$$\delta_x f = f(x), \qquad \delta = \delta_0.$$

We have

$$\hat{\delta}_x f = \delta_x \hat{f} = \hat{f}(x) = (2\pi)^{-n/2} \int_{\mathbb{R}^n} e^{-ix\cdot\xi} f(\xi)\, d\xi,$$

i.e. $\hat{\delta}_x$ is the function

$$\hat{\delta}_x(\xi) = (2\pi)^{-n/2} e^{-ix\cdot\xi}. \tag{1.1}$$

Applying formally the Fourier inversion formula we obtain for δ the representation

$$\delta(y) = (2\pi)^{-n} \int_{\mathbb{R}^n} e^{iy\cdot\xi}\, d\xi$$

which of course does not make sense since the exponential function is not integrable. However, if we put for some $b > 0$

$$\delta^b(y) = (2\pi)^{-n} \int_{|\xi| < b} e^{iy\cdot\xi}\, d\xi \tag{1.2}$$

then we have for $f \in \mathscr{S}$

$$\lim_{b \to \infty} \int_{\mathbb{R}^n} \delta^b(y) f(y)\, dy = f(0)$$

i.e. $\delta^b \to \delta$ pointwise in $\mathscr{S}'$. Hence δ^b is an approximate δ-function. From (3.19) we obtain for $l = 0$

$$\delta^b(y) = (2\pi)^{-n} \int_0^b \sigma^{n-1} \int_{S^{n-1}} e^{i\sigma y \cdot \theta}\, d\theta\, d\sigma$$

$$= (2\pi)^{-n/2} |y|^{(2-n)/2} \int_0^b \sigma^{n/2} J_{n/2-1}(\sigma|y|)\, d\sigma$$

$$= (2\pi)^{-n/2} b^n \frac{J_{n/2}(b|y|)}{(b|y|)^{n/2}} \tag{1.3}$$

where we have used (VII.3.25).

The distribution
$$\text{Ш}_h = \sum_{k \in \mathbb{Z}^n} \delta_{hk}, \quad h > 0$$
is called the shah-distribution in communication theory. To compute its Fourier transform we use the Fourier expansion of the periodic function
$$g(\xi) = \sum_l \hat{f}\left(\xi - \frac{2\pi}{h} l\right)$$
in $[-(\pi/h), \pi/h]^n$ which reads
$$g(\xi) = \sum_l \hat{g}_k e^{-ih\xi \cdot k},$$

$$\hat{g}_k = \left(\frac{2\pi}{h}\right)^{-n} \int_{[-(\pi/h), \pi/h]^n} g(\xi) e^{ih\xi \cdot k} \, d\xi$$

$$= \left(\frac{2\pi}{h}\right)^{-n} \sum_l \int_{[-(\pi/h), \pi/h]^n} \hat{f}\left(\xi - \frac{2\pi}{h} l\right) e^{ih\xi \cdot k} \, d\xi$$

$$= \left(\frac{2\pi}{h}\right)^{-n} \int_{\mathbb{R}^n} \hat{f}(\xi) e^{ih\xi \cdot k} \, d\xi$$

$$= (2\pi)^{-n/2} h^n f(hk).$$

Comparing the two expansions for g in terms of f we see that
$$\sum_l \hat{f}\left(\xi - \frac{2\pi}{h} l\right) = (2\pi)^{-n/2} h^n \sum_k f(hk) e^{-ih\xi \cdot k} \quad (1.4)$$
which holds for $f \in \mathcal{S}$. For $\xi = 0$ this is Poisson's formula
$$\hat{\text{Ш}}_{2\pi/h} = (2\pi)^{-n/2} h^n \text{Ш}_h$$
which we can also write as
$$\int f(x) \, dx = h^n \sum_k f(hk) - (2\pi)^{n/2} \sum_{l \neq 0} \hat{f}\left(\frac{2\pi}{h} l\right). \quad (1.5)$$

This can be interpreted as a representation of the quadrature error of the trapezoidal rule. For a periodic function with period a the corresponding formula reads
$$\int_{[0,a]^n} f(x) \, dx = h^n \sum_{0 \leq k < p} f(hk) - a^n \sum_{l \neq 0} c_{pl}, \quad h = \frac{a}{p} \quad (1.6)$$
where the restriction on k holds componentwise and c_l are the Fourier coefficients of f in $[0, a]$.

Now let g be an arbitrary locally integrable function with period $2a$. Then,

$g \in \mathscr{S}'$, and we claim that
$$\hat{g} = (2\pi)^{n/2} \sum_k \hat{g}_k \, \delta_{\pi k/a} \tag{1.7}$$

with $\hat{g}_k$ the Fourier coefficients of g. For the proof we apply the distribution $\hat{T}_g$ to $f \in \mathscr{S}$, substituting for g its Fourier expansion. We obtain

$$\hat{T}_g f = T_g \hat{f} = \int_{\mathbf{R}^n} g \hat{f} \, dx$$

$$= \sum_k \hat{g}_k \int_{\mathbf{R}^n} e^{i\pi x \cdot k/a} \hat{f}(x) \, dx$$

$$= (2\pi)^{n/2} \sum_k \hat{g}_k f\left(\frac{\pi}{a}k\right)$$

and this is (1.7).

Another example is the Cauchy principal value integral
$$Tf = \int \frac{f(x)}{x} \, dx \tag{1.8}$$

which can be defined for $f \in \mathscr{S}$ by either of the ordinary integrals

$$\int \frac{f(x)}{x} \, dx = \lim_{h \to 0} \int_{|x|>h} \frac{f(x)}{x} \, dx$$
$$= \int_{-\infty}^{+\infty} \frac{f(x) - f(-x)}{2x} \, dx. \tag{1.9}$$

Using the second definition we obtain for the Fourier transform of T

$$\hat{T}f = T\hat{f} = \lim_{a \to \infty} \int_{-a}^{a} \frac{\hat{f}(x) - \hat{f}(-x)}{2x} \, dx$$

$$= \lim_{a \to \infty} (2\pi)^{-1/2} \int_{-a}^{a} \int_{-\infty}^{+\infty} \frac{e^{-ix\xi} - e^{ix\xi}}{2x} f(\xi) \, d\xi \, dx$$

$$= \lim_{a \to \infty} -i (2\pi)^{-1/2} \int_{-a}^{a} \int_{-\infty}^{+\infty} \frac{\sin(x\xi)}{x} f(\xi) \, d\xi \, dx$$

$$= \lim_{a \to \infty} -i (2\pi)^{-1/2} \int_{-\infty}^{+\infty} f(\xi) \int_{-a}^{a} \frac{\sin(x\xi)}{x} \, dx \, d\xi.$$

The inner integral is bounded as a function of ξ, uniformly in a and converges pointwise to $\pi \operatorname{sgn}(\xi)$ as $a \to \infty$, except for $\xi = 0$. Letting $a \to \infty$ we thus obtain

$$\hat{T}f = -i\left(\frac{\pi}{2}\right)^{1/2} \int_{-\infty}^{+\infty} \operatorname{sgn}(\xi) f(\xi) \, d\xi$$

i.e. $\hat{T}$ is the function

$$\hat{T}(\xi) = -i\left(\frac{\pi}{2}\right)^{1/2} \operatorname{sgn}(\xi).$$

The Hilbert transform **H** is defined by $\mathbf{H}f = \frac{1}{\pi} T * f$, i.e.

$$\mathbf{H}f(x) = \frac{1}{\pi} \int_{-\infty}^{+\infty} \frac{f(y)}{x-y} \, dy. \tag{1.10}$$

Applying R4 yields

$$(\mathbf{H}f)\hat{\ }(\xi) = \frac{1}{\pi}(T*f)\hat{\ }(\xi) = \left(\frac{\pi}{2}\right)^{-1/2} (\hat{T}\hat{f})(\xi) \tag{1.11}$$

$$= \frac{\operatorname{sgn}(\xi)}{i} \hat{f}(\xi).$$

VII.2 Integration Over Spheres

In this section we collect some formulae involving integrals over S^{n-1}. Some familiarity with integration over spheres is required throughout the book.

To begin with we introduce spherical coordinates in $\mathbb{R}^n$. Let $x = (x_1, \ldots, x_n)^T \in \mathbb{R}^n$ and $x_1^2 + \ldots + x_n^2 = r^2$. Assume that $x_1^2 + \ldots + x_m^2 \neq 0$, $m = 2, \ldots, n$. Then there is a unique $\theta_{n-1} \in [0, \pi]$ such that $x_n = r \cos \theta_{n-1}$, and

$$x_1^2 + \ldots + x_{n-1}^2 = r^2 - x_n^2 = r^2 \sin^2 \theta_{n-1}.$$

Likewise, there is a unique angle $\theta_{n-2} \in [0, \pi]$ such that $x_{n-1} = r \sin \theta_{n-1} \cos \theta_{n-2}$, and

$$x_1^2 + \ldots + x_{n-2}^2 = r^2 \sin^2 \theta_{n-1} - x_{n-1}^2 = r^2 \sin^2 \theta_{n-1} \sin^2 \theta_{n-2}.$$

We continue in this fashion until we have found angles $\theta_{n-1}, \ldots, \theta_2 \in [0, \pi]$ such that, for $i = n, \ldots, 3$, $x_i = r \sin \theta_{n-1} \ldots \sin \theta_i \cos \theta_{i-1}$, and

$$x_1^2 + x_2^2 = r^2 \sin^2 \theta_{n-1} \ldots \sin^2 \theta_2.$$

Now there is a unique angle $\theta_1 \in [0, 2\pi]$ such that

$$x_1 = r \sin \theta_{n-1} \ldots \sin \theta_2 \sin \theta_1,$$
$$x_2 = r \sin \theta_{n-1} \ldots \sin \theta_2 \cos \theta_1.$$

The numbers $\theta_1, \ldots, \theta_{n-1}$ for which we now have

$$x_1 = r \sin \theta_{n-1} \ldots \sin \theta_3 \sin \theta_2 \sin \theta_1,$$
$$x_2 = r \sin \theta_{n-1} \ldots \sin \theta_3 \sin \theta_2 \cos \theta_1,$$
$$x_3 = r \sin \theta_{n-1} \ldots \sin \theta_3 \cos \theta_2,$$
$$\vdots$$
$$x_{n-1} = r \sin \theta_{n-1} \cos \theta_{n-2}$$
$$x_n = r \cos \theta_{n-1}$$

are called the spherical coordinates of x.

We want to compute the integral of a function f over S^{n-1}. Putting $x' = (x_1, \ldots, x_{n-1})^T$ we can represent the upper and lower halves $S^{n-1}_{\pm} = \{\omega \in S^{n-1} : \pm \omega_n > 0\}$ of S^{n-1} by

$$x_n = \pm \sqrt{(1 - |x'|^2)}, \quad |x'| < 1.$$

Then, with the usual definition of surface integrals,

$$\int_{S^{n-1}_{\pm}} f(x) \, dx = \int_{|x'| < 1} f(x', \pm \sqrt{(1 - |x'|^2)}) \frac{dx'}{\sqrt{(1 - |x'|^2)}}. \tag{2.1}$$

Let $\theta_1, \ldots, \theta_{n-1}$ be the spherical coordinates of x. Then,

$$\frac{\partial(x_1, \ldots, x_{n-1})}{\partial(\theta_1, \ldots, \theta_{n-1})} = \sqrt{(1 - |x'|^2)} (\sin \theta_{n-1})^{n-2} \ldots (\sin \theta_3)^2 \sin \theta_2,$$

hence

$$\int_{S^{n-1}} f(x) \, dx = \int_0^\pi \ldots \int_0^\pi \int_0^{2\pi} f(x) (\sin \theta_{n-1})^{n-2} \ldots (\sin \theta_3)^2 \sin \theta_2 \, d\theta_1 \, d\theta_2 \ldots d\theta_{n-1}. \tag{2.2}$$

In particular we obtain for the surface area $|S^{n-1}|$ of S^{n-1}

$$|S^{n-1}| = 2\pi^{n/2}/\Gamma(n/2)$$

where Γ denotes the Γ-function. For example, $|S^0| = 2$, $|S^1| = 2\pi$ and $|S^2| = 4\pi$.

The integral

$$\int_{S^{n-1}} f(\omega \cdot x) \, dx$$

for $\omega \in S^{n-1}$ does not depend on ω, so we may assume that $\omega = (0, \ldots, 0, 1)^T$. Introducing spherical coordinates $\theta_1, \ldots, \theta_{n-1}$ for x we have $\omega \cdot x = \cos \theta_{n-1}$ and

$$\int_{S^{n-1}} f(\omega \cdot x) \, dx = \int_0^\pi \ldots \int_0^\pi \int_0^{2\pi} f(\cos \theta_{n-1}) (\sin \theta_{n-1})^{n-2} \ldots \sin \theta_2 \, d\theta_1 \ldots d\theta_{n-1}.$$

The integrals over $\theta_1, \ldots, \theta_{n-2}$ add up to $|S^{n-2}|$, hence

$$\int_{S^{n-1}} f(\omega \cdot x) \, dx = |S^{n-2}| \int_0^\pi f(\cos\theta_{n-1})(\sin\theta_{n-1})^{n-2} \, d\theta_{n-1}$$

$$= |S^{n-2}| \int_{-1}^{+1} f(t)(1-t^2)^{(n-3)/2} \, dt \qquad (2.3)$$

where we have made the substitution $t = \cos\theta_{n-1}$.

Integrals over $\mathbb{R}^n$ can be expressed by integrals over spheres by introducing polar coordinates $x = r\omega$, $\omega \in S^{n-1}$:

$$\int_{\mathbb{R}^n} f(x) \, dx = \int_0^\infty r^{n-1} \int_{S^{n-1}} f(r\omega) \, d\omega \, dr$$

Similarly we write the integral over the hyperplane $x_n = s$ as

$$\int_{x_n = s} f(x) \, dx = \int_{S_+^{n-1}} f\left(\frac{s}{\omega_n}\omega\right) \frac{s^{n-1}}{\omega_n^n} \, d\omega \qquad (2.5)$$

where $s > 0$. For the proof we project the hyperplane onto S_+^{n-1} by putting $\omega = x/|x|$. The Jacobian of this projection is easily evaluated. For $l < n$ we have

$$x_l = s\omega_l/\omega_n, \quad \omega_n = \sqrt{(1 - \omega_1^2 - \ldots - \omega_{n-1}^2)}$$

hence, for $k, l < n$

$$\frac{\partial x_l}{\partial \omega_k} = \frac{s}{\omega_n}\delta_{lk} + \frac{s\omega_l\omega_k}{\omega_n^3}$$

where δ_{lk} is Kronecker's symbol. Using the formula

$$\det(I + aa^T) = 1 + |a|^2$$

where I is the unit matrix and aa^T the dyadic product, it follows that

$$\frac{\partial(x_1, \ldots, x_{n-1})}{\partial(\omega_1, \ldots, \omega_{n-1})} = \frac{s^{n-1}}{\omega_n^{n+1}}.$$

Thus, carrying out the substitution $\omega = x/|x|$ we obtain

$$\int_{x_n = s} f(x) \, dx = \int_{\omega_1^2 + \ldots + \omega_{n-1}^2 < 1} f\left(\frac{s}{\omega_n}\omega\right) \frac{\partial(x_1, \ldots, x_{n-1})}{\partial(\omega_1, \ldots, \omega_{n-1})} \, d\omega_1 \ldots d\omega_{n-1}$$

$$= \int_{\omega_1^2 + \ldots + \omega_{n-1}^2 < 1} f\left(\frac{s}{\omega_n}\omega\right) \frac{s^{n-1}}{\omega_n^{n+1}} \, d\omega_1 \ldots d\omega_{n-1}.$$

In view of (2.1) this is identical with (2.5).

Occasionally we will have to integrate over the special orthogonal group $SO(n)$, i.e. the set of real orthogonal (n, n) matrices with determinant $+1$. For this purpose we introduce the (normalized) Haar measure on $SO(n)$, i.e. the uniquely determined invariant normalized Radon measure on $SO(n)$.

Let $\theta^{m-1} \in S^{m-1}$ have the spherical coordinates $\theta_{m-1}^{m-1}, \ldots, \theta_1^{m-1}$. Then, θ^{m-1} can be obtained from the mth unit vector $e_m \in \mathbb{R}^m$ by rotations in the $x_l - x_{l+1}$ plane with angle θ_l^{m-1}, $l = m-1, \ldots, 1$. Let $u^{m-1}(\theta^{m-1})$ be the product of these rotations. We show that each $u \in SO(n)$ admits the representation

$$u = u^{n-1}(\theta^{n-1})u^{n-2}(\theta^{n-2}) \ldots u^1(\theta^1) \tag{2.6}$$

with $\theta^{m-1} \in S^{m-1}$ uniquely determined. Let $\theta^{n-1} = ue_n$. Then, $(u^{n-1}(\theta^{n-1}))^{-1}u$ leaves e_n fixed, hence

$$(u^{n-1}(\theta^{n-1}))^{-1}u = v$$

with some $v \in SO(n-1)$. Because of

$$u = u^{n-1}(\theta^{n-1})v$$

we have reduced the problem to $n-1$ dimensions. Since the case $n = 2$ is obvious, the proof of (2.6) is finished. The spherical coordinates of $\theta^{n-1}, \ldots, \theta^1$ are the Euler angles of u.

The (normalized) Haar measure on $SO(n)$ can now be defined simply as the normalized Lebesgue measure on $S^{n-1} \times \ldots \times S^1$, i.e.

$$\int_{SO(n)} f(u)\,du = \frac{1}{|S^{n-1}|\ldots|S^1|} \int_{S^{n-1}} \ldots \int_{S^1} f(u^{n-1}(\theta^{n-1})\ldots u^1(\theta^1))\,d\theta^1 \ldots d\theta^{n-1}.$$

As an immediate consequence we obtain for $\theta_0 \in S^{n-1}$ and f a function on S^{n-1}

$$\int_{SO(n)} f(u\theta_0)\,du = \frac{1}{|S^{n-1}|} \int_{S^{n-1}} f(\theta)\,d\theta. \tag{2.7}$$

Since the left-hand side is independent of θ_0 we may assume $\theta_0 = e_n$. With u as in (2.6) we get $u\theta_0 = \theta^{n-1}$, hence

$$\int_{SO(n)} f(u\theta_0)\,du = \frac{1}{|S^{n-1}|\ldots|S^1|} \int_{S^{n-1}} \ldots \int_{S^1} f(\theta^{n-1})\,d\theta^1 \ldots d\theta^{n-1}$$

$$= \frac{1}{|S^{n-1}|} \int_{S^{n-1}} f(\theta^{n-1})\,d\theta^{n-1}$$

and this is (2.7).

We use (2.7) to prove the important formula

$$\int_{S^{n-1}} \int_{\theta^\perp} f(y) \, dy \, d\theta = |S^{n-2}| \int_{R^n} |y|^{-1} f(y) \, dy. \tag{2.8}$$

For the proof we apply (2.7) to the function

$$\theta \to \int_{\theta^\perp} f(y) \, dy$$

on S^{n-1}. With $\theta_0 \in S^{n-1}$ we obtain

$$\int_{S^{n-1}} \int_{\theta^\perp} f(y) \, dy \, d\theta = |S^{n-1}| \int_{SO(n)} \int_{(u\theta_0)^\perp} f(y) \, dy \, du$$

$$= |S^{n-1}| \int_{SO(n)} \int_{\theta_0^\perp} f(uy) \, dy \, du$$

$$= |S^{n-1}| \int_{\theta_0^\perp} \int_{SO(n)} f\left(|y| u \frac{y}{|y|}\right) du \, dy$$

$$= \int_{\theta_0^\perp} \int_{S^{n-1}} f(|y|\theta) \, d\theta \, dy$$

where we have used (2.7) with θ_0 replaced by $y/|y|$. Putting $y = r\omega$, $\omega \in \theta_0^\perp \cap S^{n-1}$ yields

$$\int_{\theta_0^\perp} \int_{S^{n-1}} f(|y|\theta) \, d\theta \, dy = \int_0^\infty r^{n-2} \int_{\theta_0^\perp \cap S^{n-1}} \int_{S^{n-1}} f(r\theta) \, d\theta \, d\omega \, dr$$

$$= |S^{n-2}| \int_0^\infty r^{n-2} \int_{S^{n-1}} f(r\theta) \, d\theta \, dr$$

$$= |S^{n-2}| \int_{R^n} |x|^{-1} f(x) \, dx$$

which proves (2.8).

We conclude this section by giving quadrature rules on S^{n-1} which are exact for even polynomials of degree $2m$. For $n = 2$ we simply use the trapezoidal rule on $[0, \pi]$. We then have from (1.6)

$$\int_{S^1} f(\theta) \, d\theta = \frac{2\pi}{m+1} \sum_{j=0}^{m} f(\theta_j),$$

$$\theta_j = \begin{pmatrix} \cos \varphi_j \\ \sin \varphi_j \end{pmatrix}, \quad \varphi_j = \pi j/m+1, j = 0, \ldots, m \quad (2.9)$$

for f an even polynomial of degree $2m$. For $n = 3$ we base our quadrature rule on the nodes θ_{ji} whose spherical coordinates are (ψ_j, φ_i) where, for m odd,

$$\varphi_i = i\pi/(m+1), \quad i = 0, \ldots, m,$$

$$0 < \psi_{(m+1)/2} < \ldots < \psi_2 < \psi_1 < \pi/2,$$

$$\psi_{-j} = \pi - \psi_j, \quad j = 1, \ldots, (m+1)/2,$$

i.e. we assume the φ_i to be uniformly distributed in $[0, \pi]$ and the ψ_j to be symmetric with respect to $\pi/2$. If f is an even polynomial of degree $2m$, then f is a linear combination of terms

$$x_1^{\alpha_1} x_2^{\alpha_2} x_3^{\alpha_3}$$

where $\alpha_1 + \alpha_2 + \alpha_3$ is even and $\leq 2m$. Upon introducing spherical coordinates we get from (2.2)

$$\int_{S^2} x_1^{\alpha_1} x_2^{\alpha_2} x_3^{\alpha_3} \, dx$$

$$= \int_0^{\pi} \sin \psi \, (\sin \psi)^{\alpha_1 + \alpha_2} (\cos \psi)^{\alpha_3} \, d\psi \int_0^{2\pi} (\sin \varphi)^{\alpha_1} (\cos \varphi)^{\alpha_2} \, d\varphi.$$

In order to derive a quadrature formula for the ψ-integral we start out from the Gauss–Legendre formula of degree $m+1$. This formula reads

$$\int_{-1}^{+1} f(t) \, dt = \sum_{j=-(m+1)/2}^{(m+1)/2} A_j f(t_j), \quad j = 0 \text{ excluded}, \quad (2.10)$$

where $t_{\pm j}, t_j = -t_{-j}$ are the zeros of the Legendre polynomial P_{m+1}, and the weights $A_j = A_{-j}$ are given by

$$A_j = \frac{2}{(1 - t_j^2)(P'_{m+1}(t_j))^2},$$

Abramowitz and Stegun (1970), 25.4.29. (2.10) is exact for polynomials of degree $2m+1$, hence

$$\int_{-1}^{+1} (1-t^2)^{(\alpha_1+\alpha_2)/2} t^{\alpha_3} \, dt = \sum_{j=-(m+1)/2}^{(m+1)/2} A_j (1-t_j^2)^{(\alpha_1+\alpha_2)/2} t_j^{\alpha_3}.$$

This is a special case of (2.10) if $\alpha_1 + \alpha_2$ and α_3 are even. It is trivially satisfied, due to the symmetry of the Gaussian weights, if $\alpha_1 + \alpha_2$ and α_3 are odd. Putting $t = \cos\psi$ we finally obtain

$$\int_0^\pi \sin\psi\, (\sin\psi)^{\alpha_1+\alpha_2} (\cos\psi)^{\alpha_3}\, d\psi = \sum_{j=-(m+1)/2}^{(m+1)/2} A_j (\sin\psi_j)^{\alpha_1+\alpha_2} (\cos\psi_j)^{\alpha_3},$$

$$\psi_j = \arccos t_j, \quad j = 1, \ldots, (m+1)/2. \tag{2.11}$$

This is our quadrature rule for the ψ integral. It is exact whenever $\alpha_1 + \alpha_2 + \alpha_3$ is even and $\leq 2m$. It is interesting to study the distribution of the nodes ψ_j for m large. From Table VII.1 we see that ψ_j are almost equally distributed in $(0, \pi)$, and the weights are very close to the weights $(\pi/m+1) \sin\psi_j$ in the straightforward rule

$$\int_0^\pi \sin\psi\, f(\psi)\, d\psi \sim \frac{\pi}{m+1} \sum_{j=-(m+1)/2}^{(m+1)/2} \sin\psi_j\, f(\psi_j).$$

We conclude that for practical purposes we can replace (2.11) by the simpler rule.

$$\int_0^\pi \sin\psi\, (\sin\psi)^{\alpha_1+\alpha_2} (\cos\psi)^{\alpha_3}\, d\psi$$

$$\sim \frac{\pi}{m+1} \sum_{j=-(m+1)/2}^{(m+1)/2} \sin\psi_j\, (\sin\psi_j)^{\alpha_1+\alpha_2} (\cos\psi_j)^{\alpha_3}, \tag{2.12}$$

TABLE VII.1 Nodes and weights of the quadrature rule (2.11) for $m+1 = 16$.

j	t_j	A_j	ψ_j	$\psi_j - \psi_{j-1}$	$\dfrac{\pi}{m+1} \sin\psi_j / A_j$
1	0.09501	0.18945	1.47564		1.0317
2	0.28160	0.18260	1.28533	0.1903	1.0318
3	0.45802	0.16916	1.09503	0.1903	1.0318
4	0.61788	0.14960	0.90476	0.1903	1.0320
5	0.75540	0.12463	0.71453	0.1902	1.0323
6	0.86563	0.09516	0.52439	0.1901	1.0331
7	0.94458	0.06225	0.33450	0.1899	1.0355
8	0.98940	0.02715	0.14572	0.1888	1.0502

with the ψ_j equally distributed in $(0, \pi)$.

The φ-integral needs to be evaluated for α_3 even only since for α_3 odd our quadrature rule for the ψ-integral gives the correct value 0. Hence $\alpha_1 + \alpha_2$ is even in the φ-integral, and $(\sin \varphi)^{\alpha_1} (\cos \varphi)^{\alpha_2}$ is an even trigonometric polynomial of degree $\leq 2m$. Such a function is integrated exactly by the trapezoidal rule with the nodes φ_i, $i = 0, \ldots, m$, hence

$$\int_0^{2\pi} (\sin \varphi)^{\alpha_1} (\cos \varphi)^{\alpha_2} d\varphi = \frac{2\pi}{m+1} \sum_{i=0}^{m} (\sin \varphi_i)^{\alpha_1} (\cos \varphi_i)^{\alpha_2}$$

for $\alpha_1 + \alpha_2$ even and $\leq 2m$. Combining this with (2.11) we finally arrive at the rule

$$\int_{S^2} f(x) dx = \frac{2\pi}{m+1} \sum_{j=-(m+1)/2}^{(m+1)/2} A_j \sum_{i=0}^{m} f(\psi_j, \varphi_i) \qquad (2.13)$$

which is exact for even polynomials of degree $\leq 2m$ if the ψ_j, A_j are chosen as in (2.11). However, from a practical point of view we can as well choose equally distributed angles ψ_j with weights $A_j = (\pi/m+1) \sin \psi_j$ without much loss in accuracy.

For what is known about quadrature on S^{n-1} see Stroud (1971), Neutsch (1983), and McLaren (1963).

VII.3 Special Functions

In this section we collect some facts about well known special functions, such as Gegenbauer polynomials, spherical harmonics and Bessel functions. We give proofs only for a few results which are not easily accessible in the literature.

VII.3.1. Gegenbauer Polynomials

The Gegenbauer polynomials C_l^λ, $\lambda > -\frac{1}{2}$, of degree l are defined as the orthogonal polynomials on $[-1, +1]$ with weight function $(1-x^2)^{\lambda-1/2}$. We normalize C_l^λ by requiring $C_l^\lambda(1) = 1$. We then have

$$\int_{-1}^{+1} (1-x^2)^{\lambda-1/2} C_l^\lambda(x) C_k^\lambda(x) dx = \begin{cases} 0, & l \neq k \\ \dfrac{2^{2\lambda-1}(\Gamma(\lambda+\frac{1}{2}))^2 l!}{(l+\lambda)\Gamma(l+2\lambda)}, & l = k \end{cases} \qquad (3.1)$$

with Γ the Gamma function. For $\lambda = 0$ we have to take the limit $\lambda \to 0$. Note that due to our normalization, (3.1) and other formulas differ from the usual one as given in Abramowitz and Stegun (1970). We remark that C_l^λ is even for l even and odd for l odd.

For $\lambda = 0$ we obtain the Chebyshev polynomials of the first kind

$$T_l(x) = C_l^0(x) = \cos(l \arccos x), \quad |x| \leq 1 \qquad (3.2)$$

and for $\lambda = 1$ the Chebyshev polynomials of the second kind
$$U_l(x) = (l+1)C_l^1(x) = \frac{\sin((l+1)\arccos x)}{\sin(\arccos x)}, \qquad |x| \leq 1. \tag{3.3}$$
For $x \geq 1$ we have
$$T_l(x) = \cosh(l \operatorname{arccosh} x),$$
$$U_l(x) = \frac{\sinh((l+1)\operatorname{arccosh} x)}{\sinh(\operatorname{arccosh} x)}. \tag{3.4}$$

A simple proof of the first of these relations uses the recursion
$$T_{l+1}(x) + T_{l-1}(x) = 2xT_l(x), \qquad l = 1, 2, \ldots$$
$$T_0(x) = 1, \qquad T_1(x) = x$$
which follows immediately from (3.2) and which holds also for $x \geq 1$. Observing that
$$\operatorname{arccosh} x = \ln(x + \sqrt{(x^2 - 1)}), \qquad x \geq 1$$
we obtain for $x \geq 1$
$$T_l(x) \geq \tfrac{1}{2}(x + \sqrt{(x^2 - 1)})^l, \tag{3.5}$$
i.e. the T_l grow exponentially with l for $x > 1$.

For $\lambda = 1/2$ we obtain the Legendre polynomials
$$P_l = C_l^{1/2} \tag{3.6}$$
for which
$$|P_l(x)| \leq 1, \qquad |x| \leq 1. \tag{3.7}$$

The Mellin transform M is an integral transform on $(0, \infty)$ which is defined by
$$Mf(s) = \int_0^\infty f(x) x^{s-1} \, dx.$$
It is easily verified that
$$Mf'(s) = (1 - s)Mf(s - 1)$$
$$M(x^p f)(s) = Mf(s + p)$$
$$M(x^p f^{(p)})(s) = (-1)^p \frac{\Gamma(s+p)}{\Gamma(s)} Mf(s), \qquad s > 0 \tag{3.8}$$
$$M(f * g)(s) = Mf \cdot Mg$$
where the convolution is now
$$f * g(s) = \int_0^\infty f(r) g\left(\frac{s}{r}\right) \frac{dr}{r}.$$

From Sneddon (1972) we take the following Mellin transform pairs:

$$f(x) = \begin{cases} (1-x^2)^{\lambda-1/2} C_2^\lambda(x), & x < 1 \\ 0, & x \geq 1 \end{cases} \tag{3.9}$$

$$Mf(s) = \frac{\Gamma\left(\frac{1}{2}\right)\Gamma\left(\lambda+\frac{1}{2}\right)\Gamma(s)2^{-s}}{\Gamma\left(\frac{l+1+s+2\lambda}{2}\right)\Gamma\left(\frac{s+1-l}{2}\right)}, \quad s > l$$

$$f(x) = \begin{cases} (1-x^2)^{\lambda-1/2} C_l^\lambda\left(\frac{1}{x}\right), & x < 1 \\ 0, & x \geq 1 \end{cases} \tag{3.10}$$

$$Mf(s) = \frac{2^{s-1}\Gamma(2\lambda)\Gamma\left(\frac{s-l}{2}\right)\Gamma\left(\lambda+\frac{s+l}{2}\right)}{\Gamma(\lambda)\Gamma(s+2\lambda)}, \quad s > l$$

For $\lambda = 0$ we again take the limit $\lambda \to 0$. Note that the formulas of Sneddon (1972) have to be modified according to our normalization of the C_l^λ.

VII.3.2. Spherical Harmonics

A spherical harmonic Y_l of degree l is the restriction to S^{n-1} of a harmonic polynomial homogeneous of degree l on $\mathbb{R}^n$ (Seeley, 1966). There are

$$N(n, l) = \frac{(2l+n-2)(n+l-3)!}{l!(n-2)!}, \quad N(n, 0) = 1 \tag{3.11}$$

linearly independent spherical harmonics of degree l, and spherical harmonics of different degree are orthogonal on S^{n-1}. An important result on spherical harmonics is the Funk–Hecke theorem: for a function h on $[-1, +1]$, we have

$$\int_{S^{n-1}} h(\theta \cdot \omega) Y_l(\omega) \, d\omega = c(n, l) Y_l(\theta),$$

$$c(n, l) = |S^{n-2}| \int_{-1}^{+1} h(t) C_l^{(n-2)/2}(t)(1-t^2)^{(n-3)/2} \, dt. \tag{3.12}$$

For $n = 2$, (3.12) reads

$$\int_0^{2\pi} h(\cos(\varphi - \Psi)) e^{il\varphi} \, d\varphi = 2 \int_{-1}^{+1} h(t) T_{|l|}(t)(1-t^2)^{-1/2} \, dt \, e^{il\Psi}$$

see (3.14) below, and follows by simple substitutions from (3.2).

As a simple application we derive a pointwise estimate for the normalized spherical harmonics. Putting $h = C_l^{(n-2)/2}$ we obtain from (3.12)

$$Y_l(\theta) = \frac{1}{c(n,l)} \int_{S^{n-1}} C_l^{(n-2)/2}(\theta \cdot \omega) Y_l(\omega) d\omega,$$

$$c(n,l) = |S^{n-2}| \int_{-1}^{+1} (C_l^{(n-2)/2}(t))^2 (1-t^2)^{(n-3)/2} dt.$$

From the Cauchy–Schwarz inequality we get

$$|Y_l(\theta)|^2 \leq \left(\frac{1}{c(n,l)}\right)^2 \int_{S^{n-1}} (C_l^{(n-2)/2}(\theta \cdot \omega))^2 d\omega \int_{S^{n-1}} Y_l^2(\omega) d\omega$$

$$= \left(\frac{1}{c(n,l)}\right)^2 |S^{n-2}| \int_{-1}^{+1} (C_l^{(n-2)/2}(t))^2 (1-t^2)^{(n-3)/2} dt \int_{S^{n-1}} Y_l^2(\omega) d\omega$$

where we have used (2.3). Inserting the value of $c(n,l)$ and using (3.1) yields

$$|Y_l(\theta)|^2 \leq \frac{1}{c(n,l)} \int_{S^{n-1}} Y_l^2(\omega) d\omega, \qquad (3.13)$$

$$c(n,l) = |S^{n-2}| 2^{n-3} \left(\Gamma\left(\frac{n-1}{2}\right)\right)^2 \frac{1}{l+n/2-1} \frac{l!}{(l+n-3)!}.$$

This does not make sense for $n = 2, l = 0$, in which case we simply have $c(2,0) = 2\pi$.

For dimensions $n = 2, 3$ we shall give explicit representations of spherical harmonics. For $n = 2$ we have $N(2,l) = 2$ linearly independent spherical harmonics of degree l if $l > 0$, namely

$$Y_{l,1}(\theta) = \cos l\varphi, \quad Y_{l,-1}(\theta) = \sin l\varphi, \quad \theta = \begin{pmatrix} \cos \varphi \\ \sin \varphi \end{pmatrix} \qquad (3.14)$$

and $Y_0 = 1$. For $n = 3$ we have $N(3,l) = 2l+1$ linearly independent spherical harmonics of degree l if $l > 0$. They can be expressed in terms of spherical coordinates, see Section VII.2. We put for $\theta \in S^{n-1}$

$$\theta = \begin{pmatrix} \sin \Psi \sin \varphi \\ \sin \Psi \cos \varphi \\ \cos \Psi \end{pmatrix}, \quad 0 \leq \varphi < 2\pi, \quad 0 \leq \Psi \leq \pi$$

Then,

$$Y_{l,0}(\theta) = P_l(\cos \Psi), \quad \begin{aligned} Y_{l,k}(\theta) &= P_l^{|k|}(\cos \Psi) \cos k\varphi, \\ Y_{l,-k}(\theta) &= P_l^{|k|}(\cos \Psi) \sin k\varphi, \end{aligned} \quad 1 \leq k \leq l \quad (3.15)$$

are $2l+1$ linearly independent spherical harmonics of degree $l > 0$, and $Y_0 = 1$. The Legendre functions P_l^k are given by

$$P_l^k(t) = (-1)^k (1-t^2)^{k/2} \frac{d^k P_l}{dt^k}, \qquad 0 \le k \le l$$

with P_l from (3.6). For k even, P_l^k is a polynomial of degree l with the parity of l, while for k odd

$$P_l^k(t) = (1-t^2)^{1/2} Q_{l-1}^k(t)$$

where Q_{l-1}^k is a polynomial of degree $l-1$ with the parity of $l-1$.

VII.3.3. Bessel Functions

By J_k we denote the Bessel function of the first kind of integer order k, see Abramowitz and Stegun (1970), ch. 9. It can be defined by the generating function

$$e^{x(z-1/z)/2} = \sum_k z^k J_k(x),$$

i.e. $J_k(x)$ is the coefficient of z^k in the Laurent expansion of the left-hand side. Hence,

$$J_k(x) = \frac{1}{2\pi i} \int_C e^{x/2(z-1/z)} z^{-k-1} dz$$

where C is the circle of radius r centered at the origin. On putting $z = re^{i\varphi}$, $0 \le \varphi \le 2\pi$ this becomes

$$J_k(x) = \frac{1}{2\pi} r^{-k} \int_0^{2\pi} e^{x/2(re^{i\varphi} - r^{-1}e^{-i\varphi}) - ik\varphi} d\varphi$$

$$= \frac{1}{2\pi} r^{-k} \int_0^{2\pi} e^{x/2((r-1/r)\cos\varphi + i(r+1/r)\sin\varphi) - ik\varphi} d\varphi.$$

For $r = 1$ we obtain the integral representation

$$J_k(x) = \frac{1}{2\pi} \int_0^{2\pi} e^{ix\sin\varphi - ik\varphi} d\varphi$$

$$= \frac{i^{-k}}{2\pi} \int_0^{2\pi} e^{ix\cos\varphi - ik\varphi} d\varphi.$$

(3.16)

If $a, b \in \mathbb{R}$ and $a^2 < b^2$ we put

$$x = (b^2 - a^2)^{1/2}, \qquad r = ((b-a)/(b+a))^{1/2},$$

obtaining for $k = 0$

$$J_0((b^2 - a^2)^{1/2}) = \frac{1}{2\pi} \int_0^{2\pi} e^{-a\cos\varphi + ib\sin\varphi} \, d\varphi. \tag{3.17}$$

The Bessel functions of real order v can be obtained as Fourier transforms of Gegenbauer polynomials. More precisely we have for $\sigma > 0$ with $w(s) = (1-s^2)^{\lambda - 1/2}$

$$(wC_m^\lambda)^\wedge(\sigma) = \frac{\Gamma(2\lambda)}{\Gamma(\lambda)} (2\pi)^{1/2} 2^{-\lambda} i^{-m} \sigma^{-\lambda} J_{m+\lambda}(\sigma) \tag{3.18}$$

Gradshteyn and Ryzhik (1965), formula 7.321. For $\lambda = 0$, we take the limit $\lambda \to 0$. Combining (3.18) with the Funk–Hecke theorem (3.12) we obtain for Y_l a spherical harmonic of degree l

$$\int_{S^{n-1}} e^{i\sigma\theta \cdot \omega} Y_l(\omega) \, d\omega = (2\pi)^{n/2} i^l \sigma^{(2-n)/2} J_{l+(n-2)/2}(\sigma) Y_l(\theta). \tag{3.19}$$

For $n = 2$ this is identical with (3.16). In the evaluation of the constant we have made use of well-known formulas for the Γ-function.

We need a few results on the asymptotic behaviour of Bessel functions. The asymptotic behaviour of $J_v(x)$ as both v and x tend to infinity is crucial in the investigation of resolution. Debye's formula (Abramowitz and Stegun (1970), 9.3.7) states that $J_v(x)$ is negligible if, in a sense, $v > x$. More precisely, we have from Watson (1952), p. 255 for $0 < \vartheta < 1$

$$0 \le J_v(\vartheta v) \le (2\pi v)^{-1/2} (1-\vartheta^2)^{-1/4} \left(\frac{\vartheta e^{\sqrt{(1-\vartheta^2)}}}{1+\sqrt{(1-\vartheta^2)}} \right)^v$$

$$= (2\pi v)^{-1/2} (1-\vartheta^2)^{-1/4} (v(\sqrt{(1-\vartheta^2)}))^v,$$

$$v(t) = \left(\frac{1-t}{1+t} \right)^{1/2} e^t.$$

Using the expansion (Abramowitz and Stegun (1970), 4.1.28)

$$\ln v(t) = \tfrac{1}{2} \ln\left(\frac{1-t}{1+t} \right) + t = (-t - t^3/3 - t^5/5 - \ldots) + t$$

$$\le -t^3/3$$

for $0 \le t < 1$ we obtain

$$v(t) \le e^{-t^3/3}$$

hence

$$0 \le J_v(\vartheta v) \le (2\pi v)^{-1/2} (1-\vartheta^2)^{-1/4} e^{-(v/3)(1-\vartheta^2)^{3/2}}. \tag{3.20}$$

We see that for $\vartheta < 1$, $J_\nu(\vartheta v)$ decays exponentially as $v \to \infty$.

An asymptotic estimate for the Weber–Schafheitlin integral

$$I_{\mu\nu}(r) = \int_0^\infty J_\mu(t) J_\nu(rt)\, dt \tag{3.21}$$

for $r > 1$ and $0 \leq \nu \leq \mu$ is obtained from its representation (see Abramowitz and Stegun (1970), 11.4.34)

$$I_{\mu\nu}(r) = r^{-\mu-1} \frac{\Gamma\left(\frac{\mu+\nu+1}{2}\right)}{\Gamma(\mu+1)\Gamma\left(\frac{\nu-\mu+1}{2}\right)} F\left(\frac{\mu+\nu+1}{2}, \frac{\mu-\nu+1}{2}; \mu+1; r^{-2}\right)$$

in terms of the hypergeometric function (Abramowitz and Stegun (1970), 15.1.1)

$$F(a,b;c;z) = \frac{\Gamma(c)}{\Gamma(a)\Gamma(b)} \sum_{n=0}^\infty \frac{\Gamma(a+n)\Gamma(b+n)}{\Gamma(c+n)\Gamma(1+n)} z^n.$$

Putting

$$a = \frac{\mu+\nu+1}{2}, \quad b = \frac{\mu-\nu+1}{2}, \quad c = \mu+1$$

we obtain

$$I_{\mu\nu}(r) = r^{-c} \frac{1}{\Gamma(b)\Gamma(1-b)} \sum_{n=0}^\infty \frac{\Gamma(a+n)\Gamma(b+n)}{\Gamma(c+n)\Gamma(1+n)} r^{-2n}.$$

Using the reflection formula (see Abramowitz and Stegun (1970), 6.1.17)

$$\Gamma(b)\Gamma(1-b) = \frac{\pi}{\sin \pi b}$$

of the Γ-function we obtain

$$|I_{\mu\nu}(r)| \leq \frac{1}{\pi} r^{-c} \sum_{n=0}^\infty \frac{\Gamma(a+n)\Gamma(b+n)}{\Gamma(c+n)\Gamma(1+n)} r^{-2n}. \tag{3.22}$$

In order to estimate the sum we remark that $0 < b \leq a < c$. Choosing m such that $a+n \leq c+m < a+n+1$ we have

$$\Gamma(c+n) = (c+n-1)\ldots(c+m)\Gamma(c+m)$$
$$\geq (c+m)^{n-m}\Gamma(c+m)$$
$$\geq (a+n)^{c-a-1}\Gamma(a+n).$$

Similarly, choosing m such that $n \leq b+m < 1+n$ we have

$$\Gamma(b+n) = (b+n-1)\ldots(b+m)\Gamma(b+m)$$
$$\leq (b+n-1)^{n-m}\Gamma(1+n)$$
$$\leq (b+n)^b \Gamma(1+n).$$

Using the last two estimates in (3.22) we obtain

$$|I_{\mu\nu}(r)| \leq \frac{1}{\pi} r^{-c} \sum_{n=0}^{\infty} (a+n)^{1+a-c}(b+n)^b r^{-2n}$$

$$\leq \frac{1}{\pi} r^{-c} \sum_{n=0}^{\infty} (a+n)^{1+a-c}(a+n)^b r^{-2n}$$

$$= \frac{1}{\pi} r^{-c} \sum_{n=0}^{\infty} (a+n) r^{-2n}$$

since $c = a + b$. It follows that

$$|I_{\mu\nu}(r)| \leq (\mu+1) r^{-\mu-1} C(r) \qquad (3.23)$$

with some $C(r)$ which is a decreasing function of r.

Finally, the asymptotics of $J_\nu(t)$ as $t \to \infty$ and ν fixed is

$$J_\nu(t) = \sqrt{\frac{2}{\pi t}} \cos\left(t - \frac{\nu\pi}{2} - \frac{\pi}{4}\right) + O\left(\frac{1}{t}\right), \qquad (3.24)$$

see formula 9.2.1 of Abramowitz and Stegun (1970).

We finish this section by collecting a few integral formulas.

$$\int_0^z t^\nu J_{\nu-1}(t)\,dt = z^\nu J_\nu(z) \qquad (3.25)$$

for $\nu > 0$, $z > 0$, see Abramowitz and Stegun (1970), formula 11.3.20

$$\int_0^\infty e^{-\lambda t} t^{\nu+1} J_\nu(\rho t)\,dt = \frac{2\lambda(2\rho)^\nu \Gamma(\nu + 3/2)}{\sqrt{\pi}(\lambda^2 + \rho^2)^{\nu+3/2}} \qquad (3.26)$$

for $\lambda > 0$, $\nu \geq 0$, see Gradshteyn and Ryzhik (1965), formula 6.623.

$$\int_0^\infty J_l(t)\,dt = \begin{cases} 1, & l \geq 0, \\ (-1)^l, & l < 0, \end{cases} \qquad (3.27)$$

where l is an integer, see Abramowitz and Stegun (1970), 11.4.17.

VII.4 Sobolev Spaces

Sobolev spaces are used extensively in II.5, IV.2, V.2 and also in Chapter VI. As general reference we recommend Triebel (1978), Adams (1975). We give only a few definitions and facts which are of direct significance in our context.

The Sobolev space $H^\alpha(\mathbb{R}^n)$ or H^α of real order α is defined by

$$H^\alpha = \{f \in \mathscr{S}'(\mathbb{R}^n): (1+|\xi|^2)^{\alpha/2} \hat{f} \in L_2(\mathbb{R}^n)\}.$$

H is a Hilbert space with norm and inner product

$$\|f\|_{H^\alpha} = \left(\int_{\mathbb{R}^n} (1+|\xi|^2)^\alpha |\hat{f}(\xi)|^2 \, d\xi \right)^{1/2}, \tag{4.1}$$

$$(f, g)_{H^\alpha} = \int_{\mathbb{R}^n} (1+|\xi|^2)^\alpha \hat{f}(\xi)\overline{\hat{g}}(\xi) \, d\xi.$$

For $\alpha = 1$ we obtain from the rules R3 and R5 in VII.1

$$\|f\|_{H^1}^2 = \int_{\mathbb{R}^n} (f - \Delta f)\overline{f} \, dx$$

with Δ the Laplacian:

$$\Delta = \sum_{i=1}^n \frac{\partial^2}{\partial x_i^2}.$$

An integration by parts shows that

$$\|f\|_{H^1}^2 = \int_{\mathbb{R}^n} \left(|f|^2 + \sum_{i=1}^n \left| \frac{\partial f}{\partial x_i} \right|^2 \right) dx.$$

Thus we see that H^1 consists of the functions whose (distributional) derivatives of order ≤ 1 are in $L_2(\mathbb{R}^n)$. Likewise, H^α for $\alpha \geq 0$ an integer consists of those functions whose derivatives of order $\leq \alpha$ are in $L_2(\mathbb{R}^n)$.

If Ω is an open subset of $\mathbb{R}^n$ we put

$$H_0^\alpha(\Omega) = \{ f \in H^\alpha(\mathbb{R}^n) : \text{supp}(f) \subseteq \overline{\Omega} \}$$

where the support of $f \in \mathscr{S}'$ is the complement of the points having a neighbourhood in which f vanishes (i.e. f vanishes for all C^∞-functions with support in that neighbourhood). Note that the definition of the spaces $H_0^\alpha(\Omega)$ varies in the literature. Our spaces are the $\tilde{H}^\alpha(\Omega)$ spaces of Triebel (1978). They coincide with the usual $H_0^\alpha(\Omega)$ spaces only for $\alpha \neq k + 1/2$, k an integer. The inner product and the norm in $H_0^\alpha(\Omega)$ are those of $H^\alpha(\mathbb{R}^n)$.

An important tool in the theory of Sobolev spaces is interpolation, see Lions and Magenes (1968), ch. 1.2. Two Hilbert spaces H_0, H_1 are said to be an interpolation couple if H_1 is dense in H_0 with continuous embedding. Let S be a self-adjoint strictly positive operator in H_0 with domain H_1 such that the norms $\|f\|_{H_1}$, $\|Sf\|_{H_0}$ are equivalent on H_1. It can be shown that there is such an operator. Then we define for $0 \leq \theta \leq 1$

$$H_\theta = (H_0, H_1)_\theta = \text{domain of } S^\theta.$$

H_θ is a Hilbert space with norm

$$\|f\|_{H_\theta} = \|S^\theta f\|_{H_0}. \tag{4.2}$$

For $\theta = 0, 1$ we regain the spaces H_0, H_1. H_θ is called an intermediate or interpolation space. It can be shown that H_θ is determined uniquely by H_0, H_1 even though S is not, and the norm in H_θ is determined by (4.2) up to equivalence only. We quote a few basic facts on interpolation spaces.

LEMMA 4.1 For $0 \leq \theta \leq 1$ there is a constant $C(\theta)$ such that for $f \in H_1$ the interpolation inequality

$$\|f\|_{H_\theta} \leq C(\theta) \|f\|_{H_0}^{1-\theta} \|f\|_{H_1}^{\theta}$$

holds.

LEMMA 4.2 Let H_0, H_1 and K_0, K_1 be two interpolation couples and let H_θ, K_θ be the corresponding interpolation spaces. Let $A: H_0 \to K_0$ be a linear operator such that there are constants A_0, A_1 with

$$\|Af\|_{K_i} \leq A_i \|f\|_{H_i}$$

for $f \in H_i$, $i = 0, 1$. Then there is a constant $C(\theta)$ for each $\theta \in [0, 1]$ such that

$$\|Af\|_{K_\theta} \leq C(\theta) A_0^{1-\theta} A_1^{\theta} \|f\|_{H_\theta}$$

in H_θ. $C(\theta)$ is independent of A_0, A_1.

LEMMA 4.3 For $0 \leq \alpha \leq \beta \leq 1$ we have the reiteration property

$$(H_\alpha, H_\beta)_\theta = H_{\alpha(1-\theta) + \beta\theta}$$

for $0 \leq \theta \leq 1$, with equivalence of norms.

As an example we have, for $\alpha \leq \beta$ and $0 \leq \theta \leq 1$

$$(H^\alpha, H^\beta)_\theta = H^{\alpha(1-\theta) + \beta\theta}. \tag{4.3}$$

This follows immediately from the choice

$$(Sf)^\wedge(\xi) = (1 + |\xi|^2)^{(\beta-\alpha)/2} \hat{f}(\xi).$$

A less obvious example is

$$(H_0^\alpha(\Omega), H_0^\beta(\Omega))_\theta = H_0^{\alpha(1-\theta) + \beta\theta}(\Omega) \tag{4.4}$$

which holds for Ω sufficiently regular, e.g. $\Omega = \Omega^n$, see Triebel (1978), Theorem 4.3.2/2.

A third example is provided by the spaces $H^\alpha(\Omega)$. For α an integer ≥ 0, these spaces consist of those functions for which

$$\|f\|_{H^\alpha(\Omega)}^2 = \sum_{|k| \leq \alpha} \int_\Omega |D^k f|^2 \, dx \tag{4.5}$$

is finite. This definition extends to real non-negative orders in the following way.

For $\alpha = s + \sigma$, s an integer, $0 < \sigma < 1$, we put

$$\|f\|^2_{H^\alpha(\Omega)} = \|f\|^2_{H^s(\Omega)} + \sum_{|k|=s} \int_\Omega \int_\Omega \frac{|D^k f(x) - D^k f(y)|^2}{|x-y|^{n+2\sigma}} \, dx \, dy.$$

If Ω is sufficiently regular, then

$$H^{\alpha(1-\theta)+\beta\theta}(\Omega) = (H^\alpha(\Omega), H^\beta(\Omega))_\theta. \tag{4.6}$$

These spaces are used in Adams (1975); they agree with the $H^\alpha(\Omega)$ spaces of Triebel (1978) for Ω sufficiently regular, e.g. $\Omega = \Omega^n$. The definition (4.6) is consistent because of the reiteration property of Lemma 4.3.

The interpolation result (4.4) can be used to find equivalent norms in $H_0^\alpha(\Omega^n)$. For $\alpha \geq 0$ an integer we can expand $f \in H_0^\alpha(\Omega^n)$ in its Fourier series in $[-1, +1]^n$,

$$f(x) = (\pi/2)^{n/2} \sum_k \hat{f}(\pi k) e^{i\pi x \cdot k},$$

and we obtain from R3 of Section VII.1 and Parseval's relation

$$\|f\|^2_{H_0^\alpha(\Omega^n)} = \pi^n \sum_k (1 + \pi^2 |k|^2)^\alpha |\hat{f}(\pi k)|^2 \tag{4.7}$$

For $\alpha \geq 0$ real we define

$$\|f\|^2_{H_0^\alpha(\Omega^n)} = \pi^n \sum_k (1 + \pi^2 |k|^2)^\alpha |\hat{f}(\pi k)|^2. \tag{4.8}$$

LEMMA 4.4 The norms (4.1), (4.8) are equivalent on $H_0^\alpha(\Omega^n)$ for $\alpha \geq 0$ real.

Proof Let $0 \leq \alpha \leq \beta$ be integers. We compute a norm for

$$(H_0^\alpha(\Omega^n), H_0^\beta(\Omega^n))_\theta = H_\theta$$

by considering the operator

$$Sf(x) = (\pi/2)^n \sum_k (1 + \pi^2 |k|^2)^{(\beta-\alpha)/2} \hat{f}(\pi k) e^{i\pi x \cdot k}.$$

S is a self-adjoint operator in $H_0^\alpha(\Omega^n)$ with domain $H_0^\beta(\Omega^n)$, as can be seen from (4.7). Hence

$$\|S^\theta f\|^2_{H_0^\alpha(\Omega^n)} = \pi^n \sum_k (1 + \pi^2 |k|^2)^{\alpha(1-\theta)+\beta\theta} |\hat{f}(\pi k)|^2$$

$$= \|f\|^2_{H_0^{\alpha(1-\theta)+\beta\theta}(\Omega^n)}$$

defines a norm on H_θ. Since, by (4.4), $H_\theta = H_0^{\alpha(1-\theta)+\beta\theta}(\Omega^n)$, the lemma follows. □

The interpolation inequality in Sobolev spaces on $\mathbb{R}^n$ reads simply

$$\|f\|_{H^\gamma} \leq \|f\|_{H^\alpha}^{\frac{\beta-\gamma}{\beta-\alpha}} \|f\|_{H^\beta}^{\frac{\gamma-\alpha}{\beta-\alpha}} \tag{4.9}$$

for $\alpha \le \gamma \le \beta$. This follows from a simple application of the Cauchy–Schwarz inequality to the integral defining $\|f\|_{H^\gamma}$. For the spaces $H^\alpha(\Omega)$, $H_0^\alpha(\Omega)$ this inequality, possibly with a constant $C(\alpha, \beta, \gamma)$, follows from Lemma 4.1.

LEMMA 4.5 Let $\chi \in C_0^\infty(\mathbb{R}^n)$. Then, the map $f \to \chi f$ is bounded in H^α.

Proof For $\alpha \ge 0$ an integer, the lemma is obvious since in that case the norm in H^α can be expressed in terms of derivatives. For $\alpha \ge 0$ real, the lemma follows by applying Lemma 4.2 to the operator $Af = \chi f$ and to $H_i = K_i = H^{\beta+i}$, $i = 0, 1$ where β is an integer such that $\beta \le \alpha \le \beta + 1$. For $\alpha \le 0$ the lemma follows by duality.

In the sequel we need two embedding theorems for Sobolev spaces. The first one is the Sobolev embedding theorem, the second one the embedding theorem of Rellich–Kondrachov.

LEMMA 4.6 Let Ω be sufficiently regular, and let $\alpha > n/2$. Then, $H^\alpha(\Omega) \subseteq C(\Omega)$, and

$$\sup_{x \in \Omega} |f(x)| \le c \|f\|_{H^\alpha(\Omega)}$$

with some constant c independent of f.

For a proof see Adams (1975), Theorem 7.57. By $H^\alpha(\Omega) \subseteq C(\Omega)$ we mean that for $f \in H^\alpha(\Omega)$ there is a continuous function f^* such that $f = f^*$ a.e.

LEMMA 4.7 Let Ω be bounded and sufficiently regular, and let $\alpha > \beta$. Then, $H^\alpha(\Omega) \subseteq H^\beta(\Omega)$, the embedding being compact.

For the proof see Lions and Magenes (1968), Theorem 16.1.

We finish this section with an estimate of functions in $H^\alpha(\Omega)$ which vanish at many points in Ω.

LEMMA 4.8 Let Ω be bounded and sufficiently regular. For $h > 0$ let Ω_h be a finite subset of Ω such that the distance between any point of Ω and Ω_h is at most h. Let $\alpha > n/2$. Then there is a constant c such that

$$\|f\|_{L_2(\Omega)} \le ch^\alpha \|f\|_{H^\alpha(\Omega)}$$

for each $f \in H^\alpha(\Omega)$ vanishing on Ω_h.

Proof We carry out the proof for α not an integer and indicate the minor changes for α an integer (which in fact are simplifications) at the end of the proof.

Let $\alpha = s + \sigma$ with s an integer and $0 < \sigma < 1$. We introduce the seminorm

$$|f|^2_{H^\alpha(\Omega)} = \sum_{|k|=s} \int_\Omega \int_\Omega \frac{|D^k f(x) - D^k f(y)|^2}{|x-y|^{n+2\sigma}} \, dx \, dy.$$

Let $x_1, \ldots, x_m \in \Omega$ be such that no non-trivial polynomial of degree $\leq s$ vanishes on $x_1, \ldots, x_m$. We show that

$$\|f\|_{H^s(\Omega)} \leq c \left\{ |f|_{H^\alpha(\Omega)} + \sum_{i=1}^m |f(x_i)| \right\} \quad (4.10)$$

with some constant c independent of f. If this is not the case, then there is a sequence (f_l) in $H^\alpha(\Omega)$ such that

$$\|f_l\|_{H^s(\Omega)} = 1, \quad |f_l|_{H^\alpha(\Omega)} + \sum_{i=1}^m |f_l(x_i)| \to 0 \quad (4.11)$$

as $l \to \infty$. (f_l) is bounded in $H^\alpha(\Omega)$. Because of Lemma 4.7 we can assume that $f_l \to f$ in $H^s(\Omega)$. From the second part of (4.11) we see that f_l converges even in $H^\alpha(\Omega)$, and $|f|_{H^\alpha(\Omega)} = 0$. Hence the derivatives of order s of f are constant, i.e. f is a polynomial of degree s. Again from the second half of (4.11) we conclude with the help of Lemma 4.6 that

$$f(x_i) = \lim_{l \to \infty} f_l(x_i) = 0, \quad i = 1, \ldots, m.$$

By our choice of $x_1, \ldots, x_m$ it follows that $f = 0$. This being a contradiction to the first half of (4.11), (4.10) is established.

From (4.10) it follows that for $f \in H^\alpha(\Omega)$ with $f(x_i) = 0$, $i = 1, \ldots, m$, we have

$$\|f\|_{L_2(\Omega)} \leq c |f|_{H^\alpha(\Omega)}. \quad (4.12)$$

Applying this to the domain $h\Omega$ we obtain by a change of coordinates

$$\|f\|_{L_2(h\Omega)} \leq c h^\alpha |f|_{H^\alpha(h\Omega)} \quad (4.13)$$

if f vanishes on $hx_1, \ldots, hx_m$. The constant c in (4.13) is independent of h; in fact it is the constant in (4.12). Now we subdivide Ω into subdomains Ω_l, $l = 1, \ldots, q$, with the following properties: no non-trivial polynomial of degree $\leq s$ vanishes on $\Omega_h \cap \Omega_l$, and the diameter of Ω_l is at most $c h$ with c independent of h. Then we can apply (4.13) to each of the subdomains Ω_l, obtaining for $f \in H^\alpha(\Omega)$ vanishing on Ω_h

$$\|f\|_{L_2(\Omega_l)} \leq c h^\alpha |f|_{H^\alpha(\Omega_l)}$$

with c independent of h and f. Summing up yields

$$\|f\|_{L_2(\Omega)}^2 = \sum_{l=1}^q \|f\|_{L_2(\Omega_l)}^2 \leq c^2 h^{2\alpha} \sum_{|k| \leq s} \sum_{l=1}^q \int_{\Omega_l} \int_{\Omega_l} \frac{|D^k f(x) - D^k f(y)|^2}{|x-y|^{n+2\sigma}} dx\, dy$$

$$\leq c^2 h^{2\alpha} \sum_{|k| \leq s} \int_\Omega \int_\Omega \frac{|D^k f(x) - D^k f(y)|^2}{|x-y|^{n+2\sigma}} dx\, dy$$

$$\leq c^2 h^{2\alpha} \|f\|_{H^\alpha(\Omega)}^2.$$

This finishes the proof for α not an integer. If α is an integer, then (4.10) is replaced by

$$\|f\|_{H^{\alpha-1}(\Omega)} \leq C\left\{|f|_{H^\alpha(\Omega)} + \sum_{i=1}^m |f(x_i)|\right\}$$

with the seminorm

$$|f|^2_{H^\alpha(\Omega)} = \sum_{|k|=\alpha} \int_\Omega |D^k f(x)|^2 \, dx.$$

This is proved very much in the same way as (4.10). □

VII.5 The Discrete Fourier Transform

In this section we study the discrete analogue of the Fourier transform from a computational point of view. We use the discrete Fourier transform to compute discrete convolutions, to solve linear systems with Toeplitz structure, and to evaluate Fourier integrals.

The (one-dimensional) discrete Fourier transform of length p is given by

$$\hat{y}_k = \frac{1}{p} \sum_{l=0}^{p-1} y_l \, e^{-2\pi i k l/p}, \qquad k = 0, \ldots, p-1. \tag{5.1}$$

In view of the orthogonality relation

$$\frac{1}{p} \sum_{k=0}^{p-1} e^{2\pi i k l/p} = \begin{cases} 1, & k = 0, \pm p, \pm 2p, \ldots, \\ 0, & \text{otherwise} \end{cases}$$

we obtain immediately the discrete inverse Fourier transform

$$y_l = \sum_{k=0}^{p-1} \hat{y}_k \, e^{2\pi i k l/p}, \qquad l = 0, \ldots, p-1. \tag{5.2}$$

The evaluation of the discrete Fourier transform of length p, as it stands, requires $O(p^2)$ operations. This number can be reduced to $O(p \log p)$ by fast Fourier transform (FFT) techniques (Nussbaumer, 1982). We describe the well-known FFT algorithm of Cooley and Tukey for p a power of 2, $p = 2^m$, say.

Let $q = p/2 = 2^{m-1}$ and $w = e^{-2\pi i/p}$. Then $w^p = 1$, $w^q = -1$, and (5.1) reads

$$p \hat{y}_k = \sum_{l=0}^{p-1} y_l w^{kl}, \qquad k = 0, \ldots, p-1.$$

The basic idea in the Cooley–Tukey algorithm is to break the sum into one part with l even and the rest with l odd. This yields

$$p \hat{y}_k = \sum_{l=0}^{q-1} y_{2l} (w^2)^{kl} + w^k \sum_{l=0}^{q-1} y_{2l+1} (w^2)^{kl}$$

$$= g_k + w^k u_k, \qquad k = 0, \ldots, p-1.$$

Since $w^2 = e^{-2\pi i/q}$, g_k and u_k have period q. Hence

$$p \hat{y}_k = g_k + w^k u_k,$$
$$p \hat{y}_{k+q} = g_k - w^k u_k, \tag{5.3}$$

where k runs only from 0 to $q-1$. Since g_k, u_k can be computed by a discrete Fourier transform of length $q = p/2$ we see that the discrete Fourier transform of length p can be computed by two discrete Fourier transforms of length $p/2$, followed by $p/2$ complex multiplications and p complex additions. If this is done in a recursive way we arrive at the following number of operations: if M_m, A_m are the numbers of complex multiplications and additions, respectively, for the discrete Fourier transform of length $p = 2^m$, then

$$M_m = 2M_{m-1} + 2^{m-1},$$
$$A_m = 2A_{m-1} + 2^m$$

with $M_0 = A_0 = 0$. It follows that

$$M_m = m\,2^{m-1} = \frac{1}{2}p\,\text{ld}\,p$$
$$A_m = m\,2^m = p\,\text{ld}\,p$$

where ld is the dual logarithm. Thus the total number of operations is $O(p\,\text{ld}\,p)$ as claimed above.

There is a close connection between the discrete Fourier transform and convolutions

$$z_k = \sum_{l=0}^{p-1} x_{k-l}\,y_l, \qquad k = 0, \ldots, p-1 \tag{5.4}$$

of length p. If the sequence $(x_k)_{k \in \mathbb{Z}}$ has period p the convolution is called cyclic. In that case, the discrete Fourier transform takes (5.4) into

$$\hat{z}_k = p\hat{x}_k\,\hat{y}_k, \qquad k = 0, \ldots, p-1$$

as is easily verified. Hence cyclic convolutions can be carried out by doing two discrete Fourier transforms, followed by p complex multiplications and an inverse Fourier transform. Using FFT we need $O(p \log p)$ operations. The same applies to linear systems of the form

$$z = Xy$$

where X is a cyclic convolution, i.e.

$$X = \begin{pmatrix} x_0 & x_{p-1} & \cdots & x_1 \\ x_1 & x_0 & \cdots & x_2 \\ & & \cdots & \\ x_{p-1} & x_{p-2} & \cdots & x_0 \end{pmatrix}. \tag{5.5}$$

Equivalently, the $(k+1)$st row of X is obtained by making a ring shift in the kth row. In V.5 we apply this method to block cyclic convolutions for which the entries x_l in (5.5) are $q \times q$ matrices. In that case FFT leads to an algorithm with $O(pq^2 + pq \log p)$ operations, provided the inverses of the $q \times q$ matrices

$$\hat{x}_k = \frac{1}{p}\sum_{l=0}^{p-1} e^{-2\pi i k l/p}\,x_l$$

are precomputed and stored.

We also can deal with arbitrary convolutions in which the sequence $(x_k)_{k \in Z^1}$ is not necessarily periodic. Here we extend y_k outside $[0, p-1]$ by zero and x_k outside $[-p+1, p-1]$ by periodicity with period $2p$, the value of x_p being irrelevant. Then, the equations

$$z_k = \sum_{l=0}^{2p-1} x_{k-l} y_l, \quad k = 0, \ldots, p-1,$$

together with the (irrelevant) equations for $k = p, \ldots, 2p-1$, form a cyclic convolution of length $2p$ which can be carried out by FFTs of length $2p$, resulting in a $0(p \log p)$ algorithm for arbitrary convolutions of length p.

The matrix X of a linear system defined by an arbitrary convolution has the form

$$X = \begin{pmatrix} x_0 & x_{-1} & \cdots & x_{-p+1} \\ x_1 & x_0 & \cdots & x_{-p+2} \\ \vdots & \vdots & & \vdots \\ x_{p-1} & x_{p-2} & \cdots & x_0 \end{pmatrix}. \tag{5.6}$$

Such a matrix, whose rows are obtained by successive right shifts, is called a Toeplitz matrix. In order to handle such systems by FFT we need some preparations, see Bitmead and Anderson (1984), Brent et al. (1980) and Morf (1980).

Let M be the $p \times p$ matrix

$$M = \begin{pmatrix} 0 & \cdots & & & 0 \\ 1 & \cdot & & & \cdot \\ 0 & \cdot \cdot & & & \\ & & \cdot & & \cdot \\ \vdots & & & \cdot & \\ & & & \cdot & \\ 0 & \cdots & 0 & 1 & 0 \end{pmatrix}$$

whose only non-zero elements are in positions $(l+1, l)$, $l = 1, \ldots, p-1$. For an arbitrary $p \times p$ matrix A we define

$$\alpha_+(A) = rk(A - MAM^T),$$
$$\alpha_-(A) = rk(A - M^T AM).$$

$\alpha_+(A)$, $\alpha_-(A)$ are called the $(+)$ or $(-)$ displacement rank of A. The relations

$$A = \begin{pmatrix} a_{1,1} & \cdots & a_{1,p} \\ \vdots & \cdot & \vdots \\ a_{p,1} & \cdots & a_{p,p} \end{pmatrix}, \quad MAM^T = \begin{pmatrix} 0 & \cdots & & 0 \\ & a_{1,1} & \cdots & a_{1,p-1} \\ \vdots & \vdots & & \vdots \\ 0 & a_{p-1,1} & \cdots & a_{p-1,p-1} \end{pmatrix},$$

$$M^T AM = \begin{pmatrix} a_{2,2} & \cdots & a_{2,p} & 0 \\ \vdots & & \vdots & \vdots \\ a_{p,2} & \cdots & a_{p,p} & \\ 0 & \cdots & & 0 \end{pmatrix}$$

show that for the Toeplitz matrix X from (5.6)

$$X - MXM^T = \begin{pmatrix} x_0 & x_{-1} & \cdots & x_{-p+1} \\ x_1 & & & \\ \vdots & & 0 & \\ x_{p-1} & & & \end{pmatrix},$$

$$X - M^TXM = \begin{pmatrix} & & & x_{-p+1} \\ & 0 & & \vdots \\ & & & x_{-1} \\ x_{p-1} & \cdots & x_1 & x_0 \end{pmatrix}$$

hence $\alpha_+(X), \alpha_-(X) \le 2$.

LEMMA 5.1 If A is invertible, then

$$\alpha_+(A) = \alpha_-(A^{-1}).$$

Proof First we show that for arbitrary $p \times p$ matrices A, B,

$$rk(I - AB) = rk(I - BA). \tag{5.7}$$

In fact, if $rk(I - AB) = m$, then there are $p - m$ linearly independent vectors x_i such that $(I - AB)x_i = 0$. The vectors Bx_i must be linearly independent as well, and

$$B(I - AB)x_i = (I - BA)Bx_i = 0.$$

Hence

$$rk(I - BA) \le m = rk(I - AB).$$

Interchanging A, B we get (5.7).

Now we apply (5.7) to the matrices MA, M^TA^{-1} in

$$\begin{aligned}
\alpha_+(A) &= rk(A - MAM^T) \\
&= rk((I - MAM^TA^{-1})A) \\
&= rk(I - MAM^TA^{-1}) \\
&= rk(I - M^TA^{-1}MA) \\
&= rk((I - M^TA^{-1}MA)A^{-1}) \\
&= rk(A^{-1} - M^TA^{-1}M) \\
&= \alpha_-(A^{-1}). \quad \square
\end{aligned}$$

For x the vector $(x_0, \ldots, x_{p-1})^T$ we introduce the triangular Toeplitz matrices

$$L(x) = \begin{pmatrix} x_0 & & & 0 \\ x_1 & x_0 & & \\ \vdots & x_1 & \ddots & \\ x_{p-1} & \cdots & x_1 & x_0 \end{pmatrix}, \quad U(x) = L^T(x).$$

LEMMA 5.2 Let $x^j, y^j \in \mathbb{R}^p, j = 1, \ldots, \alpha$. Then, the following statements are equivalent:

$$A - MAM^T = \sum_{j=1}^{\alpha} x^j y^{jT}, \tag{5.8}$$

$$A = \sum_{j=1}^{\alpha} L(x^j) U(y^j). \tag{5.9}$$

Proof Putting $x_k^j = y_k^j = 0$ for $k < 0$ we have

$$(L(x^j))_{k,l} = x_{k-l}^j, \quad (U(y^j))_{k,l} = y_{l-k}^j.$$

Let

$$A = \begin{pmatrix} a_{1,1} & \cdots & a_{1,p} \\ \vdots & & \vdots \\ a_{p,1} & \cdots & a_{p,p} \end{pmatrix}$$

be the matrix (5.9). Then,

$$a_{k,l} = \sum_{j=1}^{\alpha} \sum_{i=1}^{p} x_{k-i}^j y_{l-i}^j,$$

and, with $a_{k,l} = 0$ if $k = 0$ or $l = 0$,

$$(A - MAM^T)_{k,l} = a_{k,l} - a_{k-1,l-1}$$

$$= \sum_{j=1}^{\alpha} \sum_{i=1}^{p} (x_{k-i}^j y_{l-i}^j - x_{k-1-i}^j y_{l-1-i}^j)$$

$$= \sum_{j=1}^{\alpha} \sum_{i=1}^{p} (x_{k-i}^j y_{l-i}^j - x_{k-(i+1)}^j y_{l-(i+1)}^j)$$

$$= \sum_{j=1}^{\alpha} x_{k-1}^j y_{l-1}^j$$

$$= \sum_{j=1}^{\alpha} (x^j y^{jT})_{k,l}.$$

Hence (5.8) follows from (5.9). Vice versa, let A satisfy (5.8). A is uniquely determined by (5.8) since $A - MAM^T = 0$ implies $A = 0$. On the other hand, we just showed that the matrix A from (5.9) is a solution of (5.8). Hence (5.8) implies (5.9) and the proof is complete. $\square$

LEMMA 5.3 For each $p \times p$ matrix A there are vectors $x^j, y^j \in \mathbb{R}^p$, $j = 1, \ldots, \alpha_+(A)$ such that

$$A = \sum_{j=1}^{\alpha_+(A)} L(x^j) U(y^j).$$

Proof Let B a $p \times p$ matrix with rank α, let $x^1, \ldots, x^\alpha$ be α linearly independent columns of B, and let y_k^j be the coefficient of x^j in the representation of the kth column b^k of B in terms of the vectors $x^1, \ldots, x^\alpha$, i.e.

$$b^k = \sum_{j=1}^{\alpha} y_k^j x^j, \quad k = 1, \ldots, p.$$

This means that B admits a representation

$$B = \sum_{j=1}^{\alpha} x^j y^{j\mathsf{T}}$$

in terms of α dyadic products where $y^j = (y_1^j, \ldots, y_p^j)^\mathsf{T}$. Applying this to the matrix $B = A - MAM^\mathsf{T}$ we get

$$A - MAM^\mathsf{T} = \sum_{j=1}^{\alpha_+(A)} x^j y^{j\mathsf{T}}$$

with suitable vectors x^j, y^j, and the lemma follows from Lemma 5.2.

The following theorem is our main result on inverting Toeplitz matrices.

THEOREM 5.4 *Let X be an invertible Toeplitz matrix (5.6). Then there are Toeplitz matrices L_1, L_2, U_1, U_2 such that*

$$X^{-1} = L_1 U_1 + L_2 U_2.$$

Proof According to Lemma 5.1 we have $\alpha_+(X^{-1}) = \alpha_-(X) \leq 2$. The theorem follows from Lemma 5.3. □

The significance of Theorem 5.4 lies in the fact that the linear system $Xy = Z$ can be solved by convolutions, provided the matrices L_1, U_1, L_2, U_2 are precomputed and stored:

$$y = L_1 U_1 z + L_2 U_2 z. \quad (5.10)$$

If FFT is used, this can be done with $0(p \log p)$ operations. Thus $p \times p$ systems with Toeplitz matrices can be solved with $0(p \log p)$ operations.

In V.5 we apply the algorithm (5.10) to matrices X which are block-Toeplitz, i.e. for which the entries x_l in (5.6) are $q \times q$ matrices. In this case Theorem 5.4 still holds with L_1, U_1, L_2, U_2 being block-Toeplitz as well, and the algorithm (5.10) needs $0(pq^2 + pq \log p)$ operations.

One of the main applications of the discrete Fourier transform is the approximate calculation of the Fourier transform

$$\hat{f}(\xi) = (2\pi)^{-1/2} \int_{\mathbf{R}^1} e^{-ix\xi} f(x) \, dx.$$

Assume $f = 0$ outside $[-a, a]$ and let $f_l = f(hl)$, $l = -q, \ldots, q-1$, $h = a/q$. We want to compute approximations $\hat{f}_k$ to $\hat{f}(uk)$, $k = -q, \ldots, q-1$, where $u > 0$ is the step-size in the frequency variable ξ. Discretizing the integral by the trapezoidal rule we obtain

$$\hat{f}_k = (2\pi)^{-1/2} h \sum_{l=-q}^{q-1} e^{-iklau/q} f_l, \qquad k = -q, \ldots, q-1. \tag{5.11}$$

For $u = \pi/a$ this is a discrete Fourier transform of length $2q$. Since $\hat{f}$ has bandwidth a, $u = \pi/a$ is precisely the Nyquist sampling rate for $\hat{f}$, see II.1. We see that (5.11) can be done by FFT in $0(p \log p)$ operations if the sampling in Fourier space is done at the Nyquist rate. For the error in (5.11) see Theorem III.1.3.

Sometimes (see V.2) we want to compute $\hat{f}(\xi)$ with a step-size u other than the Nyquist rate. If u is one-half of the Nyquist rate, $u = \pi/(2a)$, then we can write

$$\hat{f}_k = (2\pi)^{-1/2} h \sum_{l=-2q}^{2q-1} e^{-i\pi kl/(2q)} f_l, \qquad k = -2q, \ldots, 2q-1 \tag{5.12}$$

where f_l has been put zero for $l < -q$ and $l \geq q$ ('padding by zeros'). This amounts to doing a discrete Fourier transform of length $4q$. A more economical and more elegant procedure consists in separating odd and even k by writing

$$\hat{f}_{2k} = (2\pi)^{-1/2} h \sum_{l=-q}^{q-1} e^{-i\pi kl/q} f_l, \qquad k = -q, \ldots, q-1,$$

$$\hat{f}_{2k+1} = (2\pi)^{-1/2} h \sum_{l=-q}^{q-1} e^{-i\pi kl/q} e^{-i\pi l/q} f_l, \qquad k = -q, \ldots, q-1. \tag{5.13}$$

Now we perform two discrete Fourier transforms of length $2q$ each, one with the original data f_l, the other one with the modified data $e^{-il\pi/q} f_l$. We see that the case $u = \pi/(2a)$ (and more general, the case $u = \pi/(ma)$ with m an integer) can be handled with FFT methods as well, using $0(q \log q)$ operations.

For arbitrary step-size $u > 0$ we have to resort to a less direct method, the so-called chirp z-algorithm (Nussbaumer (1982), ch. 5.1), We write

$$-klau/q = \frac{au}{2q}(k-l)^2 - \frac{au}{2q}(k^2 + l^2)$$

in (5.11), obtaining

$$\hat{f}_k = e^{-i(au/2q)k^2} \hat{f}'_k,$$

$$\hat{f}'_k = (2\pi)^{-1/2} h \sum_{l=-q}^{q-1} e^{i(au/2q)(k-l)^2} f'_l, \qquad k = -q, \ldots, q-1, \tag{5.14}$$

$$f'_l = e^{-i(au/2q)l^2} f_l.$$

The second formula of this algorithm is a convolution of length $2q$ which can be replaced by two discrete Fourier transforms of length $4q$ each. Again we come to a $0(q \log q)$ algorithm by the help of FFT.

References

Abramowitz, M. and Stegun, I. A. (1970). *Handbook of Mathematical Functions*. Dover.
Adams, R. A. (1975). *Sobolev Spaces*. Academic Press, New York.
Altschuler, M. D. (1979). Reconstruction of the global-scale three-dimensional solar corona, in Herman, G. T. (ed.), *Image Reconstruction from Projections*. Springer.
Altschuler, M. D. and Perry, R. M. (1972). On determining the electron density distribution of the solar corona from K-coronameter data. *Sol. Phys.*, **23**, 410–428.
Amemiya, I. and Ando, T. (1965). Convergence of random products of contractions in Hilbert space. *Acta Sci. Math. (Szeged)* **26**, 239–244.
Anderson, D. L. (1984). Surface wave tomography. *Eos*, **65**, p. 147.
Anderson, T. W. (1958). *An Introduction to Multivariate Statistical Analysis*. Wiley.
Ball, J. S., Johnson, S. A. and Stenger, F. (1980). Explicit inversion of the Helmholtz equation for ultrasound insonification and spherical detection, in Wang, K. Y. (ed.), *Acoustical Imaging*, **9**, 451–461.
Bates, R. H. T., Garden, K. L. and Peters, T. M. (1983). Overview of computerized tomography with emphasis on future developments. *Proceedings of the IEEE*, **71**, 356–372.
Bates, R. H. T. and Peters, T. M. (1971). Towards improvement in tomography. *New Zealand J. Sci.*, **14**, 883–896.
Bertero, M., De Mol, C. and Viano, G. A. (1980). The stability of inverse problems, in Baltes, H. P. (ed.), *Inverse Scattering Problems*. Springer.
Bitmead, R. R. and Anderson, B. D. O. (1984). Asymptotically fast solution of Toeplitz and related systems of equations. *Linear Algebra and Applications*, **34**, 103–116.
Björck, Å. and Elving, T. (1979). Accelerated projection methods for computing pseudoinverse solutions of linear equations. *BIT*, **19**, 145–163.
Boman, J. (1984a). An example of non-uniqueness for a generalized Radon transform. Preprint, Department of Mathematics, Univ. of Stockholm.
Boman, J. (1984b). Uniqueness theorems for generalized Radon transforms. Preprint, Department of Mathematics, Univ. of Stockholm.
Bracewell, R. N. (1979). Image reconstruction in radio astronomy, in Herman, G. T. (ed.), *Image Reconstruction from Projections*, Springer.
Bracewell, R. N. and Riddle, A. C. (1956). Strip integration in radio astronomy. *Aus. J. Phys.*, **9**, 198–217.
Bracewell, R. N. and Riddle, A. C. (1967). Inversion of fan-beam scans in radio astronomy. *The Astrophysical Journal*, **150**, 427–434.
Brent, R. P., Gustavson, F. G. and Yun, D. Y. Y. (1980). Fast solution of Toeplitz systems of equations and computation of Padé approximants. *J. Algorithms*, **1**, 259–295.
Brooks, R. A. and Di Chiro, G. (1976). Principles of computer assisted tomography (CAT) in radiographic and radioisotopic imaging. *Phys. Med. Biol.*, **21**, 689–732.
Budinger, T. F., Gullberg, G. T. and Huesman, R. H. (1979). Emission computed tomography, in Herman, G. T. (ed.): *Image Reconstruction from Projections*. Springer.
Bukhgeim, A. L. and Lavrent'ev, M. M. (1973). A class of operator equations of the first kind. *Funkts. Anal. Prilozhen*, **7**, 44–53.

Buonocore, M. H., Brody, W. R. and Macovski, A. (1981). A natural pixel decomposition for two-dimensional image reconstruction. *IEEE Trans. on Biom. Eng.*, **BME-28**, 69–77.
Censor, Y. (1981). Row-action methods for huge and sparse systems and their applications. *SIAM Review*, **23**, 444–466.
Censor, Y. (1983). Finite series-expansion reconstruction methods. *Proceedings of the IEEE*, **71**, 409–419.
Censor, Y., Eggermont, P. P. B. and Gordon, D. (1983). Strong underrelaxation in Kaczmarz's method for inconsistent systems. *Num. Math.*, **41**, 83–92.
Chang, T. and Herman, G. T. (1980). A scientific study of filter selection for a fan-beam convolution algorithm. *SIAM J. Appl. Math.*, **39**, 83–105.
Cormack, A. M. (1963). Representation of a function by its line integrals, with some radiological applications. *J. Appl. Phys.*, **34**, 2722–2727.
Cormack, A. M. (1964). Representation of a function by its line integrals, with some radiological applications II. *J. Appl. Phys.*, **35**, 195–207.
Cormack, A. M. (1978). Sampling the Radon transform with beams of finite width. *Phys. Med. Biol.*, **23**, 1141–1148.
Cormack, A. M. (1980). An exact subdivision of the Radon transform and scanning with a positron ring camera. *Phys. Med. Biol.*, **25**, 543–544.
Cormack, A. M. (1981). The Radon transform on a family of curves in the plane. *Proceedings of the Amer. Math. Soc.*, **83**, 325–330.
Cormack, A. M. and Quinto, E. T. (1980). A Radon transform on spheres through the origin in $\mathbb{R}^n$ and applications to the Darboux equation. *Trans. Amer. Math. Soc.*, **260**, 575–581.
Courant, R. and Hilbert, D. (1962). *Methods of Mathematical Physics*, Volume II. Interscience.
Crowther, R. A., De Rosier, D. J. and Klug, A. (1970). The reconstruction of a three-dimensional structure from projections and its application to electron microscopy. *Proc. R. Soc. London Ser. A.*, **317**, 319–340.
Das, Y. and Boerner, W. M. (1978). On radar target shape estimate using algorithms for reconstruction from projections. *IEEE Trans. Antenna Propagation*, **26**, 274–279.
Davison, M. E. (1981). A singular value decomposition for the Radon transform in n-dimensional euclidean space. *Numer. Funct. Anal. and Optimiz.*, **3**, 321–340.
Davison, M. E. (1983). The ill-conditioned nature of the limited angle tomography problem. *SIAM J. Appl. Math.*, **43**, 428–448.
Davison, M. E. and Grünbaum, F. A. (1981). Tomographic reconstructions with arbitrary directions. *Comm. Pure Appl. Math.*, **34**, 77–120.
Deans, S. R. (1979). Gegenbauer transforms via the Radon transform. *SIAM J. Math. Anal.*, **10**, 577–585.
Deans, S. R. (1983). *The Radon Transform and some of its Applications*. Wiley.
Devaney, A. J. (1982). A filtered backpropagation algorithm for diffraction tomography. *Ultrasonic Imaging*, **4**, 336–350.
Droste, B. (1983). A new proof of the support theorem and the range characterization for the Radon transform. *Manuscripta math.*, **42**, 289–296.
Falconer, K. J. (1983). X-ray problems for point sources. *Proc. London Math. Soc.*, **46**, 241–262.
Finch, D. V. (1985). Cone beam reconstruction with sources on a curve. *SIAM J. Appl. Math.*, **45**, 665–673.
Funk, P. (1913). Über Flächen mit lauter geschlossenen geodätischen Linien. *Math. Ann.*, **74**, 278–300.
Gambarelli, J., Guerinel, G., Chevrot, L. and Mattei, M. (1977). *Ganzkörper—Computer—Tomographie*. Springer.
Gardner, R. J. and McMullen, P. (1980). On Hammer's X-ray problem. *J. London Math. Soc.*, **21**, 171–175.

Gelfand, I. M., Graev, M. I. and Vilenkin, N. Y. (1965). *Generalized functions. Vol. 5: Integral Geometry and Representation Theory*. Academic Press.

Gordon, R. (1975). Image processing for 2-D and 3-D reconstruction from projections: theory and practice in medicine and the physical sciences. Digest of technical papers, Stanford, California, August 4–7 (1975). Sponsored by the Optical Society of America.

Gordon, R., Bender, R. and Herman, G. T. (1970). Algebraic reconstruction techniques (ART) for three-dimensional electron microscopy and X-ray photography. *J. Theor. Biol.*, **29**, 471–481.

Gradshteyn, I. S. and Ryzhik, I. M. (1965). *Table of Integrals, Series, and Products*. Academic Press.

Groetsch, C. W. (1984). *The Theory of Tikhonov Regularization for Fredholm Equations of the First Kind*. Pitman.

Grünbaum, F. A. (1981). Reconstruction with arbitrary directions: dimensions two and three, in Herman, G. T. and Natterer, F. (eds), *Mathematical Aspects of Computerized Tomography*. Proceedings, Oberwolfach 1980. Springer.

Guenther, R. B., Kerber, C. W., Killian, E. K., Smith, K. T. and Wagner, S. L. (1974). Reconstruction of objects from radiographs and the location of brain tumors. *Proc. Nat. Acad. Sci., USA*, **71**, 4884–4886.

Hadamard, J. (1932). Le problème de Cauchy et les equations aux derivéees partielles linéaires hyperboliques. Herman, Paris.

Ham, F. S. (1975). Theory of tomographic image reconstruction: proof that the reconstruction matrix reduces to blockform in rotation–reflection symmetry. Report No. 75CRD205, General Electric Company Corporate Research and Development, Schenectady, NY, USA.

Hamaker, C., Smith, K. T., Solmon, D. C. and Wagner, S. L. (1980). The divergent beam X-ray transform. *Rockey Mountain J. Math.*, **10**, 253–283.

Hamaker, C. and Solmon, D. C. (1978). The angles between the null spaces of X-rays. *J. Math. Anal. Appl.*, **62**, 1–23.

Hansen, E. W. (1981). Circular harmonic image reconstruction. *Applied Optics*, **20**, 2266–2274.

Heike, U. (1984). Die Inversion der gedämpften Radontransformation, ein Rekonstruktionsverfahren der Emissionstomographie. Dissertation, Universität Münster 1984.

Helgason, S. (1965). The Radon transform on euclidean spaces, compact two-point homogeneous spaces and Grassmann manifolds. *Acta Mathematica*, **113**, 153–179.

Helgason, S. (1980). *The Radon Transform*. Birkhäuser.

Herman, G. T. and Natterer, F. (eds) (1981). Mathematical aspects of computerized tomography. *Proceedings, Oberwolfach 1980*. Springer.

Herman, G. T. and Naparstek, A. (1977). Fast image reconstruction for rapidly collected data. *SIAM J. Appl. Math.*, **33**, 511–513.

Herman, G. T. and Lent, A. (1976). Iterative reconstruction algorithms. *Comput. Biol. Med.*, **6**, 273–294.

Herman, G. T., Hurwitz, H., Lent, A. and Lung, H. (1979). On the Bayesian approach to image reconstruction. *Information and Control*, **42**, 60–71.

Herman, G. T. (1979). *Image Reconstruction from Projections*. Springer.

Herman, G. T. (1980). *Image Reconstruction from Projections. The Fundamentals of Computerized Tomography*. Academic Press.

Hertle, A. (1983). Continuity of the Radon transform and its inverse on euclidean space. *Math. Z.*, **184**, 165–192.

Hertle, A. (1984). On the injectivity of the attenuated Radon transform. *Proc. AMS*, **92**, 201–206.

Hinshaw, W. S. and Lent, A. H. (1983). An introduction to NMR Imaging: From the Block equation to the imaging equation. *Proc. of the IEEE*, **71**, 338–350.

Hoppe, W. and Hegerl, R. (1980). Three-dimensional structure determination by electron microscopy, in Hawkes, P. W. (ed.), *Computer Processing of Electron Microscope Images.* Springer.

Horn, B. K. P. (1973). Fan-beam reconstruction methods. *Proc. of the IEEE,* **67**, 1616–1623.

Hounsfield, G. N. (1973). Computerized transverse axial scanning tomography: Part I, description of the system. *Br. J. Radiol.*, **46**, 1016–1022.

Hurwitz, H. (1975). Entropy reduction in Bayesian analysis of measurements. *Phys. Rev. A.*, **12**, 698–706.

Jerry, A. J. (1977). The Shannon sampling theorem—its various extensions and applications: a tutorial review. *Proc. IEEE*, **65**, 1565–1596.

John, F. (1934). Bestimmung einer Funktion aus ihren Integralen über gewisse Mannigfaltigkeiten. *Mathematische Annalen*, **109**, 488–520.

John, F. (1955). *Plane Waves and Spherical means Applied to Partial Differential Equations.* Interscience.

Joseph, P. M. and Schulz, R. A. (1980). View sampling requirements in fan beam computed tomography. *Med. Phys.*, **7**, 692–702.

Kershaw, D. (1962). The determination of the density distribution of a gas flowing in a pipe from mean density measurements. Report A.R.L./R1/MATHS 4 105, Admiralty Research Laboratory, Teddington, Middlesex.

Kershaw, D. (1970). The determination of the density distribution of a gas flowing in a pipe from mean density measurements. *J. Inst. Maths. Applics*, **6**, 111–114.

Klotz, E., Linde, R. and Weiss, H. (1974). A new method for deconvoluting coded aperture images of three-dimensional X-ray objects. *Opt. Comm.*, **12**, 183.

Koritké, J. G. and Sick, H. (1982). *Atlas anatomischer Schnittbilder des Menschen.* Urban & Schwarzenberg, München–Wien–Baltimore.

Kowalski, G. (1979). Multislize reconstruction from twin-cone beam scanning. *IEEE Trans. Nucl. Sci.* **NS-26**, 2895–2903.

Kuba, A. (1984). The reconstruction of two-directionally connected binary patterns from their two orthogonal projections. *Computer Vision, Graphics, and Image Processing*, **27**, 249–265.

Lakshminarayanan, A. V. (1975). Reconstruction from divergent ray data. Dept. Computer Science Tech. Report TR-92, State University of New York at Buffalo.

Lax, P. D. and Phillips, R. S. (1970). The Payley–Wiener theorem for the Radon transform. *Comm. Pure Appl. Math.*, **23**, 409–424.

Leahy, J. V., Smith, K. T. and Solmon, D. C. (1979). Uniqueness, nonuniqueness and inversion in the X-ray and Radon problems. *Proc. International Symposium on Ill-posed Problems*, Newark, DE, October 1979.

Lent, A. (1975). Seminar talk at the Biodynamic. Research Unit, Mayo Clinic, Rochester, MN.

Lent, A. and Tuy, H. (1981). An iterative method for the extrapolation of band limited functions. *J. Math. Anal. Appl.*, **83**, 554–565.

Lewitt, R. M., Bates, R. H. T. and Peters, T. M. (1978a) Image reconstruction from projections: II: Modified back-projection methods. *Optik*, **50**, 85–109.

Lewitt, R. M., Bates, R. H. T. and Peters, T. M. (1978b). Image reconstruction from projections: III: Projection completion methods (theory). *Optik*, **50**, 180–205.

Lindgren, A. G. and Rattey, P. A. (1981). The inverse discrete Radon transform with applications to tomographic imaging using projection data. *Advances in Electronics and Electron Physics*, **56**, 359–410.

Lions, J. L. and Magenes, E. (1968). Problèmes aux limites non homogènes et applications. Dunod, Paris, 1968.

Littleton, J. T. (1976). *Tomography: Physical Principles and Clinical Applications.* The Williams & Wilkins Co., Baltimore.

Löw, K. H. and Natterer, F. (1981) An ultra-fast algorithm in tomography. Technical Report A81/03, Fachbereich 10 der Universität des Saarlandes, 6600 Saarbrücken, Germany.

Logan, B. F. (1975). The uncertainty principle in reconstructing functions from projections. *Duke Mathematical J.*, **42**, 661–706.
Logan, B. F. and Shepp, L. A. (1975). Optimal reconstruction of a function from its projections. *Duke Math. J.* **42**, 645–659.
Lohman, G. (1983). Rekonstruktion sternförmiger, homogener Objekte aus Projektionen. Diplomarbeit, Universität Münster.
Louis, A. K. (1980). Picture reconstruction from projections in restricted range. *Math. Meth. in the Appl. Sci.*, **2**, 209–220.
Louis, A. K. (1981a). Analytische Methoden in der Computer Tomographie. Habilitationsschrift, Fachbereich Mathematik der Universität Münster, 1981.
Louis, A. K. (1981b). Ghosts in tomography—The null space of the Radon transform. *Math. Meth. in the Appl. Sci.*, **3**, 1–10.
Louis, A. K. (1982). Optimal sampling in nuclear magnetic resonance (NMR) tomography. *Journal of Computer Assisted Tomography* **6**, 334–340.
Louis, A. K. (1983). Approximate inversion of the 3D Radon transform. *Math. Meth. in the Appl. Sci.*, **5**, 176–185.
Louis, A. K. (1984a). Nonuniqueness in inverse Radon problems: the frequency distribution of the ghosts. *Math. Z.*, **185**, 429–440.
Louis, A. K. (1984b). Orthogonal function series expansions and the null space of the Radon transform. *SIAM J. Math. Anal.*, **15**, 621–633.
Louis, A. K. (1985). Tikhonov–Phillips regularization of the Radon transform, in Hämmerlin, G. and Hoffman, K. H. (eds), *Constructive Methods for the Practical Treatment of Integral Equations*. Birkhäuser ISNM 73, 211–223.
Louis, A. K. (1985) Laguerre and computerized tomography: consistency conditions and stability of the Radon transform, in Brezinski, C.; Draux, A.; Magnus, A. P.; Maroni, P.; Rouveaux, A. (eds.): Polynomes Orthogonaux et Applications, pp. 524–531, Springer LNM 1171.
Ludwig, D. (1966). The Radon transform on euclidean space. *Comm. Pure Appl. Math.*, **19**, 49–81.
Madych, W. R. (1980). Degree of approximation in computerized tomography, in Cheney, E. W. (ed.), *Approximation Theory III*, 615–621.
Madych, W. R. and Nelson, S. A. (1983). Polynomial based algorithms for computed tomography. *SIAM J. Appl. Math.*, **43**, 157–185.
Madych, W. R. and Nelson, S. A. (1984). Polynomial based algorithms for computed tomography II. *SIAM J. Appl. Math.*, **44**, 193–208.
Markoe, A. (1986). Fourier inversion of the attenuated Radon transform. *SIAM J. Math. Anal.* to appear.
Markoe, A. and Quinto, E. T. (1985). An elementary proof of local invertibility for generalized and attenuated Radon transforms. *SIAM J. Math. Anal.*, **16**, 1114–1119.
Marr, R. B. (ed.) (1974a). Techniques for three-dimensional reconstruction. Proceedings of an international workshop, Brookhaven National Laboratory, Upton, New York, July 16–19.
Marr, R. B. (1974b). On the reconstruction of a function on a circular domain from a sampling of its line integrals. *J. Math. Anal. Appl.*, **45**, 357–374.
Marr, R. B., Chen, C. N. and Lauterbur, P. C. (1981). On two approaches to 3D reconstruction in NMR zeugmatography, in Herman, G. T. and Natterer, F. (eds), *Mathematical aspects of Computerized Tomography*. Proceedings, Oberwolfach 1980. Springer.
McLaren, A. D. (1963). Optimal numerical integration on a sphere. *Math. Comp.*, **17**, 361–383.
Morf, M. (1980). Doubling algorithms for Toeplitz and related equations. ICASSP, Denver, April 9–11, 1980.
Morse, P. M. and Feshbach, H. (1953). *Methods of Theoretical Physics*. McGraw-Hill.
Mueller, R. K., Kaveh, M. and Wade, G. (1979). Reconstructive tomography and applications to ultrasonic. *Proceedings of the IEEE*, **67**, 567–587.

Natterer, F. (1977). The finite element method for ill-posed problems. *RAIRO Anal. Numerique*, **11**, 271–278.
Natterer, F. (1979). On the inversion of the attenuated Radon transform. *Numer. Math.*, **32**, 431–438.
Natterer, F. (1980a). A Sobolev space analysis of picture reconstruction. *SIAM J. Appl. Math.*, **39**, 402–411.
Natterer, F. (1980b). Efficient implementation of 'optimal' algorithms in computerized tomography. *Math. Meth. in Appl. Sci.*, **2**, 545–555.
Natterer, F. (1983a). Computerized tomography with unknown sources. *SIAM J. Appl. Math.*, **43**, 1201–1212.
Natterer, F. (1983b). Exploiting the ranges of Radon transforms in tomography, in Deuflhard, P. and Hairer, E. (eds), *Numerical treatment of inverse problems in differential and integral equations*. Birkhäuser.
Natterer, F. (1984a). Some nonstandard Radon problems, in: Boffi, V. and Neunzert, H. (eds): *Applications of Mathematics in Technology*. Teubner.
Natterer, F. (1984b). Error bounds for Tikhonov regularization in Hilbert scales. *Appl. Anal.*, **18**, 29–37.
Natterer, F. (1985). Fourier reconstruction in tomography. *Numer. Math.* **47**, 343–353.
Natterer, F. (1986). Efficient evaluation of oversampled functions. *J. of Comp. and Appl. Math*. In press.
Neutsch, W. (1983). Optimal spherical designs and numerical integration on the sphere. *J. Comp. Phys.*, **51**, 313–325.
Nussbaumer, H. J. (1982). *Fast Fourier Transform and Convolution Algorithms*. Springer.
Papoulis, A. (1965). *Probability, Random Variables and Stochastic Processes*. McGraw-Hill.
Pasedach, K. (1977). Einsatz blockzirkulanter Matrizen zur Rekonstruktion einer Funktion aus ihren Linienintegralen. *ZAMM*, **57**, T296-T297.
Peres, A. (1979). Tomographic reconstruction from limited angular data. *J. Comput. Assist. Tomogr.*, **3**, 800–803.
Perry, R. M. (1977). On reconstructing a function on the exterior of a disc from its Radon transform. *J. Math. Anal. Appl.*, **59**, 324–341.
Perry, R. M. (1975). Reconstructing a function by circular harmonic analysis of line integrals, in Gordon, R. (ed.), *Image Processing for 2-D and 3-D Reconstruction from Projections: Theory and Practice in Medicine and the Physical Sciences*. Digest of technical papers, Stanford, California, August 4–7, 1975. Sponsored by the optical society of America.
Peterson, P. P. and Middleton, D. (1962). Sampling and reconstruction of wave-number-limited functions in N-dimensional euclidean space. *Inf. Control*, **5**, 279–323.
Pratt, W. K. (1978). *Digital Image Processing*. Wiley.
Quinto, E. T. (1980). The dependence of the generalized Radon transform on defining measures. *Trans. Amer. Math. Soc.*, **257**, 331–346.
Quinto, E. T. (1983). The invertibility of rotation invariant Radon transforms. *J. Math. Anal. Appl.*, **91**, 510–522.
Quinto, E. T. (1985). Singular value decompositions and inversion methods for the exterior Radon transform and a spherical transform. *J. Math. Anal. Appl.*, **95**, 437–448.
Quinto, E. T. (1986). Tomographic reconstruction around the beating heart, to appear in *ZAMM* 1986.
Radon, J. (1917). Über die Bestimmung von Funktionen durch ihre Integralwerte längs gewisser Mannigfaltigkeiten. *Berichte Sächsische Akademie der Wissenschaften, Leipzig, Math.—Phys. Kl.*, **69**, 262–267.
Ramachandran, G. N. and Lakshminarayanan, A. V. (1971). Three-dimensional reconstruction from radiographs and electron micrographs: application of convolutions instead of Fourier transforms. *Proc. Nat. Acad. Sci. US*, **68**, 2236–2240.

Rattey, P. A. and Lindgren, A. G. (1981). Sampling the 2-D Radon transform with parallel- and fan-beam projections. Department of Electrical Engineering, University of Rhode Island, Kingston, RI02881, Technical Report 5-33285-01, August 1981.

Romanov, V. G. (1974). Integral geometry and inverse problems for hyperbolic equations. Springer.

Rowland, S. W. (1979). Computer implementation of image reconstruction formulas, in Herman, G. T. (ed.), *Image Reconstruction from Projections*. Springer.

Schomberg, H. (1978). An improved approach to reconstructive ultrasound tomography. *J. Appl. Phys.*, **11**, L181.

Scudder, H. J. (1978). Introduction to computer aided tomography. *Proceedings of the IEEE*, **66**, 628–637.

Seeley, R. T. (1966). Spherical harmonics. *Amer. Math. Monthly*, **73**, 115–121.

Shepp, L. A. (1980). Computerized tomography and nuclear magnetic resonance. *J. Comput. Assist. Tomogr*, **4**, 94–107.

Shepp, L. A. and Logan, B. F. (1974). The Fourier reconstruction of a head section. *IEEE Trans. Nucl. Sci.*, **NS-21**, 21–43.

Shepp, L. A. and Kruskal, J. B. (1978). Computerized tomography: the new medical X-ray technology. *Am. Math. Monthly*, **85**, 420–439.

Sleeman, B. D. (1982). The inverse problem of acoustic scattering. *IMA J. Appl. Math.*, **29**, 113–142.

Slepian, D. (1978). Prolate spheroidal wave functions, Fourier analysis, and uncertainty V: The discrete case, *The Bell System Technical Journal*, **57**, 1371–1430.

Smith, K. T. (1983). Reconstruction formulas in computed tomography. *Proceedings of Symposia in Applied Mathematic (AMS)*, **27**, 7–23.

Smith, K. T. (1984). Inversion of the X-ray transform. *SIAM-AMS Proceedings*, **14**, 41–52.

Smith, K. T., Solmon, D. C. and Wagner, S. L. (1977). Practical and mathematical aspects of the problem of reconstructing a function from radiographs. *Bull. AMS*, **83**, 1227–1270.

Smith, K. T. and Keinert, F. (1985). Mathematical foundations of computed tomography *Applied Optics*, **24**, 3950–3957.

Sneddon, I. H. (1972). *The Use of Integral Transforms*. McGraw-Hill.

Solmon, D. C. (1976). The X-ray transform. *Journ. Math. Anal. Appl.*, **56**, 61–83.

Stark, H., Woods, J. W., Paul, I. P. and Hingorani, R. (1981). An investigation of computerized tomography by direct Fourier inversion and optimum interpolation. *IEEE Trans. Biomed. Engin.*, **BME-28**, 496–505.

Stonestrom, J. P., Alvarez, R. E. and Macovski, A. (1981). A framework for spectral artifact corrections in x-ray CT. *IEEE Trans. Biomed. Eng.*, **BME-28**, 128–141.

Stroud, A. H. (1971). *Approximate Calculation of Multiple Integrals*. Prentice-Hall.

Tam, K. C., Perez–Mendez, V. and Macdonald, B. (1980). Limited angle 3-D reconstruction from continuous and pinhole projections. *IEEE Trans. Nucl. Sci.*, **NS-27**, 445–458.

Tasto, M. (1977). Reconstruction of random objects from noisy projections. *Computer Graphics and Image Processing*, **6**, 103–122.

Tatarski, V. T. (1961). *Wave Propagation in a Turbulent Medium*. McGraw-Hill.

Tikhonov, A. V. and Arsenin, V. Y. (1977). *Solution of Ill-posed Problems*. Winston & Sons.

Tretiak, O. J. (1975). The point spread function for the convolution algorithm, in Gordon, R. (ed.). Image processing for 2-D and 3-D reconstruction from projections: Theory and practice in medicine and the physical sciences. Digest of technical papers, Stanford, California, August 4–7 (1975). Sponsored by the Optical Society of America.

Tretiak, O. and Metz, C. (1980). The exponential Radon transform. *SIAM J. Appl. Math.*, **39**, 341–354.

Treves, F. (1980). *Introduction to Pseudodifferential and Fourier Integral Operators, Volume 1: Pseudodifferential Operators*. Plenum Press.
Triebel, H. (1978). *Interpolation Theory, Function Spaces, Differential Operators*. North-Holland, Amsterdam.
Tuy, H. K. (1981). Reconstruction of a three-dimensional object from a limited range of views. *J. Math. Anal. Appl.*, **80**, 598–616.
Tuy, H. K. (1983). An inversion formula for cone-beam reconstruction. *SIAM J. Appl. Math.*, **43**, 546–552.
Volčič, A. (1983). Well-posedness of the Gardner–McMullen reconstruction problem. *LNM*, **1089**, 199–210.
Volčič, A. (1984). Uniqueness theorems for mixed X-ray problems of Hammer type. Preprint 1984.
Watson, G. N. (1952). *A Treatise on Bessel Functions*. University Press, Cambridge.
Wood, E. H. *et al.* (1979). Application of high temporal resolution computerized tomography to physiology and medicine, in Herman, G. T. (ed.), *Image Reconstruction from Projections*. Springer.
Yosida, K. (1968). *Functional Analysis*. Springer.
Young, D. M. (1971). *Iterative Solution of Large Linear Systems*. Academic Press.

Index

A priori information, 90, 94, 95
Abel type integral equation, 23, 24, 26
Adjoint, 18, 140
Algebraic reconstruction technique (art), 102, 137, 138, 140, 144, 160, 164, 170
Aliasing, 60, 113
Approximate delta-function, 183
Artefacts, 118, 120, 121, 159, 164, 168
Attenuated radon transform, 46, 52, 53

B-spline, 60, 107, 120, 121
Backprojection, 103, 113, 148, 151, 153
Band-limited, 54
Bandwidth, 54
Beam hardening, 3
Bessel functions, 197

Cauchy principal value, 185
Chebyshev polynomials, 154
Chirp z-algorithm, 127, 212
Collocation method, 137
Communication theory, 54, 184
Completion of data, 159, 162, 166, 168, 170, 178
Conditional expectation, 91
Cone beam scanning, 3, 147, 174
Consistency conditions, 37, 49, 159, 168
Cormack's inversion formula, 28, 155, 166
Covariance, 91
Cut-off frequency, 60

Debye's formula, 198
Diffraction tomography, 5
Digital filtering, 89
Dirac's delta-function, 183
Direct Algebraic method, 102, 146, 149, 160, 168
Discrete Fourier transform, 206
Displacement rank, 208
Distributions, 181

Divergent beam transform, 10, 33
Dual operators, 13, 47

Electron microscopy, 3
Emission CT, 4, 47
Essentially band-limited, 55
Exponential radon transform, 47
Exterior problem, 28, 30, 101, 146, 158, 166, 168

Fan-beam geometry, 82
Fan-beam scanning, 2, 10, 75, 83, 111
Fast Fourier transform (FFT), 11, 119, 120, 125, 126, 148, 164, 206, 207
Filtered backprojection, 49, 102, 103, 106, 113, 117, 128, 151, 159, 164, 168
Filtered layergram, 22, 48, 153
Filtering, 60
Fourier coefficients, 182
Fourier expansion, 184
Fourier inversion formula, 180
Fourier reconstruction, 102, 119, 120, 156
Fourier transform, 180
Funk–Hecke theorem, 195

Gamma function, 193
Gauss–Legendre formula, 191
Gegenbauer polynomials, 193
Generalized inverse, 85

Haar measure, 189
Hilbert transform, 186
Hole theorem, 30

Ideal low-pass, 60
Ill-posed, 33, 42, 85, 95, 158, 164, 166, 168
Incomplete data, 2, 85, 147, 158
Indeterminacy, 36, 90
Integral geometry, 5, 14

Interior problem, 146, 158, 169
Interlaced parallel geometry, 71, 74, 83
Interpolation of functions, 107, 108, 120, 125, 126, 127
Interpolation of spaces, 46, 60, 201, 202, 203
Inversion formulas, 18, 48, 49, 100, 102, 119, 153, 171
Isotropic exponential model, 92

Jacobi polynomials, 100

k-plane transform, 52
Kaczmarz method, 102, 128, 134, 136, 137, 139

Legendre functions, 197
Legendre polynomials, 194
Limited angle problem, 3, 158, 160, 163, 164, 166
Locality, 21, 172

m-resolving, 64
Mellin transform, 194
Mildly ill-posed, 91
Minimal norm solution, 170
Modestly ill-posed, 91

NMR imaging, 8
Normal equations, 86
Nyquist condition, 56

Optimality relation, 83, 118, 120, 127
Oversampling, 56

Parallel scanning, 2, 71, 111, 117
Parseval's relation, 183
Pet (positron emission tomography), 4, 76, 82, 83, 153
Picture densities, 94
Pixels, 137
Plancherel's theorem, 182
Poisson's formula, 184
Projection theorem, 47, 119
Pseudo-differential operators, 172

Quadrature rule, 103, 106, 190

Radar, 8
Radon transform, 9

Radon's inversion formula, 22, 151, 158, 169
Random variables, 91
Rebinning, 111
Regularization, 86, 178
Relaxation parameter, 128
Resolution, 64, 68, 71, 106, 111, 115, 116
Restricted source problem, 158
Riesz potential, 18
Rotational invariance, 146, 147, 148
Rytov approximation, 6

Sampling, 54, 71, 75, 180
Scanning geometries, 2, 71, 83, 108
Schwartz space, 9
Semi-convergence, 89, 144
Severely ill-posed, 91, 160, 163, 166
Shah-distribution, 184
Sinc function, 55
Sinc series, 57
Singular value decomposition, 85, 86, 88, 95, 100, 101, 160, 161
Sobolev spaces, 42, 92, 94, 95, 121, 200
SOR, 136
Spectral radius, 135
Spherical coordinates, 186
Spherical harmonic, 195
Stability estimate, 160, 174

Three-dimensional CT, 3, 32, 174
Tikhonov–Phillips method, 89, 91, 148, 164
Toeplitz matrix, 146, 148, 161, 164, 206, 208, 209
Tomography, 8
Transmission CT, 1
Trapezoidal rule, 56, 109, 184, 191
Tuy's condition, 174

Ultrasound CT, 4
Undersampling, 57, 118

Weber–Schafheitlin integral, 199
White noise, 91
Worst case error, 90

X-ray transform, 9

If you have any concerns about our products,
you can contact us on
ProductSafety@springernature.com

In case Publisher is established outside the EU,
the EU authorized representative is:
**Springer Nature Customer Service Center GmbH
Europaplatz 3, 69115 Heidelberg, Germany**

Printed by Libri Plureos GmbH
in Hamburg, Germany